AF342517

Advance Care Planning in the Asia Pacific

Advance Care Planning in the Asia Pacific

Editors

Raymond Han Lip Ng
Woodlands Health, Singapore

Diah Martina
Universitas Indonesia, Indonesia

Cheng-Pei Lin
National Yang Ming Chiao Tung University, Taiwan

Masanori Mori
Seirei Mikatahara General Hospital, Japan

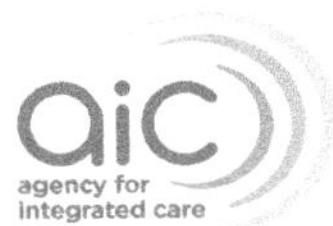

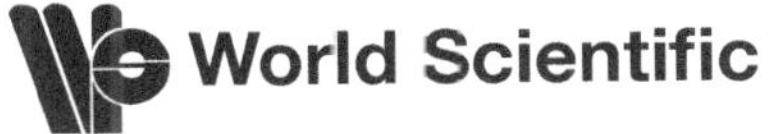

Published by

World Scientific Publishing Co. Pte. Ltd.

5 Toh Tuck Link, Singapore 596224

USA office: 27 Warren Street, Suite 401-402, Hackensack, NJ 07601

UK office: 57 Shelton Street, Covent Garden, London WC2H 9HE

Library of Congress Cataloging-in-Publication Data
Names: Han Lip Ng, Raymond, editor.
Title: Advance care planning in the Asia Pacific /
   [editor] Raymond Han Lip Ng, Woodlands Health, Singapore.
Description: New Jersey : World Scientific, [2024] | Includes bibliographical references.
Identifiers: LCCN 2023040811 | ISBN 9789811281037 (hardcover) |
   ISBN 9789811282669 (paperback) | ISBN 9789811281044 (ebook for institutions) |
   ISBN 9789811281051 (ebook for individuals)
Subjects: LCSH: Advance directives (Medical care)--Pacific Area. |
   Advance directives (Medical care)--Social aspects--Pacific Area. |
   Patient-centered health care--Pacific Area. | Medical personnel and patient--Pacific Area.
Classification: LCC R726.2 .A375 2024 | DDC 362.109182/3--dc23/eng/20231103
LC record available at https://lccn.loc.gov/2023040811

British Library Cataloguing-in-Publication Data
A catalogue record for this book is available from the British Library.

For any available supplementary material, please visit
https://www.worldscientific.com/worldscibooks/10.1142/13534#t=suppl

Desk Editors: Aanand Jayaraman/Joy Quek

Typeset by Stallion Press
Email: enquiries@stallionpress.com

Foreword

This book *Advance Care Planning in the Asia Pacific* is a seminal collection of articles that highlights the criticality of Advance Care Planning (ACP) for all of us and brings forth the perspectives, strategies, and insights in implementing and ensuring acceptance of ACP in different countries in this region. I speak on behalf of all of us in the Agency for Integrated Care that it brings tremendous pride and joy to bring this book to life for all of you.

This book unites the voices of regional experts into a singular narrative, expounding on various facets of ACP — cultural and religious consonances, practical execution, strategies for specific populations and environments, and individual narratives illuminating real-life ACP experiences.

ACP, a subject of professional and personal significance to me, has markedly evolved in Singapore's healthcare sphere over time. The evolution has been continuous, with constant improvement in ACP implementation throughout different care settings, patient groups, and the general public.

However, while ACP is vital, it needs far more attention and focus than it currently receives. In May 2023, Singapore hosted its first international ACP conference, drawing 700 delegates worldwide and sparking invigorating conversations about ACP practices.

Several writers and contributors in this publication were among those who were instrumental in sparking interest, conversation, and converts at this international ACP conference.

I would like to extend my heartfelt congratulations to the editorial team: Dr. Raymond Ng, Dr. Masanori Mori, Dr. Diah Martina, and Dr. Lin Cheng-Pei, whose foresight and commitment to the quintessential cause of ACP have resulted in this book. I am confident that their efforts manifesting in this publication will shed light on the essential aspects of ACP, acting as a guide to those who wish to understand its intricate workings and inspire the creation of more effective strategies in the Asia Pacific region in the future.

Tan Kwang Cheak
Chief Executive Officer
Agency for Integrated Care

Preface

The concept of advance care planning (ACP) arose some 50 years ago with the promise to allow competent individuals the opportunity to guide future medical decisions in the event they are incapacitated from making decisions themselves. Since then, ACP has taken root in many societies and healthcare systems, being recognised as a core tenet of person-centred care, in particular, within geriatric and palliative medicine. It has also been dogged by controversy and debates and till date, international consensus on the definition, scope, and measures of ACP remain elusive.

In practice, ACP is a complex intervention that is culture and context specific. In this day and age of fast-developing medical technologies and evolving social norms, ACP brims with both challenges and potential and a renewed understanding is needed.

This book draws contributions from various experts and endeavours to fill some of the gaps in research and scholarly articles in the current landscape of ACP implementation and practice across the Asia Pacific region. The development of ACP within the Asia Pacific region is as diverse as its histories, cultures, and contexts.

The book is divided into four sections. The first section examines the role of culture and religiosity in ACP. The second section describes real-world implementation of ACP in different sectors and countries within the Asia Pacific region. The third section sheds light on how ACP has been practised in different settings and population groups with unique needs, including during the COVID-19 pandemic. This book ends with stories of ACP from patients, caregivers, healthcare professionals, and laypeople.

This book endeavours to fill the gaps in understanding ACP in the Asia Pacific region and aspires to be a reference book across the wide spectrum of readers ranging from students, practitioners, educators, research-ers, policy makers to community advocates. We hope that it will also serve as a practical guide for many settings aspiring to start or to scale up ACP programmes.

As advocates for person-centred conversations within our own sectors, we teach that at its heart, ACP is a process embodying conversations expressing what matters to those who matter to us. In our universal endeavour to engender person-centred care in healthcare systems and a more compassionate society, we are more similar than different.

Raymond Han Lip Ng
Woodlands Health, Singapore

Diah Martina
Universitas Indonesia, Indonesia

Cheng-Pei Lin
National Yang Ming Chiao Tung University, Taiwan

Masanori Mori
Seirei Mikatahara General Hospital, Japan

About the Editors

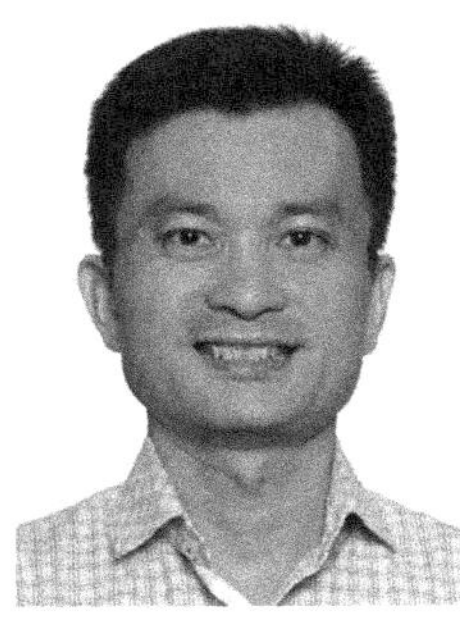

Raymond Ng is a senior consultant and the head of the Department of Palliative & Supportive Care at Woodlands Health, Singapore. He has a special clinical interest in advance care planning, palliative care in primary care, and medical education. He is dually trained in family medicine and palliative medicine. He is also a co-chair of the National Advance Care Planning Steering Committee and the course director of the graduate diploma in palliative medicine at the National University of Singapore.

Dr. Ng is an advocate for advance care planning and believes that deep within each person is a narrative that is key to person-centred care.

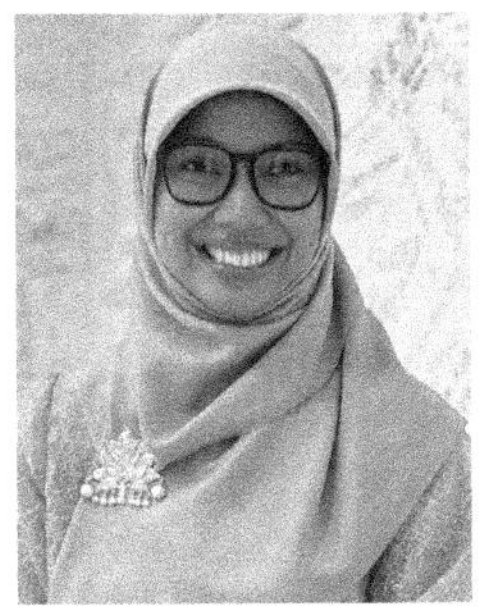

Diah Martina is a faculty member in the Division of Psychosomatic and Palliative Medicine within the Department of Internal Medicine at the Faculty of Medicine, Universitas Indonesia, Indonesia. In 2017, she completed her palliative care fellowship at the Erasmus MC Cancer Institute, supported by the ESMO Palliative Care Fellowship Award. In the same year, she became the first Indonesian recipient of the International Development and Education Award in Palliative Care (IDEA-PC) from the American Society of Clinical Oncology (ASCO). She earned her PhD from Erasmus MC University Medical Center, Rotterdam, with a dissertation on the cultural perspectives of advance care planning in Asia and

Indonesia. Dr. Martina's research interests encompass serious illness communication, culturally sensitive care and communication, spirituality, and palliative care capacity building. Engaging in international collaborations, she has contributed significantly to research on culturally sensitive serious illness communication, with over 14 publications, including the Declaration on Advance Care Planning in Asia. Actively involved in global volunteering initiatives, she has been serving as a member of the ASCO Council for the Asia-Pacific region since 2019. Recently, Dr. Martina has been involved in the advocacy effort for palliative care in Indonesia, collaborating with national stakeholders, including the Comprehensive Cancer Care of Cipto Mangunkusumo Hospital, WHO-Indonesia, and the Indonesian Ministry of Health. Following the completion of her PhD and her return to Indonesia, she assumed the role of a faculty member and facilitator for the Training for Trainers program for palliative care initiated by the Indonesian Ministry of Health for healthcare professionals across the country.

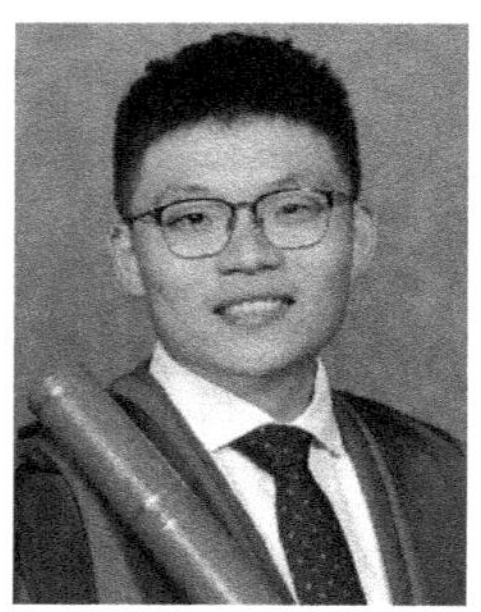

Cheng-Pei Lin is an oncology nurse and palliative care researcher from Taiwan. He is an assistant professor in nursing at the Institute of Community Health Care, College of Nursing, National Yang Ming Chiao Tung University, Taiwan. His research interests focus on end-of-life care, advance care planning, palliative care, and global palliative care evaluation. He is a member of various academic societies, including the Asia Pacific Hospice Palliative Care Network (APHN, research committee board member) and Advance Care Planning International (board member). He is the principal investigator of a project to develop an advance care planning program for the community of older people with chronic illnesses, funded by the National Science and Technology Council, Taiwan.

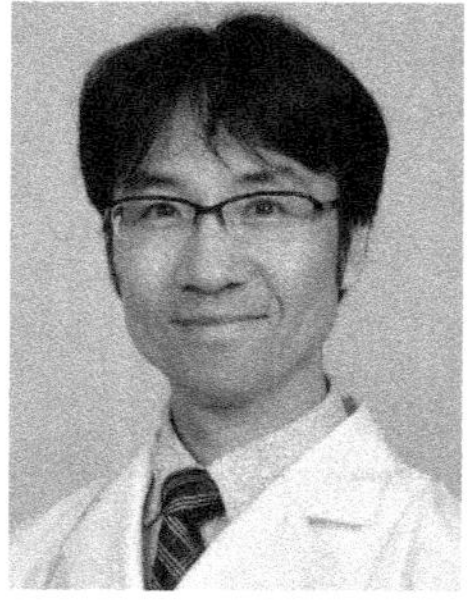

Masanori Mori is a director of the Division of Palliative and Supportive Care at Seirei Mikatahara General Hospital in Hamamatsu, Japan. His research interests include symptom management, clinician–patient communication, and advance care planning (ACP), especially in the context of Asian culture. He is the lead investigator on multiple international and national research projects, including a Delphi study on ACP in Asia and the East Asian

Cross-Cultural Collaborative Study to Elucidate the Dying Process (EASED). He has been involved in compiling the clinical practice guidelines on clinician–patient communication and ACP in Japan. He is also a member of various academic societies, including the Asia Pacific Hospice Palliative Care Network (APHN, co-vice chair).

Contents

Section 1

Culture and Religion in Advance Care Planning

Chapter 1

Culture and Advance Care Planning

Annemarie Samuels

*Institute of Cultural Anthropology and Development Sociology,
Leiden University, Leiden, The Netherlands*

The practices of palliative care and advance care planning as we currently know them in medicine have their cultural roots in the United Kingdom and the United States. Modern palliative care was developed in the 1960s and 70s in England, shaped by the work and activism of Dr. Cicely Saunders.[1] Scholars have noted how its holistic approach to the patient by interconnecting physical, social, spiritual, and psychological suffering is influenced by Anglo-Christian traditions of confession towards the end of life.[2] Advance Care Planning was developed in the United States with the aim of improving care at the end of life by discussing patient goals and wishes prior to a moment in which they may lack the capacity to decide. Although recent critiques point at the limited evidence for ACP's effectiveness[3] and its strong cultural emphasis on autonomy and self-determination that may not be suitable in diverse cultural settings,[4] the practice has also found widespread resonance and adaptation around the world.

So far, however, the overwhelming majority of studies on ACP have been conducted in the Global North. This is currently changing. Globally, scholars, policymakers, and health care workers develop approaches and practices that fit cultural ways of approaching illness, death, and dying that are quite different from those encountered by Cicely Saunders, and later developed in hospice and palliative care approaches, as well as ACP. This leads to increasing insight into cultural diversity and ACP,[5] new models for ACP in specific regions,[6] and the growing global recognition that there may be "multiple futures" for palliative care.[7]

The country-based reflections in this section add significantly to this emerging body of knowledge on ACP and cultural sensitivity, particularly in Asia. Before diving into these specific reflections, however, I will briefly reflect on scholarly approaches to the concepts of "culture" and "cultural diversity" when it comes to ACP. To do so, I borrow insights from discussions on culture in the social sciences, particularly sociology and anthropology.

Rethinking Culture

For most of the twentieth century, anthropologists and other social scientists saw culture as a specific set of customs, practices, rituals, language, and beliefs belonging to a specific group living in a specific geographical region. From the 1970s onwards, however, this notion of cultures as bounded wholes confined in place has been turned completely upside down.[8] Social scientists then started to increasingly recognize that people had always continuously been traveling and exchanging ideas and that power relations shaped interactions within and across societies. Even in the remotest villages, the socio-cultural experience of two given individuals might therefore not be entirely the same. "Culture" came to be seen as not a list of things or practices that universally applies to a given society or group and that can be described separately from actual behavior. Rather, to understand how culture shapes human behavior and interaction, it is more useful to look at the processes and practices through which individuals and collectives create and enact cultural differences or understandings — processes that always take place within structures of power.

The consequences of this move away from studying "a" culture as if separate from people's lived experiences and social inequalities and towards looking at diversity as a dynamic and interactive process that is continuously practiced and in flux, are many. We should note, for example, that it becomes impossible to speak of something like "the Indonesian culture" or "the Italian culture" because societies differ internally as much as they may differ from other societies.[8] A highly educated woman in Yogyakarta may in many ways have more in common with her counterpart in Milan than with a fisherman in Manado. This is a crucial insight for medicine, as it should caution against essentialization: a patient entering the consultation room may be related to a particular social group in society, yet this does not mean that this patient's treatment preferences necessarily align with what the health care worker may presume about this socio-cultural or religious group.[9] At the same time, seeing cultural practice as a dynamic process has taught us to understand biomedical practice itself as cultural and varying across times and places.[10] "Culturally informed care," then, as Kleinman and Benson[9] have argued, starts less from clinicians' knowledge about a particular ethnic group and more from them asking patients "what matters most to them in the experience of illness and treatment."

Cultural Diversity and ACP

This brings us to the importance of studying culturally sensitive practices of Advance Care Planning. Social scientists have long studied end-of-life care as a cultural process,[11] and recent studies show a large variety of practices in approaching death, dying, and palliative care around the world, as well as within Asia.[12,13] Such cultural variation consists for example of the extent to which people value discussing death and dying, the mode and manner of communication about serious illness and the end of life, preferences for the place of death, and the role of social and family relations in the health care process. Given this variety, and the aforementioned "Western" cultural roots of palliative care and ACP, it should not be surprising that scholars and professionals are calling for culturally sensitive practices of ACP and palliative care[14,15] and multicultural research groups.[16] They point out how it is crucial to take diverse cultural contexts and practices into account when developing locally situated ACP.

Research on cultural aspects of ACP has mostly taken place in the Global North, where ACP and palliative care have been studied in relation to ethnic and other minorities. These studies yield interesting insights, for example pointing at the importance of cultural values and spirituality, as well as differences in possibilities for accessing palliative care.[17] However, until a few years ago, studies on cultural dimensions of ACP outside of Global North settings were relatively limited.

Perspectives from Asia and the Pacific

Recent publications about ACP in Asia have started to fill this lacunae, by studying cultural dimensions of ACP and palliative care in diverse national and local settings.[5,18–20] The chapters that follow further contribute to this important development. They highlight, for example how the sensitivity of openly discussing the end of life in various Asian contexts has significant implications for ACP and the way it is adapted to work for patients and healthcare workers. In the case of Samoa, participants in a series of workshops on ACP pointed out the importance of the local value of *tausi matua*, which denotes the responsibility of family members to take care. The reliance on family members' care and decision-making is considered crucial to include in ACP implementation. Moreover, patients and family members may feel that discussing the end of life can evoke an earlier death, and health is mainly discussed within the family. These sensitivities appear crucial to be included in ACP development, as we will also see in the case of Singapore where family-centred patient care offers a promising alternative to discourses of autonomy and patient-centred care.

The case of Japan similarly shows how implicit rather than explicit communication is valued in many Asian Societies, and how family plays a crucial role in ACP. Patients' expressions of their wishes can be influenced by the cultural value of not being a burden on the family. As shown below, ACP implementation in Asia may therefore benefit from drawing on the concept of "relational autonomy", in which patients are considered as always embedded in a social network rather than singular individuals standing apart from their social relations. Yet, as the case of Japan also points out, practices of talking and not talking about dying are changing. Therefore it is crucial to keep inquiring into the patients' preferences rather than a priori assuming cultural values. This point is underscored in the case of Australia, where research emphasizes the importance of avoiding essentialist readings of preferences of cultural minority groups. Taken together, these cases not only reveal the need for creating culturally sensitive models for ACP in Asian societies, but also give important pointers for the factors to take into account in this process, including the sensitivity of discussing dying, preferences for implicit communication, the importance of the family in healthcare decision-making practices, and the cultural changes that create increasingly diverse preferences for discussing and planning care.

References

1. Clark D. (2007). From the margins to the centre: A review of the history of palliative care in cancer. *Lancet Oncology* **2007**(8): 430–438.
2. Broom A. (2015). *Dying: A Social Perspective on the End of Life*. Routledge, London.

3. Morrison R.S., Meier D.E., and Arnold R.M. (2021). What is wrong with advance care planning? *JAMA* **326**(16): 1575–1576.

4. Nguyen N., Zivkovic, T., de Haas R., and Faulkner D. (2021). Problematizing "planning ahead": A cross-cultural analysis of Vietnamese health and community workers' perspectives on advance care directives. *Qual. Health Res.* **31**(12): 2304–2316.

5. Menon S., Kars M.C., Malhotra C., *et al.* (2018). Advance care planning in a multicultural family centric community: A qualitative study of health care professionals', patients', and caregivers' perspectives. *J. Pain Symptom Manage.* **56**(2): 213–221.

6. Martina D., Geerse O.P., Lin C.-P., *et al.* (2021). Asian patients' perspectives on advance care planning: A mixed-method systematic review and conceptual framework. *Palliative Med.* **35**(10): 1776–1792.

7. Zaman S., Inbadas H., Whitelaw H., and Clark D. (2017). Common or multiple futures for end of life care around the world? Ideas from the "waiting room of history." *Social Sci. Med.* **172**: 72–79.

8. Gupta A. and Ferguson J. (1992). Beyond "culture": Space, identity, and the politics of difference. *Cult. Anthropol.* 7(1): 6–23.

9. Kleinman A. and Benson P. (2006). Anthropology in the clinic: The problem of cultural competency and how to fix it. *Plos Med.* **3**(10): 1673–1676.

10. DelVecchio-Good M.-J. (1995). Cultural studies of biomedicine: An agenda for research. *Social Sci. Med.* **41**(4): 461–476.

11. Glaser B. G. and Strauss, A. L. (1965). *Awareness of Dying*. Aldine, Chicago.

12. Banerjee D. (2020). *Enduring Cancer: Life, Death, and Diagnosis in Delhi*. Duke University Press, Durham and London.

13. Stonington S. (2020). *The Spirit Ambulance: Choreographic the End of Life in Thailand*. University of California Press, Oakland.

14. Clark D. (2012). Cultural considerations in planning palliative and end of life care. *Palliative Med.* **26**(3): 195–196.

15. Mori M. and Morita T. (2020). End-of-life decision-making in Asia: A need for in-depth cultural consideration. *Palliative Med.* DOI: 10.1177/0269216319896932.

16. Gott M., Moeke-Maxwell T., Morgen T., *et al.* (2017). Working biculturally within a palliative care research context: the development of the Te Ārai Palliative care and end of life research group. *Mortality* **22**(4): 291–307.

17. Hong M., Yi E.-H., Johnson K.J., and Adamek M.E. (2018). Facilitators and barriers for advance care planning among ethnic and racial minorities in the US: A systematic review of the current literature. *J. Immigrant Minority Health* **20**: 1277–1287.

18. Cheng H.W.B. (2018). Advance care planning in Chinese seniors: Cultural perspectives. *J. Palliative Med.* **33**(4): 242–246.

19. Martina D., Kustanti C. Y., Dewantari R., *et al.* (2022). Opportunities and challenges for advance care planning in strongly religious family-centric societies: A Focus group study of Indonesian cancer-care professionals. *BMC Palliative Care.* **21**: 110.
20. Mori M., Kuwama Y., Ashigaka T., *et al.* (2018). Acculturation and perceptions of a good death among Japanese Americans and Japanese living in the US. *J. Pain and Symptom Manage.* **55**(1): 31–38.

Chapter 2

Culture and Advance Care Planning: Perspectives from Singapore

Andy Hau Yan Ho

Psychology, School of Social Sciences,
Nanyang Technological University, Singapore
Lee Kong Chian School of Medicine,
Nanyang Technological University, Singapore

Introduction

In Singapore, a government-led, national-level Advance Care Planning programme was launched in 2011, the first of its kind in the whole of Southeast Asia. Coined "Living Matters", it was modelled after the Respecting Choices programme originally developed by the Gunderson Health Care system in Wisconsin, United States. Its goals are to empower individuals with greater autonomy in making informed end-of-life care decisions through open and honest conversations about treatment preferences between patients, their families, and their professional caregivers. Since its inauguration, more than 2,000 ACP facilitators have been trained and approximately 30,000 ACP conversations have been completed.

A national evaluation of Living Matters conducted in 2017 by my research team found that the programme was highly effective in eliciting and meeting the care preferences of patients.[1] This is particularly true for patients who wished for comfort care and no aggressive treatment with 98% care concordance, those who opted for home or hospital, or hospice care with 76% care concordance, as well as for patients who wished for strictly home care with 65% care concordance. These numbers, while encouraging, are not without caveat, as the implementation of ACP and how ACP is being perceived and received in the community have proven to be greatly challenging.[2] The reason for this is due largely in part to the complexities posed by the values, beliefs, and behaviours of the Singaporean populace, which are heavily shaped by a melting pot of cultural traditions that highlight an undercurrent of death aversion and filial piety. This chapter will examine the interplay between these key cultural idiosyncrasies with ACP practices in Singapore, and discuss the lessons learnt for enhancing ACP provision in the future.

Death Aversion

Like many countries in East Asia, where cultures are deeply rooted in the philosophies of Buddhism and Taoism, and with death often portrayed as the opposition to life or as the consequence of retribution and karma,[3] mortality has long been stigmatized in Singapore, leading to fear, anxiety, and avoidance. Death aversion is commonplace, for death is not a topic that is readily discussed in private or in the public sphere, while social connections with the dying and the bereaved are frequently restricted to close family members and healthcare teams. This is because death is deemed highly polluting, where the bad luck and ill fortune that it brings can be contaminating and passed on through sensory and physical contacts. It is against this cultural backdrop, where people often feel powerless and demoralized in the face of mortality and loss, that the Living Matters programme was born.

It is therefore not surprising that the take-up rate of ACP was extremely low in its formative years, where most patients and families were not at all ready to have any discussion about their end-of-life care as the topic carries ominous implications. Notwithstanding the death aversion of the public, healthcare workers who were trained to carry out ACP also felt uneased when called to engage in such conversations. In fact, it was discovered that of all the healthcare workers that participated in the 2017 national evaluation study, not one had completed their own ACP. And even though Living Matters was seen as a welcomed initiative that could help patients and families explore and express their needs and concerns at the end of life, the majority of healthcare workers did not feel comfortable speaking to their own family members about ACP.[2]

Filial Piety

The teachings of Confucius have deep-seated roots in all Asian societies, and many would argue that much of Singapore's national policies on ageing and family are built on the collective ideals of Confucianism. This argument holds truth when one considers that there are only two countries in the world that adopt the traditional ethics of filial piety in their national legislations to make adult children legally liable to care for their elderly parents — Singapore's Maintenance of Parent Act, and China's Law of Protection of Rings and Interest of the Aged. Such emphasis on filial traditions and family dependency has not only affected policy development but also the practice of end-of-life caregiving and decision-making.

For example, it has been reported that filial beliefs, which are exemplified through treating elders with respectful propriety and minimizing their worries, have greatly reduced the willingness of adult children to initiate ACP discussions with their elderly parents as such actions are deemed disrespectful and unfilial.[2] It has also been found that adult children often insist on withholding diagnosis and prognosis from their ailing parents to prevent them from feeling upset about their condition and impending mortality.[4] In fact, medical collusion is rampant, as healthcare workers are often requested by family caregivers not to disclose medical information to dying patients; these patients are also often barred from the care decision-making table. Even when there is no collusion and older patients are encouraged to participate in their own care decision-making process, they feel reluctant to do so and rely heavily on their families for such tasks.[5] These practices and behaviours have inevitably put a stranglehold on ACP during its inception.

Moving Forward

Despite these cultural complexities, there are clear remedies that Singapore can adopt to ensure the sustainable growth and development of ACP. First, moving beyond the notions of autonomy and patient-centred care which have dominated the Western healthcare paradigm in the twenty-first century, to that of family-centred patient care that empowers patients and family caregivers to work in reciprocal and empathic partnerships with each other and with healthcare teams to develop and achieve care goals that are based on the authentic wishes and preferences of the patient within the context of family capacity and interdependence. This requires interventions that go beyond medicine to that psychoeducation and psychotherapeutic approaches that support the exploration of dignity, legacy building, and ultimately meaning-making so that ACP conversations can emerge organically. Family Dignity Intervention is one exemplar modality that can achieve this goal.[6] Second, a holistic training programme that imparts cognitive knowledge, cultivates emotional competence, and instils interpersonal skills for working through the demanding issues of mortality among all health and social care workers can empower them to render ACP with greater authenticity and proficiency. Third, a formal life and death education curricula that target students at colleges and universities, particularly those enrolled in medicine, nursing, social work and allied health programmes, can nurture their empathic understanding of and practical competence for working with illness, death and loss. Finally, a concerted and sustained public education and publicity campaign to promote open dialogue on mortality in all facets of society can foster greater awareness and acceptance of ACP. Such an endeavour will necessitate a progression of fundamental familial values — from that of filial piety to filial compassion[7] — that it would be possible then for patients and family members to approach death-related conversations from a place of dignity and empowerment, rather than of fear and obligation.

In conclusion, ACP has become a critical component of quality palliative care in most advanced societies around the world, but it is vastly underdeveloped in many parts of Asia. The lessons learnt from Singapore's experience provide valuable insights on the implementation challenges and complexities of ACP, especially when considering the key cultural idiosyncrasies that are shared by most nations around the region. They can serve to inform the development of comprehensive and appropriate ACP programmes to empower patients' autonomy and dignity in the face of loss and mortality.

References

1.   Tan W.S., Ran B., Low C.K., Ho A.H.Y., and Car J. (2018). Using routinely collected data to ascertain concordance with advance care planning preferences. *J. Pain Symptom Manage.* **56**(5): 659–666. DOI: 10.1016/j. jpainsymman.2018.07.017.
2.   Ho A.H.Y., Lall P., Tan W.S., Patinadan P.V., Wong L.H., Dutta O., Peng W.S., Low C.K., and Car J. (2020). Sustainable implementation of advance care planning in Asia: An interpretive-systemic framework for national

development. *Palliative & Supportive Care,* **9**(1): 82–92. DOI: 10.1017/S1478951520000590.

3. Ho A.H.Y. and Chan C.L.W. (2011). Liberating bereaved persons from the oppression of death and loss in Chinese societies: Examples of the public health approaches. In S. Conway (ed.) *Governing Death and Loss: Empowerment, Involvement and Participation* (pp. 119–128). Oxford University Press, UK.

4. Dutta O., Lall P., Car J., Low C.K., and Ho A.H.Y. (2019). Patient autonomy and participation in end of life decision-making: An interpretive-systemic focus group study on perspectives of Asian healthcare professionals. *Palliative Supportive Care* **18**(4): 425–430. DOI: 10.1017/S1478951519000865.

5. Lall P., Kang N.Q.Y., Tan W.S., Dutta O., Patinadan P.V., Low C.K., Car J., and Ho A.H.Y. (2020). Competing expectations: Advance care planning from the perspectives of doctors and nurses in the South-East Asian context. *Death Stud.* DOI: 10.1080/07481187.2020.1848943.

6. Ho A.H.Y., Car J., Ho M.R., Tan-Ho G., Choo P.Y., Patinadan P.V., Chong P.H., Ong W.Y., Fan G., Tan Y.P., *et al.* (2017). A novel family dignity intervention (FDI) for enhancing and informing holistic palliative care in Asia: Study protocol for a randomized controlled trial. *Trials* **18**(1): 587. DOI: 10.1186/s13063-017-2325-5.

7. Chan C.L.W., Ho A.H.Y., Leung P.P.Y., Chochinov H.M., Neimeyer R.A., Pang S.M.C., and Tse D.M.W. (2012). The blessing and curses of filial piety on dignity at the end-of-life: Lived experience of Hong Kong Chinese adult children caregivers. *J. Ethnic Cult. Divers. Social Work* **21**(4): 277–296. https://doi.org/10.1080/15313204.2012.729177.

Chapter 3

Culture and Advance Care Planning: Perspectives from Japan

Ai Chikada

*Department of Human Health Sciences,
Graduate School of Medicine, Kyoto University, Kyoto, Japan*

Cultural Aspects

Since Confucianism and the concept of "filial piety" are ingrained in the culture of many East Asian countries, patient autonomy is consequently often strongly influenced by family values and physician authority, and the dominance of family members and physicians in patients' end-of-life decision-making has been recognized as a cultural trait in Asia.[1] Furthermore, from a cultural perspective, Asians traditionally tend to treat death as taboo and are unwilling to discuss the topic.[2] In this section, we take an example of Japanese culture to discuss the potential implications of East Asian culture to ACP.

Japan traditionally emphasizes an interactive relationship with others. In general, Japanese people do not express their preferences explicitly and expect family members and health care providers (HCPs) to make the best decision for them based on an unspoken agreement with patients.[1,3] In addition, Japanese may not share their true wishes out of consideration for the family's wishes and burdens.[1,3]

In a systematic review of Japanese papers, Chikada *et al.* reported four Japanese cultural characteristics that influence the ACP process. The first characteristic was "that Japanese people tend to avoid the explicit expression of their own preferences owing to the high-context nature of Japanese culture". Second, "Japanese people are not comfortable thinking about death and tend to defer decision-making". Third, "Families' preferences tend to be valued over patients' own owing to the family-centred culture". Finally, "Japanese people tend to refrain from explicit decision-making and place more value on harmony with families".[3] Therefore, it is necessary to respect the harmony between patient and family in patient-centred decision support when considering ACP in the context of East Asian culture.

How to Implement ACP in Clinical Practice

One of the important elements of ACP in Japan is having repetitive conversations using a patient-centred approach, including families, with the aim of creating a consensus through shared decision-making.[3] In western countries, family members participate in ACP conversations if the patient chooses, whereas in Japan, the family is usually treated as a full participant in ACP conversations from the beginning. In Japan, emphasis is placed on creating the best goals for both patients and families.[3] The family may therefore be both a facilitator and a barrier to ACP. Although there is a risk of pressure from family members, family involvement in ACP is essential because Japanese patients tend to be concerned about family opinions and potential burden in decision-making.[3,4]

To address this ethical and practical dilemma, the concept of "relational autonomy", which is a concept of autonomy that places the individual in a socially embedded network of others and the collectivist paradigm may ideally be applied to reinforce and support the patient's autonomous decision-making.[1,4] Therefore, HCPs must value a patient-centred approach while at the same time trying to maintain family harmony.[3] HCPs need to be trained in communication skills to facilitate ACP conversations among patients and families. In addition, future policies and educational programs should continue to address how to respect the patient's preferences through shared decision-making while maintaining family harmony.[1]

Importance of Understanding Values

Encouraging patients to identify their values and priorities is one of the most fundamental components of ACP. However, while recognizing that understanding cultural traits facilitates understanding of individual values, HCPs must also recognize that cultural traits do not necessarily reflect the values of all individuals and families in Japanese culture. Therefore, HCPs must be aware of the importance of respecting individual values rather than taking a stereotypical approach,[3] and strategies are needed for HCPs to encourage patients to express their values and wishes, even if they avoid asserting or explicitly stating them.[5] Takenouchi *et al.* found that the lifeline interview method (LIM) is one of the effective strategies for HCPs as an effective means of eliciting the values and priorities of patients with advanced cancer in East Asian cultures, suggesting that it can serve as a bridge for ACP conversations.[5] By detailing the ups and downs of lifelines through LIM, Asians with limited self-expression were able to articulate what matters to them, and this helped them to reconstruct their self-concept and promote autonomy.[5]

Although the topic of death tends to be taboo in Asia, the lifeline interview is a way to talk about a person's life history, expectations for the future, and thoughts about important events, rather than directly discussing life and death. In the process, patients reaffirm what matters to them and naturally discuss their preferences for current and future treatment and care, as well as life goals. Thus, for East Asians, a life review such as LIM may be an effective implicit communication approach to be used prior to a formal ACP conversation. Moreover, Japanese place a high priority on building a rapport with their healthcare providers prior to ACP conversations,[3] understanding the patient's values and what matters to them through life reviews would also contribute to building rapport.

While the concept of patient autonomy has been developing in Asia,[1] studies over the past several decades have shown that key topics such as cancer diagnosis, prognosis, ACP, and end-of-life discussions, along with traditional cultural values, are gradually shifting toward open communication.[6]

Learning Objectives
- Although there is a risk of pressure from family members on the patient's preferences, family involvement in ACP is imperative because the Japanese tend to promote autonomous decision-making in the context of relational autonomy. HCPs should help patients and families maintain harmony.

- For East Asians who tend to avoid discussing death and expressing their feelings, a life review may be an effective communication approach and contribute to building rapport with HCPs prior to a formal ACP conversation.
- The concept of patient autonomy is developing in Asia, and individual values are becoming more diverse, which makes it important to recognize the importance of respecting individual values.

References

1. Cheng S.-Y., Lin C.-P., Chan H.Y., Martina D., Mori M., Kim S.-H., and Ng R. (2020). Advance care planning in Asian culture. *Jpn. J. Clin. Oncol.* **50**(9): 976–989. https://doi.org/10.1093/jjco/hyaa131.

2. Lin C.-P., Cheng S.-Y., Mori M., Suh S.-Y., Chan H. Y.-L., Martina D., Pang W.-S., Huang H.-L., Peng J.-K., Yao C.-A., *et al.* (2019). 2019 Taipei declaration on advance care planning: A cultural adaptation of end-of-life care discussion. *J. Palliative Med.* **22**(10): 1175–1177. https://doi.org/10.1089/jpm.2019.0247.

3. Chikada A., Takenouchi S., Nin K., and Mori M. (2021). Definition and recommended cultural considerations for advance care planning in Japan: A systematic review. *Asia-Pacific J. Oncol. Nurs.* **8**(6): 628–641. https://doi.org/10.4103/apjon.apjon-2137.

4. Miyashita J., Shimizu S., Shiraishi R., Mori M., Okawa K., Aita K., Mitsuoka S., Nishikawa M., Kizawa Y., Morita T., *et al.* (2022). Culturally adapted consensus definition and action guideline: Japan's advance care planning. *J. Pain Symptom Manage.* **64**(6): 602–613. https://doi.org/10.1016/j.jpainsymman.2022.09.005.

5. Takenouchi S., Chikada A., Mori M., Tamura K., and Nin K. (2022). Strategies to understand what matters to advanced cancer patients in advance care planning: A qualitative study using the lifeline interview method. *J. Hospice Palliative Nurs.* **24**(4): E135–E143. https://doi.org/10.1097/NJH.0000000000000866.

6. Mori M., Lin CP., Cheng SY., Suh SY., Takenouchi S., Ng R., Chan H., Kim SH., Chen PJ., Yuen KK., Fujimori M., Yamaguchi T., Hamano J., Kizawa Y., Morita T., and Martina D. (2023). Communication in cancer care in Asia: A narrative review. *JCO Glob. Onco.* **9**: e2200266.

Chapter 4

Culture and Advance Care Planning: Perspectives from Australia

Craig Sinclair

*School of Psychology, University of New South Wales,
Kensington, Australia
Neuroscience Research Australia (NeuRA),
Randwick, Australia*

Across the past two decades, advance care planning (ACP) has been endorsed by professional colleges and incorporated into national quality standards for health services. The growing acceptance of ACP in Australia is seen as aligned with the value placed upon individual autonomy and person-centred care across much of Australian society. However, the expansion of ACP has raised questions about the optimal approach across Australia's ageing, geographically dispersed and culturally diverse population. This sub-chapter addresses some cultural considerations relevant to ACP policy and practice in Australia, with a focus on the First Nations and culturally and linguistically diverse (CaLD) communities, and a conclusion that inclusive, community-based initiatives are urgently needed.

Background

The Australian population is culturally diverse, with 37% of older Australians (65 years and over) being born outside Australia, and just over half of these speak a language other than English at home.[1]

Aboriginal and Torres Strait Islander peoples (hereafter respectfully referred to as Indigenous) speak over 250 unique languages and belong to many nations and tribe groups. They make up 3.8% of the Australian population, with proportionately higher rates in regional and remote areas of Australia.[2]

While modern-day Australia is culturally diverse, its society has been significantly shaped by a history of European colonisation in the late 18th century, and politically and economically motivated patterns of immigration. Up until the 1970s, the 'White Australia policy' limited migration and favoured English-speaking migrants from northern and western Europe.[3] Harmful domestic policies have resulted in dispossession and inter-generational trauma for Indigenous peoples. This history has resulted in the white and Anglo-Australian population experiencing educational, health and socio-economic privilege, creating inequities that impact health engagement and outcomes for cultural minority groups.

In addition to cultural incongruencies with the concept of ACP reported by some groups,[4] people from CaLD and First Nations communities who are potentially interested in ACP can face a range of barriers, including difficulty accessing information about routine health services, or difficulty accessing ACP resources in their preferred language/s.[5] Not surprisingly, Advance Care Planning Australia's national advance care directive (ACD) prevalence study found that older adults born outside Australia were less likely to have completed their own ACD than those born in Australia.[6]

First Nations Communities

The Indigenous peoples in Australia are custodians of the longest continuing culture in the world and practice their cultural beliefs and customs in dynamic and evolving ways. This includes practices and beliefs relating to traditional healing, end-of-life care and 'sorry business' associated with dying and grieving.[7] However the impacts of European colonisation, and damaging policies resulting in a 'Stolen Generation', have led to inter-generational trauma, loss of language and culture, along with displacement and dispossession from traditional lands. This history of colonisation means that it is especially important for any efforts to promote ACP or understand priorities for end-of-life care within Indigenous communities to use 'decolonising' approaches, which build trust, share information openly and enable community leadership and oversight.[8]

A common theme in research with Australian Indigenous communities about their priorities in end-of-life care has been connection to Country, including a desire to 'return to Country'.[9] This translates to a person's desire to receive end-of-life care in their home country, as defined through family, kinship and tribal ties. For some, this means a desire to return to specific places (which may be in regional or remote areas) prior to death, even if access to medical and care services may be limited.

While some resources do exist in Australia to guide health professionals in providing appropriate communication and culturally appropriate end-of-life care for Indigenous communities,[10] there are limited resources for servicing the diverse range of language groups spoken across Indigenous Australian communities.

Culturally and Linguistically Diverse Communities

Among the CaLD communities in Australia, a range of attitudes, experiences and barriers have been documented, reflecting the diverse backgrounds of the many cultural groups who have settled here. Communities who migrated many years ago, or who have come from countries in which English is spoken, have tended to show greater evidence of acculturation and find it easier to access information about ACP. Studies undertaken among the prominent Chinese-speaking communities in Australia have tended to show an openness to discussion about ACP, despite the recognition of traditional cultural taboos associated with talking about death.[5] A feasibility trial undertaken by Respecting Patient Choices showed that when interpreters trained in ACP were provided for Greek- and Italian-speaking hospital inpatients, they took up ACP at similar rates to English-speaking patients.[11] It has been argued that differences observed between different cultural groups should be considered not just through a lens of 'cultural difference' but also from a life-course perspective, which considers cumulative differences in access to education as a factor in attitudes towards ACP.[6]

Among the contemporary migrant population in Australia, growing populations of humanitarian refugees present an urgent need for proactive approaches which engage communities, build trust and seek co-designed approaches to ACP. However, for those who have escaped threats of poverty, war and disease, the concept of a person planning their own end-of-life care, or refusing available treatments, may also be unfamiliar or offensive.

Conclusion

Research and implementation relating to ACP among First Nations and CaLD communities in Australia is still in an early stage of development. Further work is needed, in partnership with cultural community leaders, to co-design culturally safe approaches to ACP with these First Nations and CaLD communities.

Learning Objectives

- The cultural and linguistic diversity of the Australian population means that it is important to avoid reliance on essentialist stereotypes about the attitudes or expectations of cultural minority groups with respect to advance care planning.
- A life-course perspective would consider disparities in ACP engagement between different cultural groups as the product of cumulative differences in access to education and information, not just as a product of cultural differences.
- Researchers and health service leaders should aim to engage with cultural community leaders, to understand community priorities and co-design culturally safe approaches to ACP.

References

1. Australian Bureau of Statistics. (2019). *3412.0 — Migration, Australia, 2017–18*. Australian Bureau of Statistics, Canberra. https://www.abs.gov.au/AUSSTATS/abs@.nsf/DetailsPage/3412.02017-18?OpenDocument.
2. Australian Bureau of Statistics. (2022). *Estimates of Aboriginal and Torres Strait Islander Australians*. Australian Bureau of Statistics, Canberra. https://www.abs.gov.au/statistics/people/aboriginal-and-torres-strait-islander-peoples.
3. Peters N. (2001). *Milk and Honey — But No Gold: Postwar migration to Western Australia 1945–1964*. UWA Press, Perth.
4. Zivkovic T. (2018). Forecasting and foreclosing futures: The temporal dissonance of advance care directives. *Social Sci. Med.* **215**: 16–22.

5. Yap S.S., Chen K., Detering K.M., and Fraser S.A. (2018). Exploring the knowledge, attitudes and needs of advance care planning in older Chinese Australians. *J. Clin. Nurs.* **27**(17–18): 3298–3306.
6. Sinclair C., Sellars M., Buck K., Detering KM, White BP, Nolte L., *et al.* (2021). Association between region of birth and advance care planning documentation among older Australian migrant communities: A multi-center audit study. *J. Gerontol. Series B.* **76**(1): 109–120.
7. McGrath P., Fox-Young S., and Phillips E. (2008). Insights, on aboriginal grief practices from the northern territory, Australia. *Aust. J. Primary Health.* **14**(3): 48–57.
8. Sherwood J.M. (2010). Do no harm: Decolonising aboriginal health research [Unpublished Doctor of Philosophy Thesis]. University of New South Wales, Sydney.
9. McGrath P. (2007). 'I don't want to be in that big city; this is my country here': Research findings on Aboriginal peoples' preference to die at home. *Aust. J. Rural Health* **15**(4): 264–268.
10. AGPAL Education and Training. (2021). *Gwandalan: Supporting Palliative Care for Aboriginal and Torres Strait Islander Communities.* AGPAL, Milton. https://gwandalanpalliativecare.com.au/.
11. Detering K.M., Sutton E., Fraser S., Wallis K., Silvester W., Mawren D., *et al.* (2015). Feasibility and acceptability of advance care planning in elderly Italian and Greek speaking patients as compared to English-speaking patients: An Australian cross-sectional study. *BMJ Open* **5**(8): e008800.

Chapter 5

Culture and Advance Care Planning: Samoan Perspectives from New Zealand

Eirenei Vailaau-Ah Kuoi[*] and Michelle Niukini Hendrikse[†]

*Atamu EFKS Porirua Incorporated,
Porirua, New Zealand
†Totara Hospice- POI Team,
Auckland, New Zealand

Samoa is an island nation in the South Pacific. After gaining its independence from New Zealand in 1962, Samoa and New Zealand continued to maintain strong relations through the Treaty of Friendship 1962 which helped create a path for Samoans to migrate to New Zealand for work. Samoan people have been migrating to New Zealand since the 1960s. From these initial waves of Pacific migration, diasporic waves of generations of Samoans settled in main cities within New Zealand.[1]

Fa'asamoa is essentially the Samoan way of life. It refers to the way you walk, talk and carry yourself. It is fundamentally based on *fa'aaloalo* (respect), *tautua* (service) and *alofa* (love) and these values underpin the way Samoans engage with each other. *Fa'asamoa* is built on principles of reciprocity and collective responsibility.[2] These foundational core values can help inform advance care planning (ACP) and how to effectively engage with Samoan people.

Va fealoa'i — Nurturing Relationships

Va fealoa'i refers to how Samoans develop, maintain and nurture meaningful and trusting relationships. Trust is important in the *talanoaga* (conversation) because ACP invites a person to think about potentially sensitive, emotional and difficult topics. *Va fealoa'i* is demonstrated through cultural protocols and practices whereby each person understands their place and role in relation to others. It is important to acknowledge the formal way to address an elderly person, chief or church leader as different from the way one would address an untitled young person. The language used (oratory/formal/informal) varies depending on who you are speaking to and the context of the conversation. Efi[3] describes how the use of words, language and tone is used to reiterate a sense of cultural self. The Samoan language uses allegory, allusions and metaphor in *fagogo* (fables or fairy tales), *lauga* (speeches) and a Samoan sense of self. Samoan culture privileges metaphor, allusions and allegory. In contrast, scientific discourse privileges precision and evidence[3] Documents, such as an advance care directive, and medical terminology lean more on exacting language that focuses on individual choice and autonomy. The need for "exacting" language is privileged and can be necessary to acquire health information. Exacting precise language about sensitive topics can contrast with a Samoan collective worldview, thinking and behaviour.

Va tapu'ia — Sacredness

Va tapu'ia refers to the sacred space between man and all things living and dead. *Tapu* indicates something that is subject to restrictions. The underlying sacred essence reinforces the connection or relationships with all things; God, cosmos, environment and self.[4] Any discussion regarding sensitive health issues such as future treatment options or life-sustaining treatment must therefore be facilitated with a holistic understanding of the sacredness surrounding some topics.

While it is not uncommon for Samoans to verbally discuss health, ongoing care and death with family, there are cultural differences and nuances in how Samoan people approach their health, death, and burial. Dialogue relating to death and grief for many Samoans still remains in the realm of *tapu* (sacred) or *sā* (protected).[4] Death and dying is a sensitive topic to discuss within Samoan families. Further challenges may arise when the discussion is initiated by people outside the family unit. From a palliative perspective, questions asking about wishes around death, and dying may be perceived as too direct, confrontational, invasive or too nosey. There remain superstitious beliefs around pre-empting advance discussions around one's health care, and the last stage of life, due to a fear that this may cause an earlier death to occur.

Tausi matua — Care for the Elderly

Many of the Samoan cultural values are around *tausi matua*, a widely accepted and practiced cultural belief that it is the duty of the family to care for their elderly. *Tausi matua* is considered a blessing and is a shared responsibility among family members.

Belief System Amongst Samoan People

Samoan people have a strong belief system in the sovereignty of God over life and look to God for guidance. The historical influence of Christian missionaries from the 1830s has permeated the Samoan worldview, to place trust in God to provide, for present and future needs. Advanced care planning is considerate and inclusive of a higher belief system that trusts that God is sovereign in all plans beyond this world.

Advance Care Planning — Engagement in a Samoan Church Context

In 2019, Atamu EFKS Porirua ("Atamu"), a Pacific faith-based charity in Wellington, initiated a pilot with the aim of understanding the barriers and means to engage with Samoan audiences regarding advance care planning.[5]

The pilot involved inviting predominantly elderly Samoan people, to attend one of 3 workshops delivered in *Gagana Samoa* (Samoan language). The pilot focussed on 3 main objectives.

1. Identify the barriers that prevent Samoans from accessing information about advance care planning.
2. Understand cultural influences that may affect how Samoans view end-of-life planning.
3. Develop, and test processes that can successfully engage Samoan families in advance care planning conversations.

Preparation for Engagement

Atamu facilitated workshops for three different groups of Samoan people within the same church community. A subcommittee developed an implementation plan with recommendations to translate all ACP material and ensure Samoan formal speaking protocols were adhered to. The workshops were designed with a demonstration of va fealoa'i and having respect for the va tapu'ia.

Workshop Format

Each workshop followed a similar format beginning with a prayer before formally addressing and welcoming the group. After a brief overview of ACP and why it is valuable, prepared questions were distributed to guide a *talanoa/fa'asoa* (group discussion). All verbal comments and responses were recorded and survey forms were collected at the end before concluding with a prayer and refreshments. The workshops were attended by 63 people many of whom were living at home with family and had long-term health challenges.

Emergent Themes from Workshops

Data collected from the pilot suggests that while it is not uncommon for people to discuss their health plans informally with family, more than 90% of attendees had never heard of ACP prior to attending the workshop. Clarity was provided regarding the differences between ACP and Enduring Powers of Attorney.

During the *talanoa* part of the workshops, all attendees agreed that Samoans are *tausi matua. This means that* attendees were generally confident that family carers had a strong understanding of the needs of an elderly family member. Family members who are *tausi matua* place significant importance on this responsibility and are the ones who normally accompany the elderly to required medical appointments and any other daily care requirements. Many attendees were curious as to what value an ACP would add to their lives, given their confidence that the Samoan concept of *tausi matua* was sufficient. Some expressed that *tausi matua* was not practiced in New Zealand in the same manner as younger Samoans growing up in the NZ environment due to competing priorities that make *tausi matua* in the traditional sense more difficult for them.

Most attendees indicated that the workshops were valuable, however, very few were ready to complete the ACP form. All attendees appreciated that the workshops were delivered in their own language in a safe and familiar setting (church hall). Attendees expressed the need for more conversation which should include other family members. They also provided feedback suggesting that the resources need to be developed from a Samoan perspective, rather than being a translation of an English text or worldview. This is because a strict translation of English words and ideas will not fully convey *Fa'asamoa* values as it relates to ACP.[5]

Learning Objectives

- Accessibility and dissemination of ACP resources within the Samoan community were lacking. Most people did not know about the ACP because most ACP resources were in hospitals and hospices. There were language barriers and no workshops to help people understand the information.
- There are cultural differences in how Samoans view and approach end-of-life planning. Overall, attendees preferred discussion around family members, and did not mind talking about ACP, but were not prepared to document their wishes. Some attendees did not want to burden their families unnecessarily.
- There is a need to develop and test cultural processes that successfully engage Samoan families in advance care planning conversations.

References

1. Council A. (2022). Pacific Auckland. Who are Pacific people? [cited 2023 March 29]. https://www.aucklandcouncil.govt.nz/plans-projects-policies-reports-bylaws/our-plans-strategies/auckland-plan/about-the-auckland-plan/Pages/pacific-auckland.aspx.
2. "Samoans — Culture and identity", Te Ara — The Encyclopedia of New Zealand. [Cited 2022 September 7]. https://teara.govt.nz/en/samoans/page-3.
3. Efi TATT, Suaalii-Sauni TM., Tuagalu I., Kirifi-Alai TN., Fuamatu, N. (2018). *Su'esu'e Manogi: In Search of Fragrance. Tui Atua Tupua Tamasese Ta'isi and the Samoan Indigenous Reference*. Huia (NZ) Ltd., La Vergne.

4. Seiuli B. Ua tafea le tau'ofe: Samoan cultural rituals through death and bereavement experiences. [Cited 2015]. https://researchcommons.waikato.ac.nz/handle/10289/9233.
5. ATAMU, Community workshop information ACP. 2019. [Cited 2023 March 30]. https://www.atamu.org.nz/Home.

Chapter 6

Culture and Advance Care Planning: Acculturation

Tingting Zhu[*], Diah Martina[*,†,‡,§], and Zhimeng Jia[¶,∥]

*Department of Public Health, Erasmus MC,
University Medical Center Rotterdam, Rotterdam, The Netherlands
†Department of Medical Oncology, Erasmus MC Cancer Institute,
University Medical Center Rotterdam, Rotterdam, The Netherlands
‡Division of Psychosomatic and Palliative Medicine, Department of
Internal Medicine Universitas Indonesia, Jakarta, Indonesia
§Cipto Mangunkusumo National General Hospital,
Jakarta, Indonesia
¶Temmy Latner Centre for Palliative Care,
Mount Sinai Hospital, Toronto, Canada
∥Department of Family and Community Medicine,
University of Toronto, Toronto, Canada

Introduction

Acculturation is the process of cultural and psychological change that occurs when people from unalike backgrounds come into contact with one another.[1] This encounter may result in either party accepting or dismissing the beliefs, behaviors, values, and social institutions of the others. Acculturation establishes a link between an individual's culture and the norms of a broader society.

The current approach to ACP, which originate from Western countries, places an emphasis on the completion of its documentation. (e.g., DNR, MOLST, POLST, etc.). Such an approach may result in prioritizing documentation over the conversation process.[2] This may in part explain the disproportionately low uptake of ACP among members of minoritized and marginalized cultural groups.[3] Understanding the interplay of cultural contexts in ACP could enable uptake of ACP among patients of diverse backgrounds.

Figure 1 provides the framework that outlines the many ways that individuals and groups acculturate.[4] At the individual level, the acculturation process range from assimilation (adopts the receiving culture and discards the heritage culture), separation (rejects the receiving culture and retains the heritage culture), integration (adopts the receiving culture and retains the heritage culture), and marginalization (rejects both the heritage and receiving cultures). These four acculturation processes are not static and individuals can shift between processes depending on situational factors.

The processes of acculturation intersect with ACP in two important ways: (1) an individual's cultural identity, in terms of their identification with a dominant community, influences their preferences for care (2) acculturating to ACP itself, because existing ACP practices carries an idealistic view of care planning, which values transparency, consistency, and self-advocacy amidst serious illness.

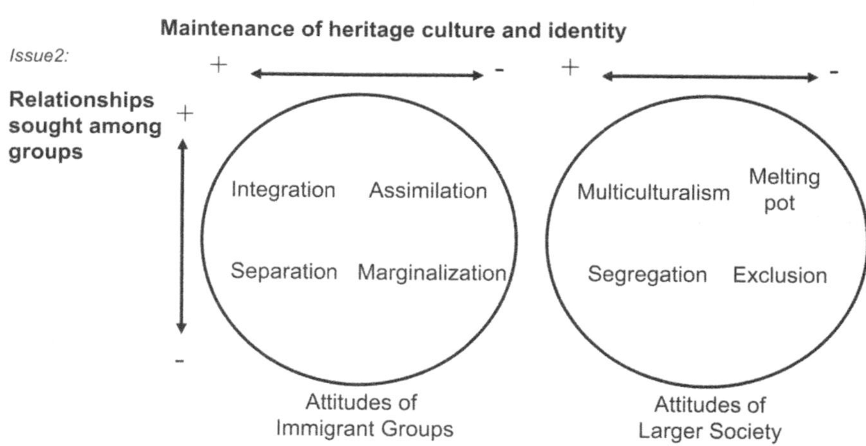

Figure 1.   Acculturation strategies in ethnocultural groups and the larger society.

Who Could be Disproportionately Burdened with Acculturation?

Minoritized groups (immigrants, migrants, cultural minorities, linguistic minorities, structurally vulnerable groups) sharing dissimilar cultural backgrounds and norms with the dominant group necessarily experience the acculturation process and might be disproportionately burdened with acculturating to the majority. We describe the acculturation process as a continuum in attempting to understand it. At one end of the continuum, people may hold tightly onto their cultural heritage and identity. On the other end, people may perceive themselves as part of the dominant culture. The processes of aligning with one's cultural heritage and with the dominant culture are fluid and can occur in parallel.

The process of ACP aims to accommodate and understand the diverse cultural background and approaches to care among patients from minoritized communities. In practice, some have found ACP irrelevant and even harmful as the enactment of ACP is perceived as incompatible with cultural traditions. Some people would wish to modify specific aspects of ACP to make them more relevant to their situation and culturally sensitive. Others, on the other hand, do not desire to keep their cultural heritage; instead, they identify as members of a larger society and perceive no hurdles to participating in ACP because it is compatible with their newly adopted cultural values and norms.

Strategies for ACP Engagement in the Context of Acculturation

A systematic review of studies among Chinese immigrants showed that there are three important factors influencing their engagement in ACP: an individual's self-perceived cultural identity, interpretation of autonomy, and interpretation of filial piety.[6] In this study, the authors showed that an individual's perception of their cultural identity may inform ACP practitioners of the individual beliefs and preferences for ACP. This creates and opportunity to allows the ACP practitioners to align ACP practices with an individual's cultural identity, values, and philosophy.

The concept of autonomy appears to be an important consideration when healthcare professionals initiate ACP conversations. For some, the idea of personal autonomy does not resonate with their daily life experiences nor was their primary consideration in the medical decision-making process. The idea of autonomy is embedded in a social network with significant others. In most cases, observing the family dynamic could help healthcare professionals understand that there is not only one means of achieving and respecting patients' autonomy.

Filial piety represents a core value that shapes family dynamics. However, it is often interpreted differently across cultures and generations. For some, meeting the need for collective identity and social expectations in a certain way is fulfilling filial piety, while for others, filial piety is manifested as understanding and supporting the wishes of elderly parents.

To better customize the varying preferences of individuals' acculturation, the many aspects of the ACP process may need to be tailored to individuals' distinct needs and values, rather than treating it as a unified process. Throughout the ACP process, great care should placed on the content and manner in which ACP is discussed.[7] These preferences may cover a range of topics, including the parties participating in the communication process and the preferred style of communication. Individuals may opt to involve patients, family members, and healthcare professionals in the communication process in different ways, and decision-making may be shared or delegated based on cultural traditions and patient preferences.[6,8] In some circumstances, cultural intermediaries, such as community leaders, religious leaders, or professional medical interpreters, may be useful in facilitating communication and ensuring that cultural traditions are respected. These stakeholders can help bridge any cultural or linguistic barriers and facilitate a culturally sensitive conversation.

Considering the parallel and intersecting processes of advance care planning and acculturation, we propose the following approach to ACP conversations:

1. Consider the degree of explicitness of communication
   When discussing challenging subjects, it is important to carefully consider each individual's preferences for the approach. People from high-context culture societies may feel more at ease if difficult topics are handled in an indirect manner (through euphemisms or metaphors). However, acculturation allows for a shift in these preferences, making it possible for an individual to favor more explicit or clear communication. Actively listening to how people choose their words

(implicit or explicit) can provide healthcare professionals with a clue as to whether it is more acceptable to commence ACP implicitly. Moreover, healthcare professionals could inquire whether individuals prefer clear and explicit information or if they feel more comfortable with less explicit ones.[9] Providing some examples may help this exploration.

2. Consideration of the importance of an individual's native language in ACP

   ACP conversations are frequently complex and nuanced, making it difficult to have such conversations in someone's second or third language. Additionally, it's not always possible to translate many expressions. Therefore, ACP may be better facilitated in one's native language, regardless of proficiency in the other languages. This highlights the importance of collaborating with trained medical interpreters in ACP, in order to act as a cultural broker or bridge in such a complex conversation. Likewise, the availability of ACP educational materials in the corresponding native language influences its uptake.

3. Consideration of the importance of a community-based approach to ACP

   An important strategy to encourage participation in ACP, particularly for people who are minorities in a multicultural society, is through a community-based approach. Because ACP is a specifically culturally relevant topic, it is critical to be able to discuss it with others who share similar cultural heritage or who are highly respected in the community.

References

1. Berry J.W. (2005). Acculturation: Living successfully in two cultures. *Int. J. Intercultural Relat.* **29**(6): 697–712.
2. Fromme E.K., *et al.* (2012). POLST Registry do-not-resuscitate orders and other patient treatment preferences. *JAMA.* **307**(1): 34–35.
3. Crooks J., Trotter, S., and Clarke, G. (2023). How does ethnicity affect presence of advance care planning in care records for individuals with advanced disease? A mixed-methods systematic review. *BMC Palliative Care.* **22**(1): 43.
4. Berry, J.W. (2003). Conceptual approaches to acculturation. In K.M. Chun, P. Balls Organista, and G. Marín (Eds.), *Acculturation: Advances in Theory, Measurement, and Applied Research* (pp. 17–37). American Psychological Association.

5. Hofstede, G., Hofstede, G. J., and Minkov, M. (2010). *Cultures and Organizations: Software of the Mind* (3rd ed.). McGraw-Hill Professional.
6. Zhu T., *et al.* (2023). The role of acculturation in the process of advance care planning among Chinese immigrants: A narrative systematic review. *Palliat Med.* **37**(8): 1063–1078. Doi: 10.1177/02692163231179255. Epub 2023 Jun 13.
7. Zwakman M., *et al.* (2021). Unraveling patients' readiness in advance care planning conversations: A qualitative study as part of the ACTION study. *Support Care Cancer* **29**(6): 2917–2929.
8. Martina D., *et al.* (2021). Asian patients' perspectives on advance care planning: A mixed-method systematic review and conceptual framework. *Palliative Med.* **35**(10): 1776–1792.
9. Back A. and Arnold R. (2009). *Mastering Communication with Seriously Ill Patients: Balancing Honesty with Empathy and Hope.* Cambridge University Press, Cambridge.

Chapter 7

Spirituality and Religion in Advance Care Planning

Kathleen Rimer

*Massachusetts General Hospital and
Hebrew Senior Life, Boston, MA, USA*

Introduction

Brenda was a 78-year-old woman who lived in a monastery (religious community) for lay and ordained people two hours from City Hospital. She first came to the hospital for a diverting ileostomy to treat her ileocolonic Crohn's disease. After two weeks in rehab, she was readmitted to the hospital with altered mental status and fever concerning for sepsis of unknown etiology. While she did not have a previous diagnosis of dementia, for two weeks in the hospital she presented with profound hypoactive delirium with disorientation, poor attention and focus, and inability to speak. Palliative care was consulted to assist with symptom management and goals of care.

Brenda's healthcare proxy was her son, Matthew, and her sister, Angela. Matthew and Angela both lived in the same monastic community as Brenda. Attending physician Dr. Engleman noted with interest Brenda and her family's religious involvement and immediately consulted with the palliative care chaplain, Rev. Sarah. Initially, as Brenda's mental status waxed and waned, Dr. Engleman wondered if prayer or religious support would feel familiar to Brenda and somehow "reach" her given that she was surely disoriented in the hospital setting.

Rev. Sarah visited Brenda that first day spoke gently with her, and offered to pray. Brenda was unable to communicate but occasionally maintained eye contact. Sarah returned the next day and met Brenda's son Matthew, who was initially reserved. Sarah suspected Brenda's family felt out of place in the hospital, and potentially misunderstood. She intended to provide hospitality to Brenda's family and communicate respect for the centrality of their religious faith (America is largely a secular country today, so being religious is more the exception than the norm). She also wanted to explore how the family's faith might impact their medical decision-making. In a conversation with Sarah, Matthew shared, "We believe God has a plan for my mom, and her vocation is not yet complete at the monastery." Matthew believed she would return to her ministry of sewing vestments, tending the community garden, and singing in the choir. At that time Matthew's main concerns were treating his mother's infection and figuring out a way for her to improve her nutrition (she had stopped eating). Rev. Sarah affirmed Matthew's thoughtfulness and relayed this information to the team. During a family meeting, Matthew and Angela opted to surgically insert a feeding tube to give Brenda's body a chance to regain some strength.

Unfortunately, Brenda's infection appeared to worsen, and the team was unable to insert the gastric tube as planned. After a week, despite treatment with comprehensive antibiotics and paracentesis, Brenda developed worsening shortness of breath and delirium and was transferred to the surgical ICU. The team was concerned that Brenda would need respiratory support to stay alive. Sarah continued to visit Angela and Matthew to offer spiritual support. During one conversation, Rev. Sarah learned that the family's perspective had shifted. "Initially we thought God still had a plan for Brenda back at the monastery. But now we are realizing that maybe God has even bigger plans for Brenda, and is calling her Home. We've decided not to intubate or resuscitate, but to focus on her comfort. We've been telling her it's ok to go to God now, to go and be at peace." Sister Angela shared, "I admit I was being selfish, wanting her to stay with me. But that's my wish, not God's, and I realize that now." Rev. Sarah prayed with Brenda's family as more members of the monastic community came to say goodbye. Brenda died peacefully, surrounded by her family and community, eleven days after being admitted to the hospital. Later, Br. Matthew sent an email to the palliative care team thanking them for their sensitive care of his mother.

> **Spirituality**: Spirituality is a dynamic and intrinsic aspect of humanity through which persons seek ultimate meaning, purpose, and transcendence and experience relationship to self, family, others, community, society, nature and the significant or sacred. Spirituality is expressed through beliefs, values, traditions, and practices.[1]
>
> **Religion**: Religion is the search for significance that occurs within the context of established institutions that are designed to facilitate spirituality.
>
> **Spiritual needs**: Needs related to a person's spirituality. Can include the need for ritual, for connection, for meaning in the face of suffering, the need for integrity, a legacy, generativity, concerns about relationships, family and/or significant others, concern or fear about dying or death.[2]
>
> **Spiritual care**: Recognition of and attention to spirituality within health care. Spiritual care relies on a multidisciplinary team (e.g., chaplains, physicians, nurses, social workers) and requires standard inclusion of a spiritual history as part of a comprehensive medical history.
>
> *—Table adapted from Balboni et al. 2022.[3]*

A diagnosis of serious illness disrupts a person's life narrative and can threaten basic assumptions about themselves and their God. Patients might ask, *"Why is this happening to me?"* and, *"What does my life mean when I cannot do what I used to do?"* or, "How will my family cope with this?" Attention to these spiritual questions by the palliative care team is an essential aspect of holistic, patient-centred care. When 1,885 seriously ill patients were asked what attributes of quality of life were most important to them as they approached death, "Being at peace with God" was ranked most important alongside "Being free from pain." This spiritual construct — being at peace — defines the quality of life for most seriously ill people nearing death.[5] How can palliative care teams address this and other spiritual needs?

Definitions

Spirituality is a dynamic and intrinsic aspect of humanity that relates to a person's quest for meaning, purpose, transcendence, and connection. Some people express their spirituality through religion; others express their spirituality through their relationships with others, creativity, nature, movement, and/or individual spiritual practices like mindfulness. Spirituality is a person's centre of connection: to themselves, to others, to

> **FICA ©Spiritual Assessment Tool [4]**
>
> **Faith (F)**: Do you have a faith tradition or religion?
>
> **Importance (I)**: How important are those beliefs to you?
>
> **Community (C)**: Do you worship in a community and is that community a regular part of your life?
>
> **Address (A)**: Is there anything I can do as your provider to take care of this important part of you?

the transcendent. As such, all patients can be the recipients of spiritual care. Common spiritual concerns that emerge during illness include the need for meaning in the face of suffering, the need for integrity, legacy and generativity, concerns about relationships, and concerns about or fear of death.[4] While the sections that follow emphasize different religious approaches to palliative care, it is important to remember that even the non-religious benefit from attention to spiritual needs by their care team.

Spiritual Screening

Early in the palliative care relationship, a provider should ask about a patient's religion or spirituality. Asking about religion or spirituality for the first time during a medical crisis can be experienced by patients as traumatic; it is better to include a spiritual screening as part of the initial patient assessment. Data suggests that when doctors engage in spiritual discussion, patients find it promotes the provision of holistic care, strengthens the doctor-patient relationship, and allows the doctor to accommodate religious beliefs in the management of their illness.[5]

Christina Puchalski created the FICA © screening tool to guide physicians in asking about religion and spirituality.[4] The tool includes four categories for inquiry: asking about a person's faith (F), the importance of their faith (I), whether they are part of a spiritual community (C), and how a provider can address or take action (A) related to any spiritual or religious needs. This simple mnemonic can assist providers in broaching the topic and works particularly well for patients who express their spirituality through traditional religious practice.

If a patient is not traditionally religious, the framework can be applied using more secular language. For example, if a patient says they do not have a religious faith, a provider can follow up with, "What are you drawing on for strength right now? What keeps you going?" A provider can ask about the important people in a patient's life, and whether a particular community is especially supportive. Finally, a provider can ask if there are ways they can support the patient's personhood. "It helps to know about you as a person, and please let us know if there are special things we can do to support you as you live with this illness."[6] Gentle, supportive inquiry strengthens the doctor-patient relationship and communicates respect and acceptance.

Impact on Advance Care Planning

When the disease progresses and treatment options are limited, many patients turn toward their faith or spirituality for guidance. The subchapters that follow review specific teachings on end-of-life care in the major world religions. Most major traditions support a patient's right to opt against futile and excessively burdensome treatment and to accept pain relief at the end of life. When physicians and interdisciplinary care teams attend to a patient's spiritual needs, patients experience higher quality of life outcomes, increased hospice utilization, and among highly religious patients, decreased aggressive care at the end of life.[3] When patients and families struggle with end-of-life decision-making due to spiritual concerns, maintaining an alliance with the family and calling in the support of a professional chaplain is critical. If a medical centre does not have access to a professional chaplain, providers can consider contacting (with permission) the patient's clergyperson to explore religious teachings on end-of-life care in conversation with the patient.

As the case in the introduction demonstrates, spiritual care is best offered by various members of the palliative care team. The physician Dr. Engleman initially learned from Brenda's family that her faith was central; the physician then contacted the palliative care chaplain. Rev. Sarah had time for daily visits with the family and served as a liaison between the family and her medical colleagues. When Matthew and Angela first opted for a feeding tube, Rev. Sarah supported them and encouraged the team to respect this decision. Using the family's language, Sarah encouraged the family to "watch and see what God would do" and pay attention to how Brenda progressed. By the time Brenda had developed irreversible sepsis, Matthew and

Angela understood God to be working in a different way with Brenda ("calling her Home"), and they changed her code status and shifted the goals of care. This process took place over eleven days. With careful, patient attention to the family's spiritual needs, the team accompanied the family as they made new meaning of Brenda's condition and accepted that she was dying.

The sections that follow elucidate different major religious teachings related to end-of-life care. Contrary to popular belief (even among believers), most major religions support advanced care planning, symptom management, and allowing for a natural death. The work of the palliative care team is to respectfully engage with patients and families around religious concerns as patients consider treatment options and preparation for death. These subchapters illustrate for providers how believers might look to their tradition for guidance. Each tradition relies on different sources of authority (catechism, scripture, precepts, teachings, and creeds), and the subchapters emphasize the diversity of practice and interpretation within them. While these guidelines about religious teachings offer helpful context and cultural framework, palliative care teams should strive to remember that every person of faith and practitioner is unique. The case studies that follow demonstrate how providers might come alongside patients and families and gently inquire about religious concerns or questions that may be causing distress, to offer sensitive, patient-centred palliative care.

References

1. Puchalski C., *et al.* (2009). Improving the quality of spiritual care as a dimension of palliative care: The report of the consensus conference. *J. Palliative Med.* **12**(10): 885–904.
2. Fitchett G., *et al.* (2020). Development of the PC-7, a quantifiable assessment of spiritual concerns of patients receiving palliative care near the end of life. *J. Palliative Med.* **23**(2): 248–253.
3. Balboni T.A., *et al.* (2022). Spirituality in Serious Illness and Health. *JAMA* **328**(2): 184–197.
4. Borneman T., Ferrell B., and Puchalski C.M. (2010). Evaluation of the FICA tool for spiritual assessment. *J. Pain Symptom Manage.* **40**(2): 163–73.
5. Steinhauser K.E., *et al.* (2000). Factors considered important at the end of life by patients, family, physicians, and other care providers. *JAMA* **284**(19): 2476–2482.
6. Best M., Butow P., and Olver I. (2016). Why do we find it so hard to discuss spirituality? A qualitative exploration of attitudinal barriers. *J. Clin. Med.* **5**(9): 77.
7. Robinson M.R., *et al.* (2016). Efficacy of training interprofessional spiritual care generalists. *J. Palliative Med.* **19**(8): 814–821.

Chapter 8

Spirituality and Religion in Advance Care Planning: Islamic Perspectives

Sakinah Alhabshi[*,†,§] and Samsiah Abdul-Majid[*,†,‡]

*Ziyara Spiritual Care, Fresno, CA, USA
†Association of Muslim Chaplains, USA
‡Westchester Medical Center, Valhalla, NY, USA
§Respect Graduate School, Bethlehem, PA, USA

Introduction

This section focuses on practical Islamic perspectives to help healthcare practitioners to understand, advocate for, and engage in ACP conversations with Muslim care-receivers. It promotes several premises that are elaborated in the following paragraphs:

First, the ACP process values Islamic worldviews, including the belief in the importance of preserving life and mitigating harm. One manifestation of this belief is through caring for the physical body as a trust (*amaanah*) from Allah, while recognizing that life ultimately resides in the soul, and that Allah has the ultimate control over how and when one dies. One's existence in this world is viewed as a test, and one's journey as a manifestation and experience of Allah's divine qualities and attributes (Qur'an 2:155, 59:22–24). The word "death" appears approximately 150 times in various conjugations throughout the Qur'an. The verses serve as a reminder to live mindfully with the limited time we have on earth, underscore the mortality that faces each person equally, and emphasize death as a transition to the infinite afterlife. This message is repeated in different variations of verses, *It is not possible for any soul to die except by the permission of God, at an appointed time* (Qur'an 3:145). Moreover, *And when I am ill, it is He who cures me; and He will cause me to die, and then bring me back to life* (Qur'an 26:80–81). Finally, *Every soul will taste death, then to Us you will (all) be returned* (Qur'an, 29:57).

Second, the ACP process respects the nuanced religious values and beliefs of individual Muslims and recognizes the tension that could arise from differences. Islamic law and objectives seek to prevent harm and bring benefit to the individual and community at large. However, conflict or confusion may surface through the differences in interpretation or definition of harm (perceived vs actual or clinical vs spiritual), misalignment in social and emotional needs or priorities, as well as diverse religious and spiritual values and beliefs. The practice of Islam is not monolithic, so it is imperative to emphasize the ACP process of respectfully exploring, affirming, and honoring nuanced values and beliefs that are important and unique to specific individuals and their loved ones.

Third, the ACP process is therefore not merely to document preferences in clinical/medical treatment for what is commonly misperceived as "preparation for imminent death." Reframing the approach to "planning for my care in advance" can reduce unintended intimidation or overwhelm, as well as help patients and their loved ones appreciate the process as just another plan of action or component of their overall holistic care.

Islamic Values/Teachings

With the above premises, we propose that three main values or teachings could facilitate understanding of the purpose and benefits of ACP conversations both for the clinician and care receiver, while also acknowledging that some Muslims may find them otherwise. The goal is not to force a mindset reframe, but rather to encourage and facilitate meaningful conversations while accompanying and addressing concerns, fears, guilt, and other tension that surface from a person's navigation of their faith journey through illness. Having said that, it is important to remain open to a spectrum of spiritual responses amidst the seemingly common ones above, including joy, affirmation of purpose, celebration, repentance, hope, reconciliation, and growth.

Value 1: Planning and Predestination: *Islamic teachings encourage planning our affairs alongside the acceptance of Allah's will and predestination.*

A prophetic tradition (*hadith*) expounding the wisdom of preparing for death may help alleviate concerns of some care-receivers that the ACP concept of future planning may be contradictory to their beliefs of God's control over life. A *hadith* narrated by Ibn 'Umar, a companion of Prophet Muhammad (*peace and blessings upon him (pbuh) — an expression of honor that Muslims use after mentioning the Prophet*), explains:

> "I was with the Prophet of God (pbuh) and a man from among the Ansar came to him and greeted the Prophet (pbuh) with salaam (peace). Then he said: *'O Prophet of Allah, which of the believers is best?'* The Prophet (pbuh) said: *'He who has the best manners among them.'* **The man then said: 'Which of them is wisest?' The Prophet (pbuh) said: 'The one who remembers death the most and is best in preparing for it. Those are the wisest'"** (Sunan Ibn Majah 4259).

Furthermore, Muslims are instructed to, *"... Consult with them (others) about matters, then, when you have decided on a course of action, put your trust in Allah: Allah loves those who put their trust in Him"* (Quran in 3:159). The ACP process can be framed as the due diligence effort (*ikhtiar*) of consulting and decision-making,[1] being forms of meritorious Islamic acts within the boundaries of a person's free will, which is then ultimately encompassed by God's will.

Value 2: Autonomy and Consultation: *Islamic teachings allow for autonomy in healthcare choices alongside consultation (istishaarah) with experts and family members.*

One saying derived from the Qur'an and *hadith* encourages autonomous decision-making by linking the invitation to rely on God's guidance alongside seeking consultation: *"He who seeks counsel from Allah (istikhaarah) will not regret it. And he who consults and seeks advice from people (istishaarah) will feel confident in the decision"* (Bukhari 7/162, Hisn Al-Muslim 74).

This approach may address concerns or fear in some patients of "doing the wrong thing", showing perceived displeasure with God's predestination by trying to control or dictate choices, resisting or expediting illness/death (to the point of worrying if certain choices amount to taking one's own life or the life of a loved one).

Muslims hold up Prophet Muhammad (pbuh) as their model. His actions during his illness and dying process spoke to the exercise of autonomy and consultation. As his illness advanced to the point that he was unable to keep moving locations comfortably, Prophet Muhammad (pbuh) consulted his family about choosing which home he wanted to remain in for care.[2] Further, when he was given some bitter-tasting medicine while he was in and out of sleep/consciousness, he awoke distraught, reminding his family that he had declined the medicine.[a] Islamic classical jurist Ibn Hajr said, *It is understood from the narration that if the sick person is cognizant and aware, he cannot be forced to take something he has prohibited, nor is he prohibited from something he has requested* (Fathul Bari, 10/167).[2] The complexities of one's situation may differ, and alternative *fatawa* (non-binding juristic opinions) on nutrition and hydration, as well as resuscitation, organ donation, or comfort care, may influence decisions. However, the emphasis of these illustrations is on the importance of a family-inclusive approach to goals of care conversations, and educating patients on their healthcare autonomy.

The family-centred approach to decision-making requires *careful consideration of family dynamics and how these may facilitate the conversation without disrupting the harmonious relationship between doctor, patient, and families.*[3] Frameworks such as the "AMEN" (A-Affirm, M-Meet, E-Educate, N-No matter what) and "NURSE" (N-Name it, U-Understand the core message, R-Respect/Reassurance at the right time, S-Support, E-Explore) communication models support clinicians in validating and responding to emotional cues.[4] Also consider clarifying the understanding and roles of healthcare proxies or surrogates in the process.

Value 3: Documenting: *Islamic teachings advise documenting important agreements in writing and/or with witnesses.*

---

[a] Sahih al-Bukhari 5709–5712: *"Aishah, wife of Prophet Muhammad (pbuh) said: "We put medicine in one side of his mouth but he started waving us not to insert the medicine into his mouth. We said, "He dislikes the medicine as a patient usually does." But when he came to his senses he said, "Did I not forbid you to put medicine (by force) in the side of my mouth?" We said, "We thought it was just because a patient usually dislikes medicine." He said, "None of those who are in the house but will be forced to take medicine in the side of his mouth while I am watching, except Al-`Abbas, for he had not witnessed your deed."* Available from: https://sunnah.com/bukhari/76.

Islamic law and ethics emphasize documenting important matters, such as a loan/debt, marriage contract, or business agreement.[b] An extract from the Qur'an 2:282, states:

> "..... You must not be against writing 'contracts' for a fixed period — whether the sum is small or great. This is more just 'for you' in the sight of Allah, and more convenient to establish evidence and remove doubts...."

Documenting generally serves two main purposes: to ensure decisions are clear and respected, as well as to prevent conflict. The ACP document specifically serves those intents as its preparation often includes conversation, open communication, and contemplation about important values and priorities. This helps preempt contestation or disagreement on what a patient's preferences were. The ACP process may be further facilitated if patients and families are informed that the document is not set in stone. Rather, it may be reviewed and revised allowing for different voices to be heard in recognition of the relational nature of decision-making. Overall, Martina *et al.* affirm that patients and families prefer to share decision-making responsibility with others to avoid regret and blame for any adverse outcomes of their decision.[1]

An Islamic legal maxim, *one must not harm others, nor cause harm to oneself,* is useful for viewing ACP as an approach to

---

[b]The Qur'an, 2:282: *"O believers! When you contract a loan for a fixed period of time, commit it to writing. Let the scribe maintain justice between the parties. The scribe should not refuse to write as Allah has taught them to write. They will write what the debtor dictates, bearing Allah in mind and not defrauding the debt. If the debtor is incompetent, weak, or unable to dictate, let their guardian dictate for them with justice. Call upon two of your men to witness. If two men cannot be found, then one man and two women of your choice will witness — so if one of the women forgets the other may remind her.1 The witnesses must not refuse when they are summoned. You must not be against writing 'contracts' for a fixed period — whether the sum is small or great. This is more just 'for you' in the sight of Allah, and more convenient to establish evidence and remove doubts. However, if you conduct an immediate transaction among yourselves, then there is no need for you to record it, but call upon witnesses when a deal is finalized. Let no harm come to the scribe or witnesses. If you do, then you have gravely exceeded 'your limits'. Be mindful of Allah, for Allah 'is the One Who' teaches you. And Allah has 'perfect' knowledge of all things."*

minimizing harm to the patient and their loved ones who may be too distressed to make challenging decisions when the patient is in critical condition or has lost capacity. In this context, "harm" includes the emotional and spiritual hardship that could surface within families through conflict and confusion. Mitigating harm and minimizing their burden is a religiously inspired demonstration of compassion for one's family, helps reduce the potential for moral distress, and facilitates the process of anticipatory grief, the grieving itself, as well as longer-term healing.

Case Example

The following example illustrates an approach that affirms a patient's religious beliefs, personal values, preferences, and concerns to arrive at a decision for an informational family meeting on ACP.

Conversation	Process / Recommendation
Muslim male, Adam, with stage II prostate cancer, COPD, and diabetes. He has been under the care of oncologist Dr. Sara (non-Muslim) for several years. Dr. Sara has been educating Adam on ACP in the past few visits, framing ACP as a process and just one part of his care plan. After some preliminaries at a recent visit:	– Culturally and linguistically relevant ACP education – AMEN/NURSE: Educate, Respect, Support, Explore – Value 1: Planning and predestination – Value 2: Autonomy and Consultation
Dr. Sara: *I remember we last discussed the benefits of including your family in our ACP conversations. I wonder if you're ready to invite them to join you at our next appointment.*	
Adam: *My children are upset. They say it's too early to talk about this "end of life" stuff when my cancer is only Stage II. I tried to explain like you said... it's not just about dying... but... *sigh**	
Dr. Sara: *It can be upsetting and confusing indeed. Can you tell me a little more about what you feel worries them most?*	– AMEN/NURSE: Affirm, Meet, Understand, Meet, Respect, Reassure, Support, Explore

(*Continued*)

Conversation	Process / Recommendation
Adam: *They associate ACP with imminent death. And they're not ready emotionally to speak about my death.* *Also, there's many complicated issues in ACP; we don't think we understand enough to make the right decision.* *And they are worried that I will not be given priority for treatment once I sign a DNR. And surrogate, who should I appoint? My son is the oldest but lives in another state, my daughter is level-headed and she lives not too far away. I don't want them to think that I favor one over the other if I choose only one surrogate.*	Adam shares his concerns. Issues identified: Misconception, fear, overwhelm, lack of clarity/understanding, the impact of making and documenting choices/ decisions, family dynamics, and expectations.
Dr. Sara: *I hear you are struggling to explain the ACP to your children, and worried about how you are going to be treated. And that you want to be fair with your children in this process.*	Affirm: joining, identifying struggles and values
Adam: *They are good to me. They want to take care of me. I don't want them to feel that they are killing me if they follow my ACP... and I don't want to break any religious rules or teachings if I choose certain decisions.*	Issues identified: Value for religious filial piety, concern on the prohibition against taking a life / causing harm.
Dr. Sara: *One of the ways we find helpful to approach the ACP process is to include the family early, and I can guide them through some of the conversations like you and I have had, to understand their values and concerns, in addition to the medical related information.* *And it doesn't have to just be one conversation and we don't have to sign anything immediately. We can arrange a Zoom call with them. Maybe we can invite our hospital Chaplain, and your family, and you can invite your Imam or Ustadz.*	Value 1: Planning and Predestination Value 2: Autonomy and Consultation. Value 3: Documenting – AMEN/NURSE: Understand, Meet, Respect, Reassure, Support, Explore – Clarifying the role/limits of physician providing general spiritual care

(*Continued*)

Conversation	Process / Recommendation
Adam: *Yes, I think it will be good to get everyone together, I can't do this alone. And yes, please include the hospital Chaplain.* *Just planning and discussing things like life machines, CPR, the food tubes, donating my organs, doesn't mean I am trying to go against Allah or rewriting my death, right?*	Responding and accepting the invitation. Feeling relief and supported. Surfacing reflection and meaning-making on life's uncertainties. Concern over denying God's predestination.
Dr. Sara: *Yes, the ACP conversations and process itself in fact helps with reflecting on important life and religious beliefs and values. We can take action to plan and document what is important to us — the way we want to live and die, within our limited human abilities — while relying on God for guidance and accepting His ultimate decision, not going against it.* *I believe that it's good practice to consult with experts and with trustworthy people on any important matter. So, I want to affirm that we are going on this ACP process with our eyes and hearts open, and involving medical and religious advisers and personal family.*	AMEN/NURSE: Affirm belief, Educate, Understand, Respect, Reassure, Support. Value 1: Planning and Predestination Value 2: Autonomy and Consultation. Value 3: Documenting Referral to an interdisciplinary team member — chaplain / religious adviser.
Adam: *Yes, it helps to know I am not alone in this confusing and scary process. I know my treatment is going well, inshaAllah (God willing), but the reality is our lives can change in a split second, even without cancer. In a funny way, being sick gives me a bonus early reminder about making the best of this temporary life!*	Relief Reflection on mortality Levity/humor in the midst of heaviness
Dr. Sara: *That is a precious reminder indeed... preparing for death and prioritizing making the best of the time we have. I'd appreciate hearing some of your hopes or reflections on your preparation, Adam.*	Affirming, inviting, no assumptions made.

(Continued)

Conversation	Process / Recommendation
Adam: *I want to be clean of impurities, to continue to pray as long as I can, and if I'm conscious, I hope to say the shahadah (testimony of faith). It would be nice if the environment is peaceful and green. I wish I can spend my last days back at my family farm, but if I'm dying at the hospital, it's okay too because I feel people are nice and caring to me here also. I want to be surrounded by the sound of the Qur'an, but not too loud... and have my family with me.*	Reflecting, sharing "what matters most" — faith, family, nature, hygiene, peace, Qur'anic recitation, leveraging on good health, legacy-building, not being a burden.
But before that day, I hope to plan more visits with my grandchildren... sponsor my family on a vacation together... sort out my finances and debt so my children don't have to worry about that. Oh, so many things, doc! May Allah make it easy for me.	
Dr. Sara: *I join you in that hope and prayer, Adam. That is a beautiful image you've described. Let's remember to document that in the ACP when we work on it.*	Affirm values and relationships. Emphasize the importance of documenting.
Dr. Sara: *And I am glad you have had a chance to discuss with your children. It looks to me they want to know more about ACP and to understand the various technicalities. And you yourself have some lingering concerns, including religious ones, as well as relationships with your children and their emotions. After the family meeting, I will be happy to facilitate further family discussions later. I am hopeful that this will make it easier for you to guide them and the hospital team on what you prefer. I will be with you all through this process, irrespective of your choices and decisions.*	Summarizing and approaching the end of the session. Plan on educating, and addressing concerns. Discussion and support continue no matter what (AMEN).

Conclusion

ACP is a process that can yield greater shared understanding and subsequent honoring of a patient/care-receiver's beliefs, values, preferences, and concerns among the triad of care-receivers, caregivers, and family. Within the context of the premises it promoted, this section offered three Islamic values/teachings that could help boost a clinician's ability to learn more from and about their patients in their ACP conversations, as well as to provide religious/spiritually-informed compassionate care.

References

1. Martina D., Kustanti C.Y., Dewantari R., Sutandyo N., Putranto R., Shatri H., and Rietjens J.A. (2022). Advance care planning for patients with cancer and family caregivers in Indonesia: A qualitative study. *BMC Palliative Care*, **21**(1): 1–12. https://doi.org/10.1186/s12904-022-01086-0.
2. Abu-Shamsieh, K. (2020) End of life care and Islamic practical theology: A case study: The dying experience of prophet Muhammad. Graduate Theological Union. https://www.proquest.com/docview/2311959676/abstract/8B8C957684CD4253PQ/1.
3. Martina D., Kustanti C.Y., Dewantari R., *et al.* (2022). Opportunities and challenges for advance care planning in strongly religious family-centric societies: A Focus group study of Indonesian cancer-care professionals. *BMC Palliative Care* **21**: 110. https://doi.org/10.1186/s12904-022-01002-6.
4. Back A., Arnold R., and Tulsky J. (2009). *Mastering Communication with Seriously Ill Patients: Balancing Honesty with Empathy and Hope.* Cambridge University Press, United Kingdom.

Chapter 9

Spirituality and Religion in Advance Care Planning: Christian Perspectives

Tia Jamir[*] and Do Bong Kim[†]

*Department of Spiritual Care and Education
Beth Israel Deaconess Medical Center, Boston, MA, USA
†Holistic Healing Institute, Sam Hospitals, Korea

The Asian Challenge: Dying Well and Advance Care Planning (ACP)

Asian cultures and countries (like many others) are facing a drastic challenge in the form of an aging and declining population, which raises questions such as, "How do we learn to die well from the slow degenerative diseases of old age? What is a good death in this context?" Interestingly, recent research demonstrates that older Asians prefer to make their own decisions after consulting adult family members.[1] The ACP discourse in the Asian milieu is an opportunity to understand the amazing technological and medicinal interventions of the 21st century. At the same time, this may be a good time to give the proper time and context for seeking epistemic humility in understanding human suffering and the human condition. To do so, however, may be beyond the limits of both science and medicine, and this is where religion has a vital role to play.

Like any other culture, Asian cultures wrestle with questions such as, "How do we live/die?" or "What is a good death?" What was once the domain of religion is now shadowed by science and/or medicine. Instead of a priest or shaman, it is now the medical professional who seems to have the authority on "how" we die.

Culture, Christianity, and the Clinic

Any culture has a porous boundary and a multivalent centre. The heart of a culture is not a solid, single core, but has within it a constant struggle for power between multiple factions to determine who will control the central values and habits of the culture (for example, medicine vs. clergy, Christian ethos vs. Asian traditional values).

Culture, in this context, is formed by external and internal *engagement* and *conflict*. One culture engages another culture — sometimes overlapping, sometimes resisting — while each culture is simultaneously struggling internally as the members of that culture vie for power and to make sense of the current moment, like making life and death decisions in an ICU. There is no longer the notion of holistic, homogeneous cultures existing in self-contained spaces. The dying process in the clinic demonstrates culture as a mixture of (many) cultures continually intersecting and evolving in a pluriform, polycentric interplay of engagement and conflict.

One of the key points is to understand and choose to privilege complexity over order and engagement over agreement. This is often hard in the clinical world where order and planned outcomes are privileged above all else. It will be helpful to know that end-of-life care is as it was 6 millennia ago, occupied by many primal emotions including disgust, fear, and anger. It is hard to tame these primal emotions.

The engagement between cultures within the same country means that the boundary of any Asian culture is not rigid and impregnable, but is a porous, semi-permeable cloud that allows the culture to intersect and interact with other competing cultures (as in Christianity vs. traditional values). This comingling at the edges often works its way into the centre of culture with the dynamic passage of time, thus creating mutations as cultures continually interact in the global arena — or in an ICU bed when loved ones are dealing with primal fears.

Furthermore, there is no one Christianity and no unified or codified belief system within Christianity. Hence, it is impossible to speak of a single Christian culture. This is not a bad thing. Christianity at its best takes shape and roots itself within a people and culture. Christian culture is not just a matter of traditions and rules, but one of style. The *what* of Christian practices may differ amongst Korean Christians, but the *how* is what characterizes them.

Christianity came to East Asia (and much of the globe), through Western missionaries. However, it is crucial to remember that Christianity, like all the major world religions, in fact, originated in Western Asia. Christians in South Korea are a vibrant minority. It is also hard to know where native Korean culture ends and where Christianity's beliefs and ritual begins.[a]

End-of-life Care and Dying Well in Asian Culture

There is great diversity within East Asian countries, cultures, and religious beliefs. At the same time, there are shared assumptions that can be traced back to a few conceptual frames of reference that are often held with unchallenged assumptions and/or as a way of life. This is how culture primarily works — the fish do not know their nose is wet. Two of the conceptual building blocks of East Asian countries are Confucianism and the concept of 'filial piety.' This means that in practice, and directly related to this section of the article, the patient's autonomy (highly assumed and privileged in the West) is consequently subordinate to family values and the physician's authority.[2,b]

---

[a]Christians, like many religious devotees, in every generation have been inspired to work with the destitute and dying. For example, Dame Cicely Saunders, the founder of the modern hospice movement was inspired and motivated by her religious pulse. This lead to the establishment of St. Christopher's Hospice in London in 1967. Both she and many of those who pioneered the subsequent expansion of hospice services were committed Christians, setting up facilities with the implicit aims of welcoming all and expressing the love of God in every aspect of patient care.

[b]Cheng *et al.*[2] Consider this: For a long time, the modern Western "enlightened" self-functions within the perspective of Cartesian dualism and understands that the only acceptable form of knowledge comes from the acquisition of scientific information through the process of empirical observation. The only thing that actually exists is that which can be observed with human senses and explained by human reason. Anything else is ignored as superstition and relegated to the private sector or disregarded altogether.

In an end-of-life scenario, the physician will often reveal the patient's poor prognosis and corresponding treatment options to a male family member, rather than to the patient. To address this ethical and practical dilemma, the concept of relational autonomy proves to be helpful in assisting Asian patients, in particular during Advance Care Planning.

Dying Well in the Christian Tradition

From a Christian perspective, it is helpful to know what Jesus said and did about the dying process. Jesus never belittled the wretchedness of death but accepted its role in the whole story of God and humanity. Even he grieved and honored the reality of death. He took moments to pause and weep — all the while knowing that he was "the Resurrection and the Life" (John 11:25). He healed the masses and wept for his friends.

Most believers ascribe to the teachings to "Turn the other cheek" (Matthew 5:39) and "Love your neighbors, as yourself" (Mark 12:31), but often find it very difficult to put into practice. Likewise, the belief in the afterlife or post-mortem life with God gives hope but the dying process remains a challenge, as the primal fear of mortality abides. Clinicians and Chaplains can be reservoirs of hope when Asian Christians are dealing with their mortality.

A familiar biblical metaphor deserves full and serious reflection here. To die is to be cut off from the living, to be cut off even from God:

> "I am overwhelmed with troubles
> and my life draws near to death.
> I am counted among those who go down to the pit;
> I am like one without strength.
> I am set apart with the dead,
> like the slain who lie in the grave,
> whom you remember no more,
> who are cut off from your care."
> (Psalms 88:3–5)

To "go down to the pit" is in some way to be at once utterly alone and with the dead which means that our goodbyes to our loved ones are final. And frankly, it's bad for us to minimize that.

But the Bible does not stop with the bad news about death. It rereads all of the above in the light of the life of Jesus. In doing so, the Bible at once recognizes the reality of the bad news and daringly asserts that it is, in God's ultimate goal, good news, such that death is no longer simply the end but is also a new beginning. The relationship changes but continues. Life after death happens. The distance between the living and the dead, ritualistically is not that far apart.

Another way to engage the dying process for the Christian is through the mystery of Baptism. Death is an identification stamped onto Christians in baptism: "Do you not know that all of us who have been baptized into Christ Jesus were baptized into his death?" (Romans 6:3). The believer's identification with Jesus, marked by baptism, means that for Christians, death is indeed the end of this life — not as an abandonment into the dark unknown but the final abandonment into the God who tasted death for all, and so removed its sting. It is the fullest abandonment into Christ, and as such, is an abandonment into Life more abundantly. Saint Paul writes, "We were buried therefore with him by baptism into death, in order that, just as Christ was raised from the dead by the glory of the Father, we too might walk in newness of life" (Romans 6:4). This abandonment of life for Life through identification with Christ begins at baptism, and carries on, in some way, forever.

Apostle Paul went on to say: "so that [we would] not grieve like the rest of mankind, who have no hope" (1 Thessalonians 4:13). Here death has a lifespan, a beginning and an end. He was acquainted with the sorrows of death and loss but learned how to orient his perspective around the story of God and everlasting life.

Christ and the Mournful Death

The good news of death is that it marks the completion of the believer's union with Christ, initiated at baptism. However, dying is hard work even for a believer. The prayer of the Christian Lord in Gethsemane is the prayer for all who die in the peace of Christ: "My Father, if it is possible, may this cup be taken from me. Yet not as I will, but as you will" (Matthew 26:3). The Gospel of Mark says that,

> They went to a place called Gethsemane, and Jesus said to his disciples, "Sit here while I pray." He took Peter, James and John along

with him, and he began to be deeply distressed and troubled. "My soul is overwhelmed with sorrow to the point of death," he said to them. "Stay here and keep watch." Going a little farther, he fell to the ground and prayed that if possible, the hour might pass from him. "Abba, Father," he said, "everything is possible for you. Take this cup from me. Yet not what I will, but what you will." (Mark 14:32–35).

And at the direst moment, when his life was slipping away, he felt abandoned by God. He stated, "My God, my God, why have you abandoned me?" (Matthew 27:46; Mark 15:34, cf. Psalm 22:1).

This anguish, fear, and troubled state of mind and soul of the Christian God when confronted by the prospect of his own encounter with death explicitly gives hope for the believers, in the face of their own or others' mortality. It will be good to remember this and remind the patient and their loved ones.

Conclusion: Applications for the Medical Practitioner

Summary

When all the medical options are at an end and when your patient and loved ones are facing the inevitable primal fear of death, what do you do? Medical professionals can, through the help of a professional chaplain, remind their Christian patients and loved ones that the prospect of dying is never undertaken without fear.

Again, we are dealing with fear and fear is a powerful force. We don't recognize the power it has over us until something draws it out, as mortality does. At its best, within Christianity, death presents us with the mystery of life held in the hands of God: A life that is not our own, that is both fragile and limited. It presents death as the great severer of all relationships. Fear of death is real, and it should not be minimized for the family/loved ones and if the patient is aware of it. This fear does not demonstrate the lack of (Christian) faith. It may demonstrate instead the presence of humanity with its myriad of emotions. Where there is much love and humanity there is also much pain; they are rather inseparable and intertwined.

Key Reminders for Practical Use

Here are some key points to remember when dealing with a Christian patient and family for ACP:

First, involve a **professional chaplain** in the discourse from the beginning, not only at the end (if they are available).

Life is a gift from God: Birth and death are part of the life processes which God has created, so we should respect them (Psalm 139:14).

Human beings are valuable because they are made in God's image: Human life possesses intrinsic dignity and value because it is created by God in his own image for the distinctive destiny of sharing in God's own life (Genesis 1:26).

The process of dying is spiritually important and should not be disrupted: The period just before death is a profoundly spiritual time. They think it is wrong to interfere with the process of dying, as this would interrupt the process of the spirit moving toward God. This is a spiritual time and what good death is. But it is hard to practice it and navigate as a family and certainly as a healthcare provider.

All human lives are equally valuable: Christians believe that the intrinsic dignity and value of human lives means that the value of each human life is identical. They don't think that human dignity and value are measured by mobility, intelligence, or any achievements in life.

In the end, rituals affirm. Rituals are a powerful human mechanism for managing extreme emotions and stress, and we should be leaning on them now as we harness the task of bringing ACP to East Asian countries and beyond.

Medicines and religions (including Christianity) have their own rituals. Rituals at their best serves both functional and utilitarian purposes. Culture, as we have seen, is a mixture of both internal engagement and conflict. Perhaps, to help our patients we can (re)learn the ancient ways of dying well, communing with the ancestors, and harnessing the ever-exciting discovery of 21st century practical medicine. If we can hold these two cultures–medicine, and religion–perhaps, we can begin to see a pattern of compassionate care done well. When the chaplain/clergy and clinician come together in the name of compassion, that is, to suffer alongside our patients in the hour of need, everyone feels heard. Our shared rituals midwife the dying process humanely in the face of primal fear for the patient/family and the health care team.

References

1. Ho L.Y.W., Kwong E.W.Y., Song M.S., Kawakami A., Boo S., Lai C.K.Y., and Yamamoto-Mitani N. (2022 December). Decision-making preferences on end-of-life care for older people: Exploration and comparison of Japan, the Hong Kong SAR and South Korea in East Asia. *J. Clin. Nurs.* **31**(23–24): 3498–3509.
2. Cheng S.Y., Lin C.P., Chan H.Y., Martina D., Mori M., Kim S.H., and Ng R. (2020 September 5). Advance care planning in Asian culture. *Jpn. J. Clin. Oncol.* **50**(9): 976–989.

Chapter 10

Spirituality and Religion in Advance Care Planning: Catholicism Perspectives

Maria Fidelis Manalo

*Section of Supportive Oncology & Palliative Care,
Augusto P. Sarmiento Cancer Institute, The Medical City,
Ortigas, Pasig City, Philippines
Department of Community and Family Medicine,
Far Eastern University-Dr. Nicanor Reyes Medical Foundation,
Fairview, Quezon City, Philippines*

Case Study: Nicole's Unwavering Trust in God

Nicole was a 31-year-old Catholic who was suffering from metastatic breast cancer. She had a challenging life, with her firstborn son, aged 7, suffering from autism and her 2nd pregnancy ending in stillbirth. Her youngest daughter was one-½-year-old.

She has had several hospitalizations recently due to the progression of her cancer which had metastasized to the lungs, liver, and bones. When the attending pulmonologist tried to have an Advance Care Planning (ACP) conversation, he started by attempting to explain Nicole's unfortunately very poor prognosis. However, her mother did not want Nicole to be fully informed about it and asserted that they believed that God would provide a miracle and she would be cured.

The attending pulmonologist then discussed Medical Orders for Life-Sustaining Treatments (MOLST). Still, he sensed they were not yet fully

---

comprehending the seriousness of Nicole's current condition. Her mother was amenable to intubation if indicated. Thus, Nicole and her family were referred to a palliative care specialist for clarification of care goals and end-of-life care and discussions. During the family meeting, the palliative care specialist showed appreciation towards what the family communicated, acknowledged their emotions with reflective summary statements, and listened carefully. However, it was made clear to the family that as difficult as talking about death may be, it is best to have the ACP conversation with Nicole herself. It was explained that it is Nicole's right to make decisions about her future care based on her values and religious beliefs. It was also clarified that if Nicole became incapacitated and unable to decide for herself, by law, her husband would be her proxy decision-maker unless she designates another person.

When the palliative care specialist had a one-on-one ACP conversation with Nicole, it turned out that she was fully aware of her poor prognosis and was calm and accepting of the terminality of her condition. She was not scared to die. All she was concerned about was the hurt that her family was experiencing and how they would be, especially her young children when she died. Nicole stipulated that she desired pain relief, IV nutrition, hydration, and spiritual care. She also confirmed her husband as her proxy decision-maker.

When asked by the palliative care specialist the reason for her strength in bearing her illness and imminent demise, Nicole said that she trusted in God's love for her and was grateful to God for everything. She also thought that God was using her as an instrument to help her family come closer to God and one another.

Nicole was hospitalized for the last time with distressing cough, breathlessness, and desaturation. As her advanced medical directives specified, intubation and cardiopulmonary resuscitation were not performed. Instead, she was given palliative sedation since she did not want to die feeling like drowning. Her family, especially her very emotional mother, eventually came to a place of acceptance of Nicole's advanced directives because of the courage Nicole showed in the face of suffering and impending death.

The Catholic Church supports the concept of advance directives. This allows individuals to name an agent to make healthcare decisions if they lose the capacity to make or express their own choices. For Roman Catholics, morally correct decisions are based on respecting the sanctity and dignity of life and acknowledging man's dependence upon God. While Catholics are not morally obligated to have advance directives, it gives Catholics a way to profess their faith and help ensure that decisions about the care they receive when they cannot speak for themselves are in accord with their religious beliefs. The Conference of Catholic Bishops of the United States and other countries urge Catholics to designate a proxy decision-maker who understands and shares Catholic values and can help apply them to the medical situation.[1]

The Catholic Guide to End-of-Life Decisions by the National Catholic Bioethics Center[2] is a brief but clear explanation of the Catholic Church's teaching on advance directives, euthanasia, and physician-assisted suicide with a glossary of terms, as well as a sample advance medical directive and health care proxy that conform to Catholic teaching on end-of-life care.

Framing Advance Care Planning (ACP) in patients' religious beliefs will help engage patients in ACP conversations. For Catholics, the first step would be to correct the occasional misconception of linking ACP with euthanasia or assisted dying.[3] Many religiously devout Catholics will not participate in ACP conversations if it's tied to euthanasia or assisted dying.

The truth that life is a precious gift from God has profound implications for the question of stewardship over human life. We are not the owners of our lives and, hence, do not have absolute power over life. We must preserve our life and use them for God's glory, but the duty to preserve life is not absolute.[1] Death is a reality that will come inexorably at any moment. Death is neither to be feared and avoided at all costs nor to be sought and directly procured.

A truly Catholic Advance Medical Directive addresses five fundamental principles,[4] which are expounded in the Catechism of the Catholic Church (CCC).[5] The religious beliefs and values which are facilitators to advance care planning conversations are:

1. **Desire for Pain Relief:** The use of painkillers to alleviate the suffering of the dying, even at the risk of shortening their days, can be morally in conformity with human dignity if death is not willed as an end or a means but only foreseen and tolerated as inevitable. Palliative care is a special form of disinterested charity. As such, it should be encouraged. (CCC, no. 2279)

2. **Assessing the Proportionality of Life-Sustaining Medical Treatments:** Decisions to administer, refuse, or discontinue life-sustaining treatment should be based on proportionality. Individuals

are required to preserve life using proportionate means, which, in the patient's judgment, offer a reasonable hope of benefit and do not entail an excessive burden or impose excessive expense on the family or the community. One is not obligated to pursue or continue life-sustaining treatments considered burdensome, dangerous, extraordinary, or disproportionate to the expected outcome, i.e., its risks or burdens are disproportionate to its expected benefits. Here one does not will to cause death; one's inability to impede it is merely accepted. The patient should make the decisions if he is competent and able or, if not, by those legally entitled to act for the patient, whose reasonable will and legitimate interests must always be respected. (CCC, no. 2278).

3. **Providing Nutrition and Hydration (Food and Water):** The failure to provide a patient with nutrition and hydration — to end the patient's life or accelerate the patient's death — constitutes euthanasia and is always wrong, even when nourishment must be provided by artificial means. However, their administration should be suspended when nutrition and hydration no longer benefit the patient because they cannot absorb or metabolize them. In this way, one does not unlawfully hasten death but respects the natural course of the critical or terminal illness.[4]

4. **Prohibiting Euthanasia:** Direct euthanasia is morally unacceptable. Euthanasia is understood as an action or an omission which, of itself or by intention, causes death so that all suffering may, in this way, be eliminated. Euthanasia's terms of reference are to be found in the intention of the will and the methods used. Euthanasia constitutes a murder gravely contrary to the human person's dignity and respect due to the living God, his Creator. (CCC, no. 2277).

5. **Providing for Spiritual Care:** When Catholics are in the final stages of a terminal illness or injury or when death is imminent, they should be informed of this so that they may prepare themselves for death. They need to be attended by a Catholic priest to receive the sacraments (Reconciliation, Holy Eucharist, and the Anointing of the Sick) that prepare them for the heavenly homeland. (CCC, no. 1525). The grace of the Anointing of the Sick has as its effects: the uniting of the sick person to the passion of Christ for his good and that of the whole Church; the strengthening, peace, and courage to endure in a Christian manner the sufferings of illness or old age; the forgiveness of sins, if the sick person was not able to obtain it through the sacrament of

Penance; the restoration of health, if it is conducive to the salvation of his soul; and the preparation for passing over to eternal life. (CCC, no. 1532). In addition, the Church offers those who are about to leave this life the Eucharist as viaticum, the seed of eternal life and the power of resurrection. (CCC, no. 1524).

Most Christian faiths, and some strains of Orthodox Judaism, accept the possibility of a miracle.[6] This religious belief is a possible barrier to prognostic understanding and ACP conversations. By definition, religious belief in miracles refers to the expectation that because of some divine intervention, events may unfold in ways that defy the natural or expected order of things to be more in one's favor. This belief may be uniquely associated with more favorable expectations of one's prognosis than general religiousness because the latter may manifest in a variety of ways, including unfavorable disease expectations (e.g., "if dying from this illness is part of God's plan for me, I am okay with that").[7]

Patients who reported belief in the divine intervention were less likely to engage in advance care planning or to have a living will. Belief in divine intervention, turning to a higher power for strength, support, and guidance, and using spirituality to cope with a serious illness like cancer was associated with a preference for cardiopulmonary resuscitation, mechanical ventilation, and hospitalization in a near-death scenario.

Engaging patients and families who anticipate miraculous healing involves exploring the meaning and significance of a miracle, providing a balanced, nonargumentative response, and negotiating patient-centred compromises while conveying respect for patient spirituality and practicing good medicine. Such an approach, tailored to the specifics of each family, can be effective in helping a family come to a place of acceptance about the impending death of their loved one.[6]

The Judeo-Christian moral tradition teaches and explains that human life is a gift of a loving God.[8] This tradition further values and respects the life of every human being because each human being is made in the image and likeness of God. Therefore it has a special value and significance. Catholic Christians believe that each person has come from God and will return to God — in God's time and in God's way.[9]

It is not always easy for Catholic patients, families, or healthcare agents to apply the principles of proportionality to a particular situation. Some, at the conservative end of the spectrum, might be so concerned about avoiding euthanasia by omission that they may choose overly burdensome care.[3] Consultation with medical advisors is almost always required to evaluate potential benefits, burdens, and risks. Consultation with competent Catholic chaplains and spiritual advisors may help patients, families, or healthcare agents arrive at objective and honest decisions.

It is essential for healthcare professionals to have a basic understanding of the moral principles and teachings on the Christian meaning of pain, suffering, death, and the afterlife to facilitate advanced care planning. Devout Catholics' beliefs and values help them cope with their illness positively.

During Advance Care Planning, when healthcare workers honestly discuss prognosis and end-of-life care preferences, patients are given time to prepare for their death and be at peace with God and everyone else. All these lead devout Catholics to face death calmly, trusting Almighty God. Their only request from physicians is to help them be as pain-free and comfortable as possible. In line with their advance medical directives, when death is imminent, the Catholic chaplain gives them the Sacraments of the Catholic Church (Reconciliation, Holy Eucharist, and the Anointing of the Sick). At the same time, their families keep prayerful vigil beside the dying Catholic, reciting the Holy Rosary and other devotional prayers.

Learning Objectives
- Advance care planning aims to discover and record the patient's wishes for the end of life. Therefore, healthcare professionals must understand Catholic moral principles and teachings informing Catholic patients' decision-making to facilitate advanced care planning.
- Discussions about advance medical directives with Catholics should address five fundamental principles: (1) the desire for pain relief, (2) assessing treatments as either ordinary or extraordinary, (3) providing nutrition and hydration, (4) prohibiting euthanasia, and (5) providing for spiritual care.
- Physicians may find it very challenging to have ACP discussions with patients and families expecting a miraculous recovery. Thus, it is crucial to explore the meaning and significance of a miracle, provide a balanced, nonargumentative response and negotiate patient-centred compromises while conveying respect for patient spirituality and practicing good medicine.

References

1. United States Conference of Catholic Bishops. (2018 June). *Ethical and Religious Directives for Catholic Health Care Services*, (6th edn.). Digital Edition.
2. National Catholic Bioethics Center. (2011). *A Catholic Guide to End-of-life Decisions*. NCBC, Philadelphia, PA. https://www.ncbcenter.org/store/catholic-guide-to-end-of-life-decisions-english-pdf-download (Accessed 2023 January 21).
3. Pereira-Salgado A., Mader P., O'Callaghan C., Boyd L., and Staples M. (2017 December 28). Religious leaders' perceptions of advance care planning: A secondary analysis of interviews with Buddhist, Christian, Hindu, Islamic, Jewish, Sikh and Bahá'í leaders. *BMC Palliative Care* **16**(1): 79.
4. Morrow P. (2013 November). The catholic living will and healthcare surrogate: A teaching document for evangelization, and a means of ensuring spirituality throughout life. *Linacre Q* **80**(4): 317–322.
5. Catechism of the Catholic Church (CCC). (1997). Revised in accordance with the official Latin text promulgated by pope John Paul II, Vatican City: Libreria Editrice Vaticana. https://www.vatican.va/archive/ENG0015/__P2I.HTM (Accessed 2023 January 9).
6. DeLisser H.M. (2009 June). A practical approach to the family that expects a miracle. *Chest* **135**(6):1643–1647.
7. George L.S., Balboni T.A., Maciejewski P.K., Epstein A.S., and Prigerson H.G. (2020 February 15). "My doctor says the cancer is worse, but I believe in miracles" — When religious belief in miracles diminishes the impact of news of cancer progression on change in prognostic understanding. *Cancer* **126**(4): 832–839.
8. *Congregation for the Doctrine of the Faith Letter Samaritanus Bonus (Good Samaritan) on the Care of Persons in the Critical and Terminal Phases of Life*. Libreria Editrice Vaticana, Vatican City, 2020.
9. Catholic Dioceses of Arlington and Richmond. (2014). Catholic advance medical directives. https://vacatholic.org/wp-content/uploads/2017/05/Advance-Medical-Directive-booklet.pdf (Accessed 2023 January 9).

Chapter 11

Spirituality and Religion in Advance Care Planning: Hindu Perspectives

Seema Rajesh Rao[*,†,‡] and Srinagesh Simha[*,‡,¶]

*Karunashraya Institute for Palliative Care Education and Research (KIPCER), Bangalore Hospice Trust — Karunashraya, Bangalore, Karnataka State, India
†Cancer Treatment Centers Program, Lien Collaborative for Palliative Care and Asia Pacific Hospice Palliative Care Network, Singapore
‡School of Medicine, Cardiff University, Cardiff, UK
¶Adjunct Faculty, Department of Palliative Medicine and Supportive Care, Kasturba Medical College and Hospital, Manipal, Manipal Academy of Higher Education, Manipal, Karnataka State, India

Introduction

Death is a universal phenomenon. It is influenced by cultural and religious worldviews. Each religion understands and addresses the concept of suffering, death and dying differently. Rituals surrounding death and dying vary. Some communities bury, some cremate, and others embalm or preserve the dead. Religious beliefs inform and influence an individual's illness experience and healthcare decisions. Religion and rituals are important, especially when patients are nearing end-of-life. To provide culturally competent care, healthcare providers must understand their patients' ethnocultural and religious beliefs.

Advance care planning (ACP) is a process of communicating and documenting an individual's current and future end-of-life-care preferences. It is a communication contract between the patient, family, and healthcare providers. It ensures patients receive medical care concordant with their values, life goals, and preferences. When patients cannot make informed medical decisions due to disease progression, an ACP provides the framework for the way forward for healthcare providers and caregivers. Spirituality and religion influence how individuals cope with suffering, view autonomy, and prepare for and accept death and dying. ACP tailored to unique beliefs and practices of the patient's culture improves the quality of death and dying. This section explores the views of suffering, death and dying in Hinduism and informs healthcare providers about how religious values and beliefs can impact ACP conversations.

The Basic Tenets of Hinduism

Hinduism is the third-largest religion in the world and one of the oldest. It is often referred to as a 'way of life'. It is predominantly practised in the Indian subcontinent and Asia. A substantial population of Hindus also live in Australia, North America, Europe and Africa. Hinduism is henotheistic. Hindus believe in one Supreme God, the *Brahman,* but also acknowledge the existence of other deities. Hinduism is borne out of the synthesis of diverse regional schools of thought, beliefs, traditions, and philosophies. While engaging in end-of-life conversations with Hindu patients and families, healthcare providers need to acknowledge this diversity and elicit the specific beliefs and practices of the individual.[1]

The cycle of birth (rebirth), life, and death is one of the basic tenets of Hinduism. This creation, preservation, dissolution, and recreation cycle is called *samsara*. The physical body perishes when an individual dies, but the *atman*, the soul, is eternal.[2]

> "As a person sheds worn-out garment and wears new ones, likewise, at the time of death, the soul casts off its worn-out body and enters a new one." (Bhagavad Gita 2.22)

The atman either reunites with *Brahman* (the Supreme God) to attain the ultimate liberation or transmigrates into a new body. All living organisms pass through the cycle of *samsara* until they attain *moksha*.[1] The cycle of samsara is illustrated in Figure 1.

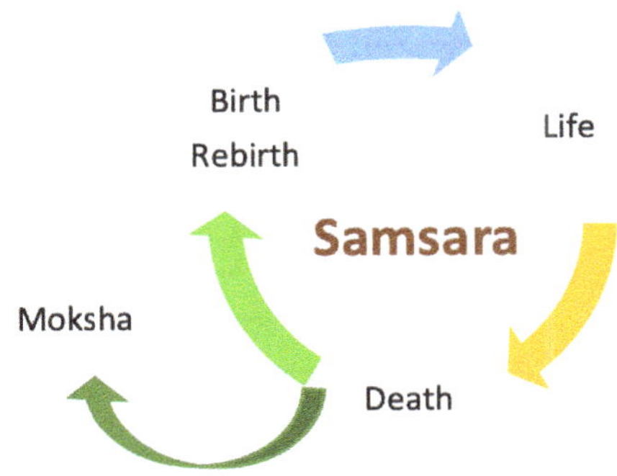

Figure 1.   The cycle of Samsara.

Hindus believe in *Karma*, the causal law of the Universe. *Karma* states that the quality of an individual's future existence is determined by their actions. A morally good act produces positive consequences, while a bad act produces negative consequences.[2] Individuals with good *karma* have a more fortunate existence, while bad *karma* attracts suffering and distress. Belief in *karma* strongly influences a Hindu's attitude towards life. Life events are viewed as a result of one's past and current *karma*.[2]

Hinduism describes four goals (*purusarthas*) as essential for all human beings', emotional well-being and spiritual development.[2] *Dharma* is righteousness, the moral and ethical values that oversee human existence. *Artha* is the pursuit of economic prosperity, while *kama* is the pursuit of pleasure of the senses. As per Hindu belief, the proper pursuit of wealth and pleasure is vital to well-being but should be done within the ambit of *dharma,* which provides the moral and ethical framework for pursuing these goals.[2] The final goal of human life is *moksha*, that is, liberation from the cycle of *samsara*.[1]

According to Hinduism, humans are bound by certain personal and collective obligations. This concept of human indebtedness (*Rna*) is unique to Hindu tradition. Righteous living involves fulfilling obligations towards God, sages (gurus), ancestors (family), other humans, and all living beings. As per the Hindu worldview, these obligations override personal rights and freedom. Spiritual distress arises from an inability to fulfil one's obligations. In Hinduism, the human lifespan is divided into 4 stages (*Ashrama*), with set ethical guidelines, duties, responsibilities, and goals for each stage. Though these stages are generally linear, a spiritually awakened soul can directly enter into the *sannyasa* stage after the acquisition of the requisite knowledge (*Brahmacharya*). The details of the 4 *ashramas* are given in Table 1.

Table 1.   The stages of human life.

Sl No	Ashrama or Stage	Age (Years)	Description	Purusarthas
1	Brahmacharya (Student Life)	Up to 24	• Student stage • Duty — acquisition of knowledge • Practise of celibacy	• Living a life of Dharma
2	Grihastha (Household Life)	24–48	• Married Life • Duty — maintaining a household • Material attachment to one's life	• Living a life of Dharma • Pursuing Artha and Kama
3	Vanaprastha (Retired Life)	48–72	• Retirement stage • Duty — pursuit of wisdom • Gradual withdrawal from worldly affairs • Handing over control to progeny	• Living a life of Dharma • Moving towards Moksha
4	Sannyasa (Renounced Life)	72+ or anytime	• Ascetic stage • Duty — non-attachment to material pursuits • Renunciation of material desires	• Living a life of Dharma • Devoted to Moksha

In Hinduism, death is not the end, but a point where the soul transitions from one life to another after shedding the mortal body. A good death in Hinduism involves dying in a conscious state, with the right thought in mind, in the right place (preferably home), at an auspicious time, with the worldly duties completed and karmic debts repaid, surrounded by family and friends. Vegetarianism, ritualistic fasting, meditation, and chanting/singing are some rituals followed in preparation for dying. After-death rituals are paramount in Hinduism, conducted by the eldest male member of the family. The after-death rituals are described in Table 2. Bodies are cremated and rituals continue for one year. Fulfilling the rituals is one of the obligatory duties of the family members. Unnatural and unprepared deaths, occurring in unsuitable places, are termed bad deaths. They are believed to bring unfortunate consequences for the family. Family members need to perform retributive rituals to offset the effects of bad death.

Table 2.   After-death rituals in Hinduism.

- The body is bathed by the eldest male member of the family
- The body is placed on the floor with the head facing north
- The eyes are closed. Small cotton buds are placed into the nose and ear orifices. The big toes are tied together with a piece of cloth and a lamp is lit near the head of the deceased body, which is dressed in a white cloth
- Water from the river Ganga and sacred Tulsi is placed into the deceased mouth
- The deceased body is carried to the crematorium in a bamboo stretcher
- Cremation is done within 24 hours primarily by the eldest son
- No food is cooked or eaten until the cremation is complete. Once the cremation is done, the house is cleaned and purified as per tradition. All family members have a bath and food is cooked in the house
- The rituals continue for 13 days — a period of impurity is observed by all family members during this period
- The ashes are immersed in a holy river (preferably Ganges)
- A period of mourning and remembrance continues for one year

The Concept of Advance Care Planning in Hinduism

About 94% of the global Hindu population lives in India. Advance care planning is a relatively new concept in India, with its adoption and implementation still in the early stages. Poor awareness among healthcare providers and patients and the absence of appropriate legal and ethical frameworks have hindered the uptake of ACP in India.[3] Much of the literature on how Hindu beliefs influence ACP is sourced from the immigrant population in developed countries. In a study determining the rate of completion of advance directives among American Hindus, 9% had completed advance directives, 44% expressed a desire to complete them, and 4% did not want to have these conversations.[4] These figures are below the national average of 37% in the United States.[4] Attitudes regarding ACP are influenced by an individual's religion, race, and cultural values.

Death is viewed benevolently in Hinduism, as an opportunity to move towards liberation.[2] Death occurs once the *karmic* debts are repaid and an individual's obligations are fulfilled. Hindus believe death should neither be prolonged nor accelerated, as both incur *karmic* debts.[2] Euthanasia, assisted dying, and suicide are considered as bad deaths.[5] Autopsy and organ donation are believed to interfere with the transmigration of the soul.[5] Hindus are receptive to forgoing life-sustaining interventions (intubation, nasogastric tube feeding, cardiopulmonary resuscitation, anti-biotics, etc.) when illness is terminal and futility evident. In places where life-sustaining therapies are initiated, the healthcare provider is viewed as the karmic tool carrying out a preordained fate.[4] This passive acceptance of death, with belief in destiny and karma, facilitates conversations regarding death and dying. The low completion rate of advance directives is attributed to the reluctance to interfere with a preordained destiny.[4] In addition, it is suggested that ACP, with a focus on the physical body and its functions, may not resonate with the Hindu population, where the main focus is on purifying the soul for a better rebirth.[2,5]

Hindus believe pain and suffering result from inappropriate thoughts, words, or actions (bad *karma*) of the past or the current lifetime.[2] Physical suffering is an accepted form of redemption in Hinduism. Self-willed death by voluntary cessation of eating and drinking is an accepted practice among many Hindus.[2,6] It allows an individual to atone for past sins and progress on the spiritual path. Some Hindus endure pain and distressing symptoms stoically, refusing medications that cloud the mind, including opioids.[4,6] Hindus believe that thoughts at the time of death determine where an individual is reincarnated, preventing discussions regarding terminal sedation.[4]

Healthcare provider attitudes also impact patient choices regarding end-of-life care.[1] Interestingly, a study of physicians in the United States showed that Hindu physicians were four times more likely to object to terminal sedation than their counterparts from other religious back-grounds.[6] Many Indian families place implicit trust in doctors and rely on them for healthcare decisions. In such instances of deferred autonomy, a healthcare provider's attitude towards ACP and end-of-life discussions influence patient choices.[4]

Connectedness with family and community is an important compo-nent of spiritual well-being in Hinduism.[2] Filial responsibilities and kin-ship ensure that decisions are made collectively, with multiple family members involved in the decision-making process.[2] Many Hindu families protect their loved ones by not disclosing complete information regarding the disease.[2] In Western cultures, individual autonomy is the norm. The doctor's ethical duty is to obtain informed consent regarding life-sustain-ing interventions from the affected individual when they are mentally capable.[4] In India, nearly one-third of the patients in palliative care are unaware of their prognosis.[1,2] In such a scenario, conversations regarding living wills and advance directives become redundant. Healthcare decisions are made by the head of the family; either a senior family member (mostly male), the oldest son, or the husband.[4,6] In a Hindu household, elderly family members are respected and valued, with the oldest son obligated to care for them. When an adult offspring is involved in decision-making, filial piety impacts decisions regarding life-sustaining treatment.[6] In addition, the emotional stress and conflict involved in such decisions deter the completion of ACP.[4] When end-of-life care decisions are made collectively, conflicting views regarding care from different family members, faith in traditional systems of medicine, and geographical distance hinder the completion of advance directives.[4] If applicable, a durable power of attorney is a viable option in these circumstances.[4]

One of the important barriers to the effective implementation of ACP is a lack of awareness.[3] In an observational study 70% of Canadian South Asian adults of Hindu origin lacked an understanding of palliative care, ACP, and its benefits.[4] This lack of understanding resulted in aggressive treatments at the end of life. For many Hindus in developed countries, the cultural and language barriers and the isolation they experience in an alien healthcare system hinder end-of-life care discussion.[4,6]

Religious beliefs influence how individuals cope with illnesses and impact attitudes towards death and dying. Healthcare providers must be mindful of providing culturally-competent care. Initiating conversations about ACP with Hindu families should involve a family-oriented approach, with clinicians proactively eliciting the patient's and family's communication and information preferences, and involving the family in the decision-making process. When communication conundrums like collusion exist, clinicians must carefully assess and signpost goals that are mutually acceptable to healthcare providers, patients and families alike.[4]

Conclusion

Advance care planning improves the quality of death and dying. It is an important component of quality end-of-life care. Religious and cultural perspectives can hinder or facilitate end-of-life conversations. Death preparation in Hinduism primarily focuses on spiritual aspects rather than physical aspects. Collective decision-making is the norm among Hindu families. Healthcare providers must proactively explore patients' and their families' unique beliefs and practices, and address their healthcare wishes appropriately. A family-centred, culturally-competent care can increase the acceptance of ACP among the Hindu population.

Learning Objectives

- Hinduism promotes acceptance of death and preparation for dying.
- There is poor acceptance of advance care planning among Hindus.
- A belief that death is preordained, reluctance to interfere with the dying process, collective decision-making, and lack of awareness are some of the barriers for advance care planning.
- To improve acceptance of ACP, healthcare providers need to be mindful of the specific ethno-cultural and religious practices of Hindus, and explore and address the specific concerns.

References

1. Viswanath V., and Rao S.R. (2021). Palliative care: The Hindu perspective. In Benton K.D. and Pegoraro R. (eds.), *Finding Dignity at the End of Life A Spiritual Reflection on Palliative Care*, (1st edn.). Routledge, New York.
2. Rao S.R., Viswanath V., and Simha S. (2022). Spiritual healing in cancer care: A Hindu perspective, In Silbermann M. and Berger A. (eds.), *Global Perspectives in Cancer Care: Religion, Spirituality, and Cultural Diversity in Health and Healing*, (1st edn.). Oxford University Press, New York, pp. 229–239.
3. Gursahani R., Mani R.K., and Simha S. (2019). Making end-of-life and palliative care viable in India: a blueprint for action. *Natl. Med. J. India* **32**(3): 129–133. https://doi.org/10.4103/0970-258X.278684.
4. Doorenbos A.Z. and Nies M.A. (2003 Jan). The use of advance directives in a population of Asian Indian Hindus. *J. Transcult. Nurs.* **14**(1): 17–24. DOI: 10.1177/1043659602238346. PMID: 12593266.
5. Thrane, S. (November 2010). Hindu end of life: Death, dying, suffering, and Karma. *J. Hospice Palliative Nurs.* **12**(6): 337–342. DOI: 10.1097/NJH.0b013e3181f2ff11.
6. Chakraborty R., El-Jawahri A.R., Litzow M.R., Syrjala K.L., Parnes A.D., and Hashmi S.K. (2017 October). A systematic review of religious beliefs about major end-of-life issues in the five major world religions. *Palliative Support Care* **15**(5): 609–622.

Chapter 12

Spirituality and Religion in Advance Care Planning: Buddhism Perspectives

Lee Chung Seng

Palliative Medicine, Tan Tock Seng Hospital, Singapore

Case Scenario 1

TH was a 35 years old Buddhist doctor who was diagnosed to have metastatic gastric cancer with liver metastasis. He was married with a 3 years old son. Despite undergoing multiple courses of chemotherapy treatment, his condition continued to deteriorate. Being a medical professional and a practising Buddhist, he knew that death was inevitable and he had a frank discussion with his medical oncologist. As the palliative chemotherapy was no longer effective, his main priorities were being comfortable and able to spend time with his family at home. He was referred to the hospice home care team helped to titrate the medications for symptom control and provided psycho-emotional support for the family. He was able to spend the last few weeks of his life at home with his loved ones and was able to practice meditation and chanting with the guidance of a religious teacher and spiritual friends. He passed away peacefully in the presence of his loved ones in his bedroom.

Case Scenario 2

Mdm. T was a 71 years old lady who suffered from chronic kidney disease. Her condition was worsening and she would need dialysis to sustain her life. She was a divorcee with three children. She lived with her second son in his 4-room HDB flat. The patient was a housewife and depended on her children financially.

She was admitted due to fluid overload, severe itch due to uraemia, poor appetite and generalized fatigue. Her renal physician initiated the discussion on dialysis. She was consistent that she did not want dialysis due to financial concerns and that the dialysis would affect her lifestyle. On the other hand, the children were very supportive and wanted her to go through the dialysis. She was subsequently referred to a palliative care physician to establish the goal of care and manage her symptoms.

The palliative care physician explored the spirituality of Mdm T and initiated an ACP discussion. Mdm T was a staunch Buddhist. She was actively involved in Buddhist community activities. The Buddhist rituals such as going to temples and prayers were important to her. She felt that the dialysis was just adding to her suffering (discomfort) and that it prolonged her life unnecessarily. She was aware that without dialysis she would likely have a shortened lifespan. She would rather have a shortened lifespan than suffer the inconvenience and side effects of dialysis. She opted for conservative management of her end-stage renal failure and symptom management for the complications of her uraemia. She hoped to minimize blood tests and admissions to the hospital, and was against going to ICU and HD. She would prefer her symptoms to be managed in a home setting and spend her last days at home with her family.

With regards to financial concerns, she did not want to burden the family with debts. She knew that they could approach National Kidney Foundation for assistance with her dialysis fees but she still declined dialysis.

The palliative care physician then facilitated a family discussion together with the patient. The children subsequently accepted the patient's decision to decline dialysis. The patient was subsequently referred to hospice home care and passed away peacefully at home 4 months later.

Introduction to Buddhism

One fundamental belief in Buddhism is that all unenlightened beings will experience continual cycles of rebirth (Samsara). Existence as a sentient being, will inadvertently be associated with experiences of suffering (Dukkha), owing to the natural degradation of all experiences — in particular, experiences which are pleasant and desirable. The form of rebirth one undertakes is influenced by karma, which is the natural law of cause and effect. By this law, wholesome actions will lead to wholesome rebirths, while unwholesome actions will lead to unwholesome rebirths.

An individual can be freed from this cycle of endless rebirths by pursuing the training taught by the Buddha and through attaining the state of Nibanna (liberation). For the yet unenlightened, the state of a person's mind at the point of death directly conditions his next rebirth. This mental state is influenced by the wholesome and unwholesome karma he accumulated over his lifetime, as well as by his environment before he dies. For this reason, some Buddhist patients request to be alert and have a clear mind at the time of death, so that they may proactively direct their mind towards wholesome thoughts.

The Buddhist scriptures provide ethical principles regarding what constitutes wholesome and unwholesome actions. Lay Buddhists are encouraged to undertake five precepts, which form the foundation of a moral life. The spirit of the first precept lies with respect for life or non-harming and prohibits the killing of living things. This precept is often deliberated when Buddhists need to make end-of-life care decisions.

Advance Care Planning (ACP)

Buddhists are often reminded that death is certain, though the time of death is uncertain. As such, they are encouraged to prepare for our own deaths. Advance care planning is one of the ways to prepare for one's death. By making one's decision on medical care known to their loved ones, they can then act on his/her behalf in the event that one loses his mental capacity.

The discussion of ACP can be based on the Buddhist principle of skilful speech, which involves speech that is factual, helpful, kind and timely.[1]

1. Is the fact provided during the ACP discussion truthful? Is there any coercion?
   When a physician communicates with a patient and family, the medical facts will need to be provided truthfully for the ACP discussion. One will need to be mindful of any undue influences by the family on the medical decision made by the patient.
2. Is the ACP discussion helpful to the person? Is he prepared to talk about it?
   It is important to ensure that the patient is prepared to talk about advance care planning. It will be detrimental if the discussion is initiated when the patient is not willing.

3. Is the discussion conducted in a kind manner, allowing the person to talk about what he is ready to share?

    During the facilitation of ACP discussion, the physician can gently explore the patient's understanding of own health condition, providing the person the space to share one's emotions, values and healthcare preferences in a "safe" environment.

4. Is the discussion being conducted at the right time? Is the person and loved ones prepared to discuss ACP? Is there enough time set aside for the discussion?

    It is important to set aside adequate time for the ACP discussion. If the ACP could not be completed within the allocated time, one can schedule another meeting to complete the discussion. It is encouraged to review the ACP regularly, especially when there is an occurrence of a new healthcare event.

Buddhists' View on Euthanasia

From the Buddhist perspective, both euthanasia and assisted suicide are disallowed as they violate the first precept of respecting life or non-harm. Killing is one of the four most serious offences under the monastic code (Vinaya) and will lead to a monk's lifetime expulsion from the monastic community.[2] Five conditions need to be fulfilled to constitute a breach of this precept — (i) a human being as a victim; (ii) the knowledge that the victim is a human; (iii) the intention to end life; (iv) effort made to end life; (v) and death resulting from the aforementioned effort.

The violation of this Vinaya rule, in relation to euthanasia and abetment of suicide is depicted in the excerpt from a commentary below:

> "Should any monk intentionally deprive a human being of life, or look about for a knife-bringer [to help him end his life], or eulogise death, or incite [anyone] to death saying 'My good man, what need have you of this evil, difficult life? Death would be better for you than life,' — or who should deliberately and purposefully in various ways eulogise death or incite [anyone] to death: he is also one who is defeated [in the religious life], he is not in communion."

(Buddhaghosa as cited in Harvey, 2011, p. 289)[3]

From the Buddhist's perspective, must life be preserved at all costs?
It is important to recognise that the violation of the first precept will necessarily comprise an explicit intent to end life. Hence a patient who "makes death his aim" and act to end his life would breach this precept. However, this does not mean that Buddhism advocates that life must be preserved at all costs. A terminally ill patient, who accepts the inevitability of his death and witnesses a high carer burden, may forego medical treatment to allow a natural progression of his illness.

> "But in the case of a patient who has suffered a long time with a serious illness, the nursing monks may become weary and turn away in despair thinking 'when will we ever cure him of this illness?' Here it is legitimate to decline food and medical care if the patient sees that the monks are worn out and his life cannot be prolonged even with intensive care."
>
> Samantapasadika, volume 2, p 467

Herein, the patient wishes to live but accepts that further life-prolonging treatment would be futile and excessively burdensome to caregivers. Forgoing treatment under such circumstances is legitimate. This is aligned with the core tenets of Buddhist teachings, which emphasize the impermanence of life and expound the development of wisdom and equanimity towards death.

Buddhism does not believe there is a moral obligation to preserve life at all costs. Death cannot be postponed forever, and Buddhists are encouraged to be mindful and prepare for it. To seek to prolong life beyond its natural span when no remedy is in sight is a denial of the reality of human mortality. In Buddhism, this intent arises from delusion (Moha) and excessive attachment (Tanha).

From a physician's perspective, rather than embarking on a series of piecemeal treatments which would not produce a net improvement in a terminally ill patient's overall condition, it would often be appropriate to allow events to run their own courses. In such cases, it is justifiable to forego treatment that is futile or overly burdensome when weighed against a dismal clinical prognosis.

Buddhists' Perspective on Death and Organ Donation

According to Buddhist teachings, death occurs when the body is bereft of three things: vitality (Ayu), heat (Usma), and sentiency (Viññana). From a metaphysical perspective, death occurs with the cessation of the life faculty that a person carries. However, the exact moment of death would not be identifiable using modern instruments, under both of these definitions.

However, this should not pose a barrier towards organ donation in our modern world. Firstly, organ donation is arguably one of the most benevolent acts of gifting a person can perform for another. Organ donation has been described as "an extremely positive action, since it stems from a genuinely compassionate wish to benefit others". Thus, we could approach the topic of organ donation via the fact that the person is cultivating great compassion to offer part of his body for the sake of others.

Secondly, organ donation is frequently performed after a clinical diagnosis of brain death — this translates to an inability of the brainstem to perform life-sustaining functions such as independent breathing. Hence the forgoing of futile interventions, including mechanical ventilation, would be permissible as discussed in earlier sections.

Palliative and Hospice Care

Compassion for the sick and dying plays an important role in Buddhist practice. The Buddha is frequently quoted to have said "whoever who would tend to me, should tend to the sick." In the Suttas, the Buddha personally tended to the needs of his critically ill disciples. This includes nursing the wounds of a monk whose generalised pustular eruptions were so severe his friends abandoned him. The Buddha boiled water and washed the dying monk with his own hands, then cleaned and dried his robes. On another occasion, the Buddha encountered a monk stricken with severe dysentery, who laid on robes soiled in urine and excrement. He washed and tended to the sick monk before he enumerated the qualities that should be present in a good nurse.

These noble qualities include being competent to administer medicine, discerning what is agreeable to the patient and what is not, keeping away what is disagreeable and giving only what is agreeable, and acting out of compassion rather than for the sake of remuneration. He should also not feel repulsion towards saliva, phlegm, urine, stools, sores, etc. Additionally, he should be capable of exhorting and encouraging the patient with noble teachings. These attributes remain relevant to palliative healthcare professionals today.

Palliative and hospice care should be supported and provided to all patients. Buddhists can also use this journey to change the view on death from seeing it as the end of life to "an elongated interval to be experienced, studied, and used for inner wisdom". The patient who is facing the reality of death can use this opportunity to understand the nature of existence. For health care providers who frequently address this suffering, they should use this opportunity to acquire inner wisdom.

Learning Objectives
- Buddhism teaches that death is an integral part of life. As such, Buddhists are encouraged to be prepared for death. Advance care planning is one of the ways to prepare for one's death.
- Euthanasia is rejected by most Buddhists as it violates the First Precept, which prohibits intentional killing.
- The withdrawal of medical intervention when death is imminent and the care-giver burden is high is ethically permissible.
- Palliative healthcare professionals should aspire to develop professional competencies, compassion towards the dying, as well as the ability to provide good spiritual care.

References

1. Nyanaponika T. and Bodhi B. *Numerical Discourses of the Buddha. An Anthology of Suttas from Anguttara Nikaya.* Vistaar Publications, New Delhi.
2. Keown D. (1998–1999). Suicide, assisted suicide, and euthanasia: A Buddhist perspective. *J. Law Relig.* **13**: 385–405.
3. Harvey P. (2011). *An Introduction to Buddhist Ethics: Foundations, Values and Issues.* Cambridge University Press, Cambridge, UK.

Section 2

Real World Implementation of Advance Care Planning

Chapter 13

Role of Different Stakeholders (Patients, Family Caregivers, and Healthcare Staff) in Advance Care Planning

Shao-Yi Cheng

Department of Family Medicine, College of Medicine and Hospital, National Taiwan University, Taipei, Taiwan

Introduction

Taiwan is the first Asian country to legalize the Natural Death Act. It is specifically stipulated to respect the will of terminally ill patients during medical treatment and honor their rights. It was launched in 2000 and amended in 2013 and allows the physician to withhold or withdraw life-sustaining treatment based on the will of the patient to achieve a good death. However, it only benefits a limited number of patients and many details are not specified. The advance directives (AD) completion rate has been relatively low in Taiwan compared to Western countries since the approval of the Natural Death Act. The Patient Right to Autonomy Act goes one step further to ensure patient autonomy, honoring their rights to a good and natural death and promoting harmonious physician–patient relationships.[1] This Act was passed by the Legislative Yuan in Taiwan at the end of 2016 and enacted on January 6, 2019. It advocates AD through the process of advance care planning (ACP) consultation and is aimed at persons under any of the following clinical conditions: patients diagnosed with terminally-ill diseases, with irreversible coma, in a vegetative state, with terminal dementia, and incurable diseases. Before signing the law, through the mandatory process of ACP conducted by the medical team with the patient and family, the patient may decide whether to continue the medical treatment to prolong life or not when terminally ill and evaluate available options. During the ACP process, the patient designates a medical surrogate. A patient may consequently express his/her decision on the medical treatment, while artificial nutrition and hydration can become comatose after a thorough discussion with the medical team. In this chapter, we would specifically discuss the role of each stakeholder in the ACP.

ACP in Asian Culture

From a policy perspective, the advocacy for ACP is a means to honor patient autonomy. Recently, international Delphi consensus studies were conducted in the US and Europe to develop a definition of ACP and the recommendations for its application.[2] ACP was defined as the ability to enable individuals to define goals and preferences for future medical treatment and care, to discuss these goals and preferences with family and healthcare providers, and to record and review these preferences if appropriate. Sudore *et al.* conducted a series of extensive studies on ACP in the US. They defined[3] and measured the outcome of ACP[4]; how to best engage ACP in different populations such as older adults, people with chronic illnesses, the homeless, and prisoners. She also investigated the obstacles to promoting ACP; designed the web-based tool "PREPARE" to facilitate the implementation of ACP; conducted randomized controlled trials (RCTs) to demonstrate the efficacy of ACP for the public and patients with cancer, and investigated the utilization of ACP on electronic records for emergency physicians and safety for patients.

However, these studies were mainly conducted in Western countries. End-of-life communication in Asian countries such as Japan, Korea, and Taiwan is usually rare and only the end-of-life care preferences of a few patients can be honored.[5] Since most East Asian countries are influenced by the Confucianism and concept of "filial piety (a virtue and primary duty to respect and care for parents and senior relatives)", patient autonomy is consequently subordinate to family values and physician authorities. The dominant role of family members and physicians during the end-of-life decision-making of a patient is recognized as a cultural feature in Asia. Physicians often disclose the poor prognosis of patients and corresponding treatment options to the male family member, rather than the patient him/herself when the patient may be unable to psychologically accept the disease prognosis. To address this ethical and practical dilemma, the concept of "relational autonomy" and the collectivism paradigm may be ideally used to assist Asian people, especially older adults, to share their preferences for future care and decision-making on certain clinical situations with their families and important others. The definition and recommendations for ACP, therefore, need to be re-evaluated and redefined to be culturally specific for Asian societies. In 2019, six Asian countries published a declaration of ACP on the definition and delineation of the roles of stakeholders from a cultural context.[6]

ACP in Taiwan

Taiwan is the first Asian country to legalize the Patient Right to Autonomy Act following the Natural Death Act in 2000. The Natural Death Act guarantees dying patients the right to withhold and withdraw life-sustaining treatment (LST); however, because the family can decide for the patient and the context is limited to LST, the Act comes into play only when the patient is imminently dying.

The Patient Right to Autonomy Act goes one step further compared to the Natural Death Act. It applies to healthy people with mental capacity, the content includes issues related to artificial hydration and nutrition as well as LSTs, and it can be amended only by the patient.

Since ACP consultation is mandatory to sign AD, the minimum eligible age for the consultation is 20 years or above and lowered to 18 years since 2023. ACP consultation is a clinical feature of ACP in Taiwan. During the ACP consultation clinics, patients meet the medical team in the company of at least one relative with or without the medical surrogate. A medical surrogate is defined as someone who has no conflict of interest with the patient such as an organ transplant donor and excludes a successor to the patient. The medical team will discuss in detail the possible LSTs and artificial hydration and nutrition under any one of the five clinical conditions with the patients for at least an hour. The medical team usually comprises a medical doctor, a nurse, and a social worker/psychologist. In Taiwan, although most healthcare services are covered by the National Healthcare Insurance (NHI), the ACP services are not yet supported by the NHI system. Therefore, ACP participants need to pay an out-of-pocket fee of approximately 115 USD for the ACP consultation. If there is a second person who wishes to consult the medical team, such as a family member, there would be a concession charge of 82 USD for the second person, and so on. A unified AD form would be completed to record the end-of-life care preferences of the patient if appropriate. After the informed AD consent is signed by two witnesses, the form will be uploaded and stored in an online electronic platform and reported on the personal healthcare intelligent card. Thereafter, all hospitals in Taiwan would acknowledge that the patient has completed the AD and will act accordingly. Additionally, to facilitate the signing of AD since 2020, hospitalized patients may consult the ACP staff to complete the AD. During the COVID-19 pandemic, we applied online consultation to assist the public with the completion of the AD since 2022. As of March 2023, nearly 234 hospitals across Taiwan have provided ACP consultation clinics. Consequently, around 46,000 people have signed up for AD.

Roles of Stakeholders

Individuals

From an individual perspective, a patient should be informed of the right to decide on future medical care, including the legal options or guidelines of life-sustaining medical treatment (e.g., cardiopulmonary resuscitation, intubation, antibiotics, blood transfusion, renal dialysis, artificial nutrition, and hydration) when becoming terminally ill. Before such decision-making, patients should receive sufficient medical information, including prognosis from clinicians. ACP should be conducted when the person has decisional capacity. Patients are advised to appoint a family member(s) (or a person important to the patient) in advance as representatives to speak on behalf of the patient based on the preferences of the patient, should they be at some point unable to make their own decisions.[6]

A systemic review of the perspectives on ACP of Asian patients showed a willingness influenced not only by their knowledge of their disease and ACP but also by their beliefs regarding: (1) its consequences; (2) whether the concept was in accordance with their faith and wishes of their families or physicians; and (3) the presence of barriers. Essential considerations for the engagement of patients include preferences (1) for being actively engaged or delegating autonomy to others; (2) the timing, and (3) whether the conversations would be documented.[7] In Taiwan, before initiating the law, a study showed that most of the AD (95%) were signed by caregivers. More specifically, higher education level; cancer diagnosis; having family members, care homes, friends, or maids as primary caregivers; and patients knowing about their poor prognosis were associated with a higher likelihood of signing the ADs.[8]

A mixed cross-cultural study was conducted between Japan and Taiwan on the timing of initiating ACP and found that (of 700 respondents) 72% (of 365) of respondents in Japan and 84% (of 335) in Taiwan ($P < 0.001$) accepted the discussion before the illness.[9] In Japan, factors associated with the willingness before illness were younger age and rejection of life-sustaining treatments; while in Taiwan, older age, stronger social support, and rejection of life-sustaining treatments were the main factors. Four main categories of attitudes were extracted: the most common welcomed discussion as a wise precaution; responses in this first category outnumbered the preference for the postponement of discussion until imminent end-of-life, acceptance of the universal inevitability of death, and preference for a discussion from a healthcare providers' initiative. A recent large-scale study revealed the prevalence of older female patients who did not have an appointed surrogate decision-maker had a higher intention of not receiving life-sustaining treatment (LST) or artificial nutrition and hydration (ANH) under the five specified clinical and disability conditions.[10] The study implies that most patients are willing to begin discussion before their health is severely compromised; nevertheless, as of 2023, only 46,000 eligible people signed AD which is far under the expectation.

Family Members

It is necessary to acknowledge the importance of family members and the emotional environment of the patient, especially in Asia. The needs of the family members and close caregivers throughout the illness must be recognized and attended to. The family members are encouraged to participate in advanced care planning discussions between the patient and clinicians, as the patient may lose decisional capacity with disease progression. Family members are expected to remind, help, and/or accompany the patient to share their preferences for future medical care, and consider advance directives, if appropriate, through ACP when one of the family members is diagnosed with an incurable disease.[6]

Family members play a crucial part in the engagement of ACP in Asia. Since most East Asian countries are influenced by Confucianism and the concept of 'filial piety (a virtue and primary duty to respect and care of parents and senior relatives),' patient autonomy is consequently subordinate to family values and physician authority. The dominance of family members and physicians during the EOL decision-making of a patient is recognized as a cultural feature in Asia. The concept of "relational autonomy" and the collectivism paradigm may be used to assist Asian people, especially older adults, to share their preferences on future care and clinical situations with their families and important others.

Healthcare Professionals

To ensure quality care and informed decision-making, clinicians should discuss with patients and their family members the medical conditions and future care based on the readiness of the patient. As preferences can change over time, clinicians should assist patients in sharing their preferences regarding care and conduct regular ACP discussions as needed, and document the contents of each discussion. Further, the team should provide care consistent with the preferences of the patient such as facilitating the wishes to die at home if applicable and possible. The medical care team members must actively remind patients, especially those with terminal illnesses, to consider advance directives through ACP and choices of life-sustaining medical treatments (e.g., cardiopulmonary resuscitation, intubation, antibiotics, blood transfusion, renal dialysis, artificial nutrition, and hydration). Social workers may help arrange places of care and/or services based on patient preferences and assist them and their families to register and complete advance directives through available resources such as ACP clinics as per local and legal jurisdiction.[6]

In Taiwan, physicians and nurses at ACP clinics can explain to the patient and family members the definitions and spectrum of life-sustaining treatment, followed by a discussion on artificial nutrition and hydration. Artificial nutrition and hydration present a special ethical dilemma, especially in Asia. A national cohort study revealed that more than half of terminally ill dementia patients received tube feeding.[11] Recently, cross-cultural, multicenter research demonstrated that moderate artificial hydration is beneficial to the quality of dying and death to those in the palliative care unit.[12] Any issues related to psychosocial care could be answered by a psychologist or social worker.

Since cross-cultural studies have shown that the public would like to discuss ACP as early as possible when they are non-frail, physicians and other medical specialties should proactively raise this topic whenever possible.

Educators

From a cultural perspective, Asians traditionally regard death as a taboo and are reluctant to face and discuss the topic. Therefore, it is crucial to provide clinicians and the public with appropriate learning opportunities about dying and issues that arise during illnesses involving decisional capacity. Thanatology and ethics should also be included at all levels of education, especially for medical professionals. Professionals ought to take responsibility to better educate physicians, nurses, and other healthcare professionals with the necessary skills to improve the quantity and quality of meaningful ACP discussions.[6]

Education, not only for medical students but also for the public is vital to campaign for ACP; unfortunately, it is not prevalent nor included in all medical curricula. Future reforms should view this as an indispensable part of medical education. In addition, ACP education within a community should be encouraged to break up the taboo. Using multimedia as an educational tool, studies have shown a high percentage of community-dwelling elderly selecting palliative care at the end of life and completion of AD after a community interventional program. Participants in the intervention group also had a positive change in knowledge, subjective norms, perceived behavioral control, and behavioral intention of ACP for advanced dementia.[13]

Researchers

More research and guidelines in the fields of ACP and palliative care are warranted to serve as references for various stakeholders such as clinicians, educators, and policymakers for future implementation throughout Asia. The strategies for conversation and culturally sensitive models of advance care planning delivery should be a research priority before their implementation in clinical settings.[6]

In Taiwan, numerous studies and ongoing trials have been focusing on barriers and facilitators of willingness to visit ACP clinics and complete

AD. More emphasis should be placed on effective interventions to promote the completion of AD and cross-cultural comparisons in the future.

Policymakers

Governments, health insurers, and healthcare organizations should secure appropriate funding and support for ACP. In addition, patient autonomy-related laws should recognize the ACP process (such as surrogate decision-making and advance directives) as a legally binding guide in medical decision-making.[6]

The low completion rate of AD in Taiwan has consequently generated many problems. From a policy perspective, simplifying the procedures, reimbursing the consultation fees, and promoting ACP in communities' long-term care facilities are top priorities. The Legislative Yuan in Taiwan has held several public hearings on the current situation and provided suggestions to improve ACP have formulated strategies for its promotion.

Conclusion

Taiwan has been a pioneer in the campaign for patient autonomy for the terminally ill in Asia due to the implementation of the Natural Death Act, the Patient Right to Autonomy Act, and unique features such as ACP clinics. The roles and tasks of stakeholders are well defined; nevertheless, more efforts should be directed toward the low AD completion rate. Education should be prevalent for both medical professionals and the public on thanatology. More community engagement is expected. In addition, the process of ACP consultation and AD completion should be simplified. Lastly, ACP consultation fees should be completely or partially waived and priorities set. In summary, ACP should be more accessible after the endeavor of individuals, family members, medical professionals, educators, researchers, and policymakers.

Acknowledgement

We are grateful for the support from the Department of Family Medicine, National Taiwan University Hospital.

References

1. Cheng S.Y., Lin C.P., Chan H.Y., Martina D., Mori M., Kim S.H., and Ng R. (2020 September 5). Advance care planning in Asian culture. *Jpn. J. Clin. Oncol.* **50**(9): 976–989.

2. Rietjens J.A.C., Sudore R.L., Connolly M., van Delden J.J., Drickamer M.A., Droger M., *et al.* (2017 September). Definition and recommendations for advance care planning: An international consensus supported by the European Association for palliative care. *Lancet Oncol.* **18**(9): e543–e551.

3. Sudore R.L., Lum H.D., You J.J., Hanson L.C., Meier D.E., Pantilat S.Z., *et al.* (2017 May). Defining advance care planning for adults: A consensus definition from a multidisciplinary Delphi panel. *J. Pain Symptom Manage.* **53**(5): 821–832.e1.

4. Sudore R.L., Heyland D.K., Lum H.D., Rietjens J.A.C., Korfage I.J., Ritchie C.S., *et al.* (2018 February). Outcomes that define successful advance care planning: A Delphi panel consensus. *J. Pain Symptom Manage.* **55**(2): 245–255.e8.

5. Lin C.P., Cheng S.Y., and Chen P.J. (2018 July 20). Advance care planning for older people with cancer and its implications in Asia: Highlighting the mental capacity and relational autonomy. *Geriatrics (Basel).* **3**(3): pii: E43.

6. Lin C.P., Cheng S.Y., Mori M., Suh S.Y., Chan H.Y., Martina D., *et al.* (2019 October). Taipei declaration on advance care planning: A cultural adaptation of end-of-life care discussion. *J. Palliat Med.* **22**(10): 1175–1177.

7. Martina D., Geerse O.P., Lin C.P., Kristanti M.S., Bramer W.M., Mori M., *et al.* (2021 December). Asian patients' perspectives on advance care planning: A mixed-method systematic review and conceptual framework. *Palliative Med.* **35**(10): 1776–1792.

8. Chang H.Y., Takemura N., Chau P.H., and Lin C.C. (2022 October 12). Prevalence and predictors of advance directive among terminally ill patients in Taiwan before enactment of Patient Right to Autonomy Act: A nationwide population-based study. *BMC Palliative Care.* **21**(1): 178.

9. Miyashita J., Kohno A., Cheng S.Y., Hsu S.H., Yamamoto Y., Shimizu S., *et al.* (2020 July). Patients' preferences and factors influencing initial advance care planning discussions' timing: A cross-cultural mixed-methods study. *Palliative Med.* **34**(7): 906–916.

10. Liu C.J., Yang C.Y., Hsieh M.H., Liu C.K., Chen M.C., Huang S.J., *et al.* (2022 December 2). Advance care planning among adult patients and their end-of-life care preferences. *Omega (Westport).* 302228221143687.

11. Chen P.J., Liang F.W., Ho C.H., Cheng S.Y., Chen Y.C., Chen Y.H., and Chen Y.C. (2018 March). Association between palliative care and life-sustaining treatments for patients with dementia: A nationwide 5-year cohort study. *Palliative Med.* **32**(3): 622–630.

12. Wu C.Y., Chen P.J., Cheng S.Y., Suh S.Y., Huang H.L., Lin W.Y., Hiratsuka Y., Kim S.H., Yamaguchi T., Morita T., Tsuneto S., Mori M., and EASED Investigators. (2022 April 15). Association between the amount of artificial hydration and quality of dying among terminally ill patients with cancer: The East Asian collaborative cross-cultural study to elucidate the dying process. *Cancer* **128**(8): 1699–1708.
13. Chiu Wu C.H., Perng S.J., Shi C.K., and Lai H.L. (2020 August). Advance care planning and advance directives: A multimedia education program in community-dwelling older adults. *J. Appl. Gerontol.* **39**(8): 811–819.

Summary box

1. ACP consultation is team-based and multidisciplinary.
2. ACP consultation should be proactive.
3. ACP should be conducted when the person has decisional capacity.
4. Family members are expected to remind, help, and/or accompany the patient to share his or her goals and preferences for future medical care, and consider advance directives, if appropriate, through the process of ACP.

Chapter 14

Ethics & Law on Advance Care Planning: A Perspective from Singapore

Sumytra Menon[*] and Chua Shumin Eunice[†]

*Centre for Biomedical Ethics, Yong Loo Lin School
of Medicine, National University of Singapore, Singapore
†Department of General Medicine,
Tan Tock Seng Hospital, Singapore

Background

Population and Culture

Singapore is a small island state with a multi-ethnic and multi-religious population of 5.5 million. The main ethnic groups are Chinese (74.3%) alongside Malays, Indians, and other minorities. As for religious beliefs, Singaporeans identified as Taoists, Christians, Buddhists, Muslims, Hindus, as well as other religions, although some have no religion.[1] Singapore has a family-centric society, which probably stems from the Confucian values of the ethnic Chinese-majority population where the focus is more on the family rather than the individual. So, family members are expected to be the first line of emotional, financial, and social support for their loved ones. These expectations are also reflected in Singapore's social policies. For example, adult children are expected to take care of their elders, and this can even be enforced through laws such as the Maintenance of

Parents Act, where parents can seek an order requiring their children to provide them with a basic level of financial assistance.[2] Support from the community and various government agencies is regarded as the last resort. Due to these sociocultural norms and social policies, many individuals are conditioned to consider the effect of any healthcare decisions they make on their family members. These family members may also exert some influence, which may be wanted or unwanted, and positive or negative, on the individual when making decisions.

The population in Singapore is rapidly ageing and the size of nuclear families decreasing.[3] So, the family's resources and support for the older person may increasingly become limited. Consequently, family members may be influenced by practical matters in making care decisions. For example, the individual may prefer to continue living at home as they age whereas the family may wish to admit them to a nursing home because there is no caregiver to tend to them at home. It is challenging to respect the wishes of these individuals, especially if they are living in a multi-generational home with their relatives. The individual may feel unwanted by their family whereas the family is probably worried they are unable to care for the individual when they are out to work all day.

While advance care planning is not only about death and dying, making future healthcare plans may be perceived to lead to such topics, which are considered taboo subjects by many Singaporeans.[4] This is largely due to cultural and religious beliefs that view death as a sensitive and solemn topic. Some healthcare professionals may even have reservations about starting the discussion with their patients and family, fearful of causing offence and affecting the therapeutic relationship. Family members may be fearful of initiating discussions on end-of-life wishes with the patient to avoid causing anxiety and to help them maintain a positive outlook. These social and cultural norms may make it challenging for patients to engage in advance care planning discussions due to resistance and discomfort with end-of-life matters.

Types of Advance Care Plans

In Singapore, advance care plans (ACPs) can be made by individuals who are mentally competent. Often, the ACP will be conducted by a trained facilitator in a healthcare facility, and those present include the person/patient and loved ones they select to be part of the ACP conversation. There are three types of ACP in Singapore — the General ACP, Disease-Specific ACP, and Preferred Plan of Care (PPC). The General ACP is meant for individuals who are generally healthy, and it usually states their preference for care if struck with an unexpected and catastrophic condition resulting in a long-term loss of mental capacity, e.g., serious brain damage. The Disease-Specific ACP is for patients with specific conditions such as chronic kidney failure, and the conversations with the facilitator are tailored to suit the trajectory of their disease. The PPC is conducted with patients who are estimated to have about one year left to live and is focused on end-of-life decisions.

Ethical Principles

The main ethical principles in advance care planning are autonomy and beneficence.

Autonomy

The individual's values, beliefs, culture, and healthcare preferences are explored during the advance care planning process. To the extent possible, these values and preferences should be respected and used to guide making healthcare decisions when the individual loses mental capacity. During the advance care planning discussions, if individuals request inappropriate treatment, the healthcare professionals should explain why the request is inappropriate, address any concerns and offer alternatives. This active engagement provides constructive and respectful support, to foster the individual's autonomy in considering their preferences. A relational framing of autonomy recognizes the important role that family members and healthcare professionals can have in fostering the individual's autonomy. This could be achieved through respectful and constructive checking of the basis of individuals' expressed preferences and the alignment of these preferences with their deeper values and broader goals. Furthermore, it minimizes situations where individuals select preferences that are clinically inappropriate and which healthcare professionals are not obliged to provide just because it was earlier selected. Therefore, the advance care planning discussion is a suitable opportunity to elicit the individual's rationale for requesting that treatment, and correcting any misconceptions that they might have. Of course, it is critical that healthcare professionals provide the necessary information regarding the benefits and risks of treatment, including alternative options, to guide the patient in making an informed decision. Treatment options offered should still be based on professional judgment and adhere to accepted practices.

Healthcare professionals must be sensitive to balance promoting the individual's autonomy while trying to also manage the family's expectations. The individual is invited to select one or more loved ones to participate in the advance care planning conversations, and these persons are usually family members. Sometimes, families try to "protect" their elderly relatives from anxiety and distress by requesting that if the prognosis is dire, the healthcare professionals should not disclose it to the patient. While such requests are borne out of good intentions, healthcare professionals are strongly discouraged from participating in such "collusion" with the family unless withholding the information is necessary to prevent the patient from suffering very serious harm, and guidance on managing such situations has been promulgated through ethical guidelines.[5] Engaging in such practices make it almost impossible to conduct advance care planning conversations since the individuals are not apprised of their actual medical condition and/or prognosis.

Beneficence

Healthcare professionals are obliged to maximise benefits and minimise harms when caring for patients, and this is usually reflected through providing care and treatment that is in their best interests. Sometimes, individuals have healthcare preferences that others do not perceive are in their best interests. For example, someone with cancer may refuse chemotherapy even though the treatment may extend their life for a few years. Many healthcare professionals and the patient's loved ones may be uncomfortable with this refusal and attempt to gently persuade the patient to receive chemotherapy. The patient however may have their own reasons to refuse chemotherapy. If their reasons are due to a misconception or misunderstanding, the healthcare professional can make clarifications, and this may affect the patient's decision. Ultimately, the decision of a competent patient should be respected. Subsequently, if the patient loses capacity to decide on treatment, it could be argued that the healthcare professionals can now decide for the patient instead and provide chemotherapy since it is in the patient's best interests. It would be disrespectful for the patient to receive chemotherapy when they earlier specifically refused it, and it would not be in their best interests since the patient already clearly expressed their wishes and refused chemotherapy. This approach is concordant with the Singapore Mental Capacity Act (MCA), which lays out the test for best interests, and which will be discussed further below.[6]

The Law

Legal System

Singapore has a common law system, which consists of two strands that are intended to complement each other. The first strand is the written law (called statutes or Acts), which are passed in Parliament. The second strand may be described as judge-made law, which are decisions made by judges in court cases when two or more parties have a dispute, and judgments are typically published to explain the law and reasons for the court's decision. Decisions made by the court in cases cannot contradict statutes, and laws made in court cases can be overridden subsequently by statute.

Advance Medical Directive Act

Singapore has a law on advance medical directives called the Advance Medical Directive Act (AMDA), which was passed by Parliament in 1996.[7] The AMDA applies to directives that have been made using a specific form laid out in the AMDA's regulations. It allows someone who is at least 21 years old and who has the mental capacity, to sign this form to withhold or withdraw extraordinary life-sustaining treatment at a time in the future if three doctors have certified they are terminally ill and are at imminent death. An Advance Medical Directive made under the AMDA will take precedence over an ACP if the ACP also includes preferences on extraordinary life-sustaining treatment.

Advance Care Plans

Singapore does not have a statute for advance care planning. The ACP forms used by healthcare institutions in Singapore state that they are not legal documents and are a guide when making treatment decisions for patients who have lost capacity. This statement is made with reference to the MCA, which intends for doctors to be the final decision-makers for life-sustaining treatment or treatment to prevent serious deterioration for patients who lack the capacity to decide instead of the donee of a lasting power of attorney (if one was appointed to make healthcare decisions under the MCA).[8] Any decision taken on behalf of patients who lack the mental capacity to decide must be made in their best interests in accordance with section 6 of the MCA. The best interests test requires the decision-maker to consider various factors including the patient's past and present wishes, values, beliefs and culture, and the views of the patient's loved ones and caregivers.

Individuals making advance care plans using the above-mentioned ACP forms, or those that make their own ACPs or advance medical directives not using the AMDA (hereinafter referred to as common law directives) may be intended by their makers to bind doctors and their loved ones when making healthcare decisions on their behalf should they lose capacity in the future. There have been no cases in Singapore which have addressed the legal status of such common law directives and whether or to what extent they may bind others. Some healthcare professionals may consider the lack of a statute or court judgment on common law directives to be an advantage since it may permit them to exercise more latitude when interpreting a common law directive. Conversely, other healthcare professionals may consider it a hindrance because it lacks legal certainty.

Conclusion

ACP facilitators and healthcare professionals should be guided by the ethical principles of autonomy and beneficence when conducting ACP conversations. Patients' preferences and values should be elicited to promote their autonomy while trying to also manage the family's expectations in our family-centric society. Ethical tensions may also arise if patients' wishes clash with their families or healthcare professionals' expectations. While ethics and law are closely connected, the application of law is not just black and white and requires interpretation. Furthermore, the law does not contain written solutions to ethical dilemmas. Therefore, practical ethical reasoning, alongside knowledge of the law is required to evaluate ethical issues and value conflicts in ACP.

References

1.   Census of Population 2020 Statistical Release 1: Demographic Characteristics, Education, Language and Religion. Department of Statistics, Ministry of Trade & Industry, Republic of Singapore. https://www.singstat.gov.sg/-/media/files/publications/cop2020/sr1/cop2020sr1.ashx.

2. Maintenance of Parents Act 1995. Cap 167B. 2020 Rev Ed Sing. https://sso.agc.gov.sg/Act/MPA1995.

3. Population in Brief 2022. National Population and Talent Division, Strategy Group, Prime Minister's Office, Singapore Department of Statistics, Ministry of Home Affairs, Immigration & Checkpoints Authority & Ministry of Manpower. https://www.strategygroup.gov.sg/files/media-centre/publications/Population-in-Brief-2022.pdf.

4. Menon S., Kars M.C., Malhotra C., *et al.* (2018 August). Advance care planning in a multicultural family centric community: A qualitative study of health care professionals', patients', and caregivers' perspectives. *J. Pain Symptom Manage.* **56**(2): 213–221.e4. https://doi.org/10.1016/j.jpainsymman.2018.05.007.

5. Singapore Medical Council. (2016). *Handbook on Medical Ethics*. C5.2. https://www.healthprofessionals.gov.sg/docs/librariesprovider2/guidelines/2016-smc-handbook-on-medical-ethics---(13sep16).pdf.

6. Mental Capacity Act 2008. Cap 177A. 2020 Rev Ed Sing. Available at: https://sso.agc.gov.sg/Act/MCA2008.

7. Advance Medical Directive Act 1996. Cap 4A. 2020 Rev Ed Sing. Available at: https://sso.agc.gov.sg/Act/AMDA1996.

8. Singapore Parliamentary Debates, Official Report (2008 September 15). Vol 85 (Vivian Balakrishnan, Minister for Community Development, Youth and Sports).

Chapter 15

Advance Care Planning in Hong Kong*

Carmen W. H. Chan, Yong-Feng Chen,
and Helen Y. L. Chan

*The Nethersole School of Nursing, Faculty of Medicine,
The Chinese University of Hong Kong,
Hong Kong SAR, China*

Introduction

Advance care planning (ACP) is a process of communication among a patient, his/her family members and healthcare professionals regarding future care in the event of losing mental capacity.[1] It has been developed over 30 years as a potential solution to promote goal-concordant care in patients' last phase of life.[2] In this paper, we provide an overview of ACP development in Hong Kong and the challenges encountered in its implementation. Then, we share some of our work in promoting ACP in Hong Kong over the past two decades.

---

*Re-published with permission from special issue of ZEFQ journal; "Advance Care Planning around the World: Evidence and Experiences, Programmes and Perspectives".

An Overview of ACP Development in Hong Kong

Hong Kong faces the challenges brought by an ageing population and increased prevalence of chronic diseases, with 80% of deaths each year occurring in people aged 65 years or older.[3] However, many people have unrealistic expectations about treatment efficacy.[4] The phenomenon of overtreatment and medicalisation of death neither improves the quality of end-of-life care for patients nor satisfaction with care amongst bereaved families. Disputes within families or between healthcare professionals and families, which result in a sense of guilt, regret, grievance and complaints, are often reported.[5]

There has been growing recognition amongst healthcare providers of the need to promote the concept of engaging patients in planning for their end-of-life care. A number of non-governmental organizations, community organizations and professional organizations have launched various ACP programmes in hospital, community care and long-term care settings on their own initiatives.[6] In particular, The Hong Kong Jockey Club Charities Trust has invested substantial funding to support ACP development in community care settings and care homes[7] and capacity building[8,9] in the past few years.

At the policy level, the Hong Kong Hospital Authority has developed specific guidelines and a template form for guiding clinicians in conducting ACP, in addition to guidelines on Do-Not-Attempt Cardiopulmonary Resuscitation (DNACPR) and updated the Guidelines on Life-sustaining treatments for severely ill patients. The government also launched a public consultation on legislation for advance directives that was conducted in 2019.[10] Yet, the impacts of these policies on the clinical practices have not been studied systematically.

Challenges in ACP Implementation in Hong Kong

ACP emphasizes in-depth discussions about values, needs, and goals of care, as well as preparing advance directives.[11] Studies have shown that ACP can strengthen patients' autonomy and satisfaction with care, improve compliance with patients' end-of-life wishes, and reduce the net costs of care.[12–15] However, ACP is complex because it involves a range of behaviours, such as recognizing the need, seeking information, reflecting on own values, communicating with others, and documentation, of a process of change.

Inadequate Preparation for Public

The findings of our population survey showed that the majority of people in Hong Kong are not familiar with the concept of ACP.[16] Many family members felt obliged to try every means to maintain the patient's life, regardless of the cost. Due to poor communication about patients' values about care, patients' preferences for how they would like to live out their final stage of life are often overlooked.[6] Failure to provide an opportunity for open communication about ACP may result in dying people being forced to receive aggressive, yet futile, treatments even if they would prefer comfort measures.

Talking about end-of-life matters has been regarded as a curse and thereby became a cultural taboo in the community.[4,17,18] Such avoidance had even diffused into daily life. For example, the number "four" which has the same pronunciation as death is avoided in the block numbers on an estate or in the floor number of a building. It is not uncommon for patients, family members, and even healthcare professionals to try to avoid conversations about dying.[19,20]

In contrast, several local studies found that older people and terminally ill patients appreciated the opportunity to share their views about end-of-life care and funeral arrangements.[21,22] The bereaved families also wished to receive more information about the patient's prognosis and care at an earlier time to support them in preparing EOL care for their sick relatives.[5]

Inadequate Preparation for Healthcare Professionals

As over 90% of deaths occur in acute care settings, it is commonly assumed that healthcare providers, especially doctors and nurses, are responsible for initiating ACP in both palliative care and non-palliative care units.[4,23] There remains a strong belief in society that medical doctors are authoritative in treatment decisions and thus paternalism still prevails.

While healthcare providers are expected to serve as both initiators and decision coaches in the ACP process,[23] relevant education is limited.[24] Hence, most of them are hesitant to initiate the conversation because they perceive themselves as having poor skills to bring up conversations, lacking knowledge about symptom management, and facing time constraints due to heavy clinical workloads.[20,25] These issues are also common in other cultures and countries.[18,24,26–28]

Strengthening Public Education

Our team is amongst the first in the local community to promote ACP. Here, we shared four dimensions of our work, as follows.

Promotional Activities

We have designed a program to raise public awareness about ACP and advocate for their right to autonomy in the choice of preferred end-of-life care.[22] We conducted eight roadshows to promote public awareness of ACP. Five of the eight roadshows were held in hospital lobbies, with the remaining three taking place in malls or community centres. The roadshow activities included handing out health promotion pamphlets and VCDs and small-group discussions about perceptions of life and death. The objectives were to educate the general public about palliative care and ACP and to enroll 100 palliative care patient dyads (the patient and their families) for extensive ACP support. In total, 2,817 participants in the eight roadshows received pamphlets, VCDs, and booklets that raised their awareness of ACP.

Use of Multimedia Means

To sustain the effects of the promotional campaign, we continuously developed various kinds of educational materials, including a pamphlet, poster, booklet, board game, website, videos and video decision aid for wider access.[22,29,30] These materials contain information about cultural views of life and death, concepts and procedures used in ACP, and interviews with celebrities who have experienced the loss of family members. The materials are used to continue raising public awareness in hospitals, communities, and non-governmental organizations.

Capacity Building

Skill training workshops to train nurses, doctors, and medical social workers were also provided.[22] This workshop covered the management of symptoms, psychosocial interventions, and a detailed discussion of ACP. We integrated lectures, role play, and case scenarios to teach these healthcare professionals about death education and preparation (i.e., identifying preferences and valuing end-of-life care, preparing the AD document). They were encouraged to be volunteer counsellors to work with participants who accepted the idea of ACP. The healthcare professionals who participated in the workshop perceived the workshop to be well-organized and to have successfully boosted their capacity to apply ACP knowledge in palliative care settings.[22] They particularly appreciated the role play and case discussions, which showed real-world applications of ACP knowledge.

ACP Implementation

An 8-week home-based palliative care program for 108 end-stage cancer patients and their families was launched.[22] They participated in intensive discussions about ACP with trained healthcare professionals. These discussions covered identifying a healthcare proxy, potential scenarios involving death and dying, the benefits and drawbacks of medical interventions, priorities and spiritual values when undergoing life-sustaining treatment, arrangements for the afterlife, perceptions of advance directives, and discussions with families about their responsibilities when making medical decisions for their loved ones. In the end, all of the 108 patients demonstrated improved comprehension and acceptance of ACP. Their hospital readmission rates dropped from 53% to 23%, monthly hospital stays were reduced from 8.5 days to 1.4 days, and quality of life was improved at the end of the program and 3 months after the program ended.[22] In addition, our other studies that evaluated ACP showed that the process addressed patients' existential distress, increased their readiness for ACP behaviours without causing stress or anxiety, and improved the dyadic concordance in EOL care preferences.[31–33]

Development of an Evidence-based Professional Training Program

Healthcare professionals are a crucial part of educating the public and patients in the end-of-life stage about ACP and putting it into practice. Based on the experiences drawn from our previous works, we conducted a systematic review to identify effective components in educational programs for preparing healthcare providers in various disciplines to be ACP facilitators.[34] For our review, we selected 10 studies from 4,025 articles published before July 2018 and available on eight databases. These studies were conducted in Korea, Canada, Australia, the UK, and the US. The participants included nurses, physicians, and medical students. The primary focus of the training programs was communicating about ACP and the needs and experiences of patients in the ACP process. All of the training programs used instructional sessions, and some used additional discussion, role play, and advanced technologies (i.e., audio-visual materials, online tutorials, and e-simulations with interactive patients). The programs were implemented in a variety of formats, such as short courses (2-day retreat/16-hour curriculum), as a series (twice a week for 4 weeks, 60 min per session), lunch conferences (two 60-min sessions), and morning sessions (six 60-min sessions). The participants identified role play, case-based discussions, and interactive mini-lectures as their preferred modes of learning.

All of these training programs showed positive results, including significant improvements in participants' ACP knowledge, confidence, positive attitude toward shared decision-making, and communication skills when discussing end-of-life issues. However, the methodological quality of these training programs was suboptimal; two had strong ratings, two had moderate ratings, and six had weak ratings as assessed by the Effective Public Health Practice Project (EPHPP) appraisal tool. Rigorous studies are needed to prove their effectiveness.

Way Forward

The definition of a "good death" varies amongst individuals, thus effective communication is required to achieve goal-concordant care. Using multi-media and web-based techniques to create a sustained ACP training program for busy healthcare providers will improve the quality of people's end-of-life care. Although the findings of our studies suggested that ACP is feasible and acceptable in Hong Kong, its impact on healthcare utilization has not been much studied. In addition, more sustainable training programs based on scientific approaches are needed to improve healthcare providers' ability to practice ACP in non-palliative care settings and to enhance public awareness and acceptance of ACP.

References

1. Lin C.P., Cheng S.Y., Mori M., Suh S.Y., Chan H.Y., Martina D., *et al.* (2019). Taipei declaration on advance care planning: A cultural adaptation of end-of-life care discussion. *J. Palliative Med.* **22**(10): 1175–1177.

2. Morrison R.S., Meier D.E., and Arnold R.M. (2021). What's wrong with advance care planning? *JAMA.* **326**(16): 1575–1576.

3. Hospital Authority Head Office (2012). *Strategic Service Framework for Elderly Patients.* Hospital Authority, Hong Kong.

4. Chan H.Y.L., Lee D.T.F., and Woo J. (2019). Diagnosing gaps in the development of palliative and end-of-Life care: A qualitative exploratory study. *International Journal of Environmental Research and Public Health.* **17**(1): 151.

5. Chan H.Y.L., Lee L.H., and Chan C.W.H. (2013). The perceptions and experiences of nurses and bereaved families towards bereavement care in an oncology unit. *Supportive Care Cancer.* **21**(6): 1551–1556.

6. Chan H.Y.L., Chung C.K., Tam S.S., and Chow R.S. (2021). Community palliative care services on addressing physical and psychosocial needs in people with advanced illness: A prospective cohort study. *BMC Palliative Care.* **20**(1): 143.

7. Chan H.Y.L., Chan C.N., Man C.W., Chiu A.D., Liu F.C., and Leung E.M. (2022). Key components for the delivery of palliative and end-of-life care in care homes in Hong Kong: A modified Delphi study. *International Journal of Environmental Research and Public Health.* **19**(2): 667.

8. Xiu D., Chow A.Y.M., and Chan I.K.N. (2021). Development and psychometric validation of a comprehensive end-of-life care competence scale: A study based on three-year surveys of health and social care professionals in Hong Kong. *Palliative Support Care* **19**(2):198–207.

9. Wong K.T.C., Chow A.Y.M., and Chan I.K.N. (2022). Effectiveness of educational programs on palliative and end-of-life care in promoting perceived competence among health and social care professionals. *Am. J. Hosp. Palliative Care* **39**(1): 45–53.

10. Food and Health Bureau. (2020). End-of-life care: Moving forward (Legislative Proposals on Advance Directives and Dying in Place) Consultation Report. Hong Kong.

11. Reynolds K.S. (2004). End-of-life care in nursing home settings (unpublished PhD thesis). The University of North Carolina, Chapel Hill.

12. In der Schmitten J., Lex K., Mellert C., Rothärmel S., Wegscheider K., Marckmann G. (2014). Implementing an advance care planning program in German nursing homes: Results of an inter-regionally controlled intervention trial. *Deutsches Arzteblatt Int.* **111**(4): 50–57.

13. Hammes B.J., Rooney B.L., and Gundrum J.D. (2010). A comparative, retrospective, observational study of the prevalence, availability, and specificity of advance care plans in a county that implemented an advance care planning microsystem. *J. Am. Geriatrics Soc.* **58**(7): 1249–1255.

14. Detering K.M., Hancock A.D., Reade M.C., and Silvester W. (2010). The impact of advance care planning on end of life care in elderly patients: Randomised controlled trial. *BMJ* **340**: c1345.

15. Klingler C., In der Schmitten, J., and Marckmann G. (2016). Does facilitated advance care planning reduce the costs of care near the end of life? Systematic review and ethical considerations. *Palliative Med.* **30**(5): 423–433.

16. Chan C.W.H., Wong M.M.H., Choi K.C., Chan H.Y.L., Chow A.Y.M., Lo R.S.K., and Sham M.M.K. (2019). Prevalence, perception, and predictors of advance directives among Hong Kong Chinese: A population-based survey. *International Journal of Environmental Research and Public Health.* **16**(3): 365.

17. Chan C.W.H., Choi K.C., Chan H.Y.L., Wong M.M.H., Ling G.C.C., Chow K.M., *et al.* (2019). Unfolding and displaying the influencing factors of advance directives from the stakeholder's perspective: A concept mapping approach. *J. Adv. Nurs.* **75**(7): 1549–1562.

18. Cheng S.Y., Lin C.P., Chan H.Y., Martina D., Mori M., Kim S.H., *et al.* (2020). Advance care planning in Asian culture. *Jpn. J. Clin. Oncol.* **50**(9): 976–989.

19. Wan Z., Chan H.Y.L., Chiu P.K.C., Lo R.S.K., Cheng H.-L., Leung D.Y.P. (2022). Experiences of older adults with frailty not completing an advance directive: A qualitative study of ACP conversations. *Int. J. Environ. Res. Public Health* **19**(9): 5358.

20. Chan C.W.H., Wong M.M.H., Choi K.C., Chan H.Y.L., Chow A.Y.M., Lo R.S.K., *et al.* (2019). What patients, families, health professionals and hospital volunteers told us about advance directives. *Asia Pac. J. Oncol. Nurs.* **6**(1): 72–77.

21. Nan K., Lai R.Y.-K., and Chan H.Y.-L. (2023). Decision control preference for end-of-life care among older adults. *Geriatrics Gerontol. Int.* **23**(2): 151–152.

22. Chan C.W., Chui Y.Y., Chair S.Y., Sham M.M., Lo R.S., Ng C.S., *et al.* (2014). The evaluation of a palliative care programme for people suffering from life-limiting diseases. *J. Clin. Nur.* **23**(1–2): 113–123.

23. You J.J., Downar J., Fowler R.A., Lamontagne F., Ma I.W., Jayaraman D., *et al.* (2015). Barriers to goals of care discussions with seriously ill hospitalized patients and their families: A multicenter survey of clinicians. *JAMA Internal Med.* **175**(4): 549–556.

24. Mills J., Kim S.H., Chan H.Y.L., Ho M.H., Montayre J., Liu M.F., *et al.* (2021). Palliative care education in the Asia Pacific: Challenges and progress towards palliative care development. *Progr. Palliative Care* **29**(5): 251–254.

25. Chan H.Y.L., Kwok A.O.L., Yuen K.K., Au D.K.S., and Yuen J.K.Y. (2020). Association between training experience and readiness for advance

care planning among healthcare professionals: A cross-sectional study. *BMC Med. Edu.* **20**(1): 451.

26. Duke G. and Thompson S. (2007). Knowledge, attitudes and practices of nursing personnel regarding advance directives. *Int. J. Palliative Nur.* **13**(3): 109–115.

27. Rietze L. and Stajduhar K. (2015). Registered nurses' involvement in advance care planning: An integrative review. *Int. J. Palliative Nur.* **21**(10): 495–503.

28. McCourt R., James Power J., and Glackin M. (2013). General nurses' experiences of end-of-life care in the acute hospital setting: A literature review. *Int. J. Palliative Nur.* **19**(10): 510–516.

29. Liu L., Chan H.Y.L., Ho T.C.-K, Chow R.S.K., Li M.M.Y., Cheung E.W.S., *et al.* (2023). A serious game for engaging older adults in end-of-life care discussion: A mixed method study. *Patient Edu. Couns.* **113**: 107787.

30. Lai J.C. and Chan H.Y. (2023). A video decision aid for advance care planning among community-dwelling older chinese adults: A cluster randomized controlled Trial. *J. Palliative Med.* **26**(5): 637–645.

31. Chan H.Y.L. and Pang S.M.C. (2010). Let me talk — An advance care planning programme for frail nursing home residents. *J. Clin. Nur.* **19**(21–22): 3073–3084.

32. Chan H.Y.L., Ng J.S.C., Chan K.S., Ko P.S., Leung D.Y., Chan C.W.H., *et al.* (2018). Effects of a nurse-led post-discharge advance care planning programme for community-dwelling patients nearing the end of life and their family members: A randomised controlled trial. *Int. J. Nur. Stud.* **87**: 26–33.

33. Yeung C.C., Ho K.H., and Chan H.Y.L. (2023). A dyadic advance care planning intervention for people with early-stage dementia and their family caregivers in a community care setting: A feasibility trial. *BMC Geriatr.* **23**(1): 115.

34. Chan C.W.H., Ng N.H.Y., Chan H.Y.L., Wong M.M.H., and Chow K.M. (2019). A systematic review of the effects of advance care planning facilitators training programs. *BMC Health Ser. Res.* **19**(1): 362.

Chapter 16

Advance Care Planning in Malaysia*

Zee Nee Lim[†], Wan Jun Ng[‡], and Chee Chan Lee[§]

[†]*Hospis Malaysia, Kuala Lumpur, Malaysia*
[‡]*Queen Elizabeth Hospital, Kota Kinabalu, Malaysia*
[§]*Tunku Azizah Hospital, Kuala Lumpur, Malaysia*

Background of the Health Care System

Malaysia, an upper middle-income country,[1] has a total population estimated to be 33 million in the fourth quarter of 2022.[2] The Malaysian healthcare system comprises mainly of public sector health services, which are tax-funded, government-run services, as well as fee-for-service private sector health services.[3]

Malaysia has a dual burden of disease, with rising rates of non-communicable diseases (NCDs) as well as persistent problems with infectious diseases, particularly tuberculosis and dengue.[4] In addition, Malaysia is now an ageing society, with 7.3% of the total population aged 65 and over.[2] In a population study to estimate future projections of adult palliative care needs in Malaysia, it is estimated that there will be a 240% increment in the year 2030 compared to 2014, with the highest needs among the age group[3] 80-year-olds.[5] In a cross-country comparison of expert assessments of the quality of death and dying, Malaysia ranked 62 out of

---

*Re-published with permission from special issue of ZEFQ journal: "Advance Care Planning around the World: Evidence and Experiences, Programmes and Perspectives".

81 countries.[6] This brings to the fore the poor end-of-life care delivery in the country.

Studies have shown that the elderly population in Malaysia is receptive to the concept of advance directives (AD) and advance care planning (ACP).[7,8] Potential advantages of ACP implementation in Malaysia could include less aggressive medical care near death, earlier hospice referrals, improved bereavement experience of families as well as positively impacting the quality of end-of-life care.[9–11]

Policy or Legislative Efforts/Milestones

There is currently no legislation on AD or ACP in Malaysia.[12,13] In the absence of a legislative framework, the author explored the possibility of relying on Malaysia's code of medical ethics and guidelines to guide advance decisions but also discussed how it remained unclear how these guidelines could be effectively carried out in clinical practice.[12]

In the Malaysian Medical Association's code of medical ethics, it is stated that in the context where death is imminent and curative or life-prolonging treatment is futile, one should always take into consideration any advance directives and the wishes of the family.[14] This may be problematic from the ethical viewpoint. Firstly, AD or ACP plays a very limited role in the context where death is imminent. Priority should shift to goals of care discussion whereby palliative care is the only acceptable way. Secondly, the wishes of the family may not necessarily reflect the patient's preferences.

On the other hand, in the Malaysian Medical Council Guideline on the consent for the treatment of patients, it states that "a medical practitioner should refrain from providing treatment or perform any procedure if there is an unequivocal written directive by the patient that such treatment or procedure is not to be provided in the circumstances which now apply to the patient".[15] This has broader coverage and is potentially useful in ACP development and implementation because it is not limited to a situation when death is imminent.

As for policy development, the national palliative care policy and strategic plan 2019–2030 states that community participation in advance care planning is recommended in strategy no.6: "Encourage Community Participation in the Provision and Promotion of Palliative Care for the Nation".[16] However, there was no further information on how this is going to be implemented.

Definition(s) and Model(s) of ACP Used

There is no consensus definition of ACP in Malaysia. However, local studies' use of ACP concept to shape their research work is consistent with a multidisciplinary Delphi panel consensus definition of ACP for adults,[17]; with the aim to ensure people receive medical care that is consistent with their values, goals and preferences during serious and chronic illness.[18,19]

Education Training on Healthcare Professionals in ACP

An Example of ACP Training Programme in Sabah

The ACP training programme in Sabah, a Malaysian state occupying the northern part of the island of Borneo, targets healthcare professionals. The training module covers the what, why, who, when and how of ACP in 2 concise lectures, followed by ACP demonstration and role plays. Every participant will be given the opportunity to conduct ACP discussion. Participants are also expected to submit two completed ACP forms from the cases used in role-play in order to receive course completion certificate and badge.

Four ACP training sessions have been conducted since its inception, initially virtually during COVID times which later became hybrid sessions. A total of 92 doctors have been trained so far. 97% of participants gained solid knowledge and 93% had confidence in conducting ACP after the training. 90% of them considered changing their old practice and 96% would recommend the training to other colleagues. [W.J. Ng, personal communication, 2023 March 29].

An Example of ACP Training Programme for Paediatric Healthcare Professionals

In the year 2019, the head of all paediatric departments from the Ministry of Health in Malaysia met to discuss formalizing and standardizing ACP discussion amongst paediatric healthcare professionals. This ACP form is now included in the handbook of children's palliative care Malaysia.[20] Paediatric doctors undergoing palliative care training will be trained in ACP. The ACP training programme is also being introduced to other paediatric departments in stages. [C.C. Lee, personal communication, 2023 March 27].

Examples of Institutional Implementation

The ACP programme in Sabah was started in September 2021 by the palliative care unit in Queen Elizabeth Hospital. The programme targeted at clinicians consists of 3 parts: a standardized ACP form endorsed at the state hospital level, a conversation guide sheet, and a half-day training module. It is hoped that the ACP programme will eventually be advocated at the state level where patients with life-limiting illnesses can be further empowered in their care. [W.J. Ng, personal communication, 2023 March 29].

Research Agenda on ACP

The published research on ACP to date mainly focuses on attitude and perception,[7,8,22] development and validation of the ACP questionnaire,[19] validation of malay ACP questionnaire,[21] measuring educational impact on ACP[18] as well as legal[12,13] and the religious perspectives[22] on advance medical directives.

Future research should be nationally driven. Firstly, a research committee that includes the patient and public should be set up to identify a list of ACP research topics. Subsequently, a focus group to determine the priority of ACP research topics can be done. We may also want to explore collaborations with neighboring countries to advance and influence ACP development in Malaysia.

Patient and Public Involvement in Research and Development of ACP

Patient and public involvement in ACP is still limited. There have been efforts by civil society organizations and advocacy groups to raise awareness about ACP by hosting informational events, but there is no direct involvement of the public in planning and developing research in ACP.

Addressing Diversity and Vulnerabilities Regarding ACP Access and Use

Malaysia is a multi-cultural, multi-ethnic country, largely comprised of Malays (69.4%), Chinese (9.7%), Indians (4%), indigenous groups (11.9%) and others (5%).[2] Linguistic diversity and cultural factors may impact consultation and communication processes.[23] Therefore, it is important to recognize that different beliefs and practices regarding end-of-life care may impact ACP. This was shown in a local study describing view of fifteen older Malaysians whereby some wanted to leave matters to fate or God, or leave it to their children to decide.[8] However, another local cross-sectional study assessing the attitude, knowledge and practice of community-dwelling adults regarding ACP did not find any association with religion.[22]

A recent nationwide health literacy survey in 2019 showed that limited health literacy groups were prevalent amongst older age groups, lower education levels and lower household income.[24] These individuals may be at risk of not fully understanding their options for end-of-life care. In addition, vulnerable groups such as individuals with dementia or other conditions leading to cognitive impairment may not have the ability to make decisions for themselves.

To address these vulnerabilities, it is important to provide accessible resources on ACP which are culturally and linguistically appropriate. It may also be necessary to provide additional support for individuals with cognitive impairment, involving family members or other trusted individuals in the decision-making process.

Main Challenges and Barriers

1. Awareness and understanding of ACP: studies have consistently demonstrated lack of awareness and knowledge of ACP amongst adults in Malaysia.[8,18,22] Patients with lack of knowledge of ACP are less likely to engage in ACP discussions.[25] In addition, public education to promote ACP is lacking nationally. In fact, systematic reviews have shown that public education can improve ACP receptivity by empowering people to better cope with uncertainty and set goals for future care.[26]

2. Health system policies: ACP implementation is currently being led at the institutional level. However, the success in implementing ACP at an institutional level is influenced by many factors, including supportive culture for end-of-life care; administrative support for the coordination, monitoring and accessing records; manpower and staff preparation; time and resources devoted to ACP.[26] Educational policies and standardized training programmes across different healthcare

settings are also needed to equip healthcare professionals with the necessary skill set to work with patients in meeting their ACP needs. Ideally, ACP needs to be supported by strong policy initiatives at a national level.

3. Legislative framework: Some common law examples from Australia and Singapore reveal an approach that favours regulation in governing advanced medical decisions.[13] While regulation promotes clarity, there are limitations in the statutory approach. A medical law framework that upholds a person's right to autonomy in Malaysia may not be compatible with certain subgroups of patients who prefer families and healthcare professionals to make decisions or leaving it up to God to decide.[7,8,21]

Conclusion

It is evident that there is much to learn nationally and internationally about ACP before any decision on the implementation of ACP is made in Malaysia. ACP is a public health issue and requires a concerted effort of all stakeholders, including Government agencies, academic institutions, and non-government organizations to raise public awareness. More research is needed to shape the future direction of ACP development in Malaysia.

Acknowledgement

I would like to thank Dr Wan Jun Ng and Dr Chee Chan Lee for their contributions.

References

1. The World Bank. https://www.worldbank.org/en/country/malaysia/overview#:~:text=As%20an%20upper%20middle%2Dincome,income%20and%20developed%20nation%20status (Accessed 2023 March 28).
2. Department of Statistics Malaysia Official Portal https://www.dosm.gov.my/v1/index.php?r=column/pdfPrev&id=VndFcmkvVTZoVTNYOTN2MzRtNy9zQT09 (Accessed 2023 March 21).
3. World Health Organization institutional repository for information sharing. Malaysia health system review. https://apps.who.int/iris/handle/10665/206911 (Accessed 2023 March 22).

4. Malaysia health systems research volume I. https://www.moh.gov.my/moh/resources/Vol_1_MHSR_Contextual_Analysis_2016.pdf (Accessed 2023 March 22).

5. Yang S.L., Woon Y.L., Teoh C.C.O., *et al.* (2022). Adult palliative care 2004–2030 population study estimates and projections in Malaysia. *BMJ Supportive Palliative Care* **12**: e129–e136. http://dx.doi.org/10.1136/bmjspcare-2020-002283.

6. Finkelstein E.A., Afsan B., Goh C., Baid E., *et al.* (2022). Cross country comparison of expert assessments of the quality of death and dying 2021. *J. Pain Symptom Manage.* **63**(4): e419–e429. https://doi.org/10.1016/j.jpainsymman.2021.12.015.

7. Koh T.L., Lei C.S., Tajudin T.R., and Abdulshakur Z. (2017). Advance directives among elderly population: A Malaysian experience. *J. Indian Acad. Geriatr.* **13**: 62–67.

8. Htut Y., Shahrul K., and Poi P.J.H. (2007). The views of older Malaysians on advanced directive and advanced care planning. *Asia-Pac J. Public Health* **19**(3): 58–67.

9. Sudore R.L. and Fried T.R. (2010 August 17) Redefining the "planning" in advance care planning: Preparing for end-of-life decision making. *Ann. Intern. Med.* **153**(4): 256–261. DOI: 10.7326/0003-4819-153-4-201008170-00008.

10. Detering K.M., Hancock A.D., Reade M.C., and Silvester W. (2010 March 23). The impact of advance care planning on end of life care in elderly patients: Randomised controlled trial. *BMJ,* **340**: c1345. DOI: 10.1136/bmj.c1345.

11. Brinkman-Stoppelenburg A., Rietjens J.A.C., and van der Heide A. The effects of advance care planning on end-of-life care: A systematic review. *J. Palliative Med.* 2014: **28**(8): 1000–1025. DOI: 10.1177/0269216314526272.

12. Tan M.K.M. (2018). Considerations for introducing legislation on advance decisions in Malaysia. *Asian Bioethics Rev.* **10**: 87–92. https://doi.org/10.1007/s41649-018-0048-x.

13. Chan H.Y. (2019). Regulating advance decision-making: Potential and challenges for Malaysia. *Asian Bioethics Rev.* **11**: 111–122. https://doi.org/10.1007/s41649-019-00078-2.

14. Malaysian Medical Association Code of Ethics. https://mma.org.my/web/wp-content/uploads/MMA_ethicscode.pdf (Accessed 2023 March 3).

15. Malaysian Medical Council Guideline. https://mmc.gov.my/wp-content/uploads/2019/11/Consent_Guideline_21062016.pdf (Accessed 2023 March 3).

16. National Palliative Care Policy and Strategic Plan 2019–2030. https://www.moh.gov.my/moh/resources/Polisi/BUKU_NATIONAL_PALLIATIVE_CARE_POLICY_AND_STRATEGY_PLAN_2019-2030.pdf (Accessed 2023 March 1).

17. Sudore R.L., Lum H.D., You J.J., Hanson L.C., *et al.* (2017 May). Defining advance care planning for adults: A consensus definition from a multidisciplinary delphi panel. *J. Pain Symptom Manage.* **53**(5): 821–832. DOI: 10.1016/j.jpainsymman.2016.12.331.

18. Hing (Wong) A, Loh E.C., Tan L.P., Ng K.P., *et al.* (2016). Clinical Impact of Education provision on determining advance care planning decisions among end stage renal disease patients receiving regular haemodialysis in University Malaya Medical Centre. *Indian J. Palliative Care* **22**: 437–445. DOI: 10.4103/0973-1075.191788.

19. Lai P.S.M., Mudri S.M., Chinna K., and Othman S. (2016). The development and validation of the advance care planning questionnaire in Malaysia. *BMC Med. Ethics* **17**: 61 DOI: 10.1186/s12910-016-0147-8.

20. Lee C.C. and Tan C.E. Handbook of Children's Palliative Care Malaysia. https://www.moh.gov.my/index.php/database_stores/attach_download/681/169 (Accessed 2023 March 10).

21. Lim M.K., Lai P.S.M., Wong P.S., Othman S., *et al.* (2021). Validation of the psychometric properties of the malay advance care planning questionnaire. *BMC Palliative Care* **20**: 109 https://doi.org/10.1186/s12904-021-00790-7.

22. Alias F., Kassim P.N.J., and Abdullah M.N. (2022 December 32). Understanding advance medical directives from the Malaysian and Islamic law perspectives. *Malays. J. Islamic Sci.* 17–39.

22. Lim M.K., Lai P.S.M., Lim P.S., Wong P.S., *et al.* (2022). Knowledge, attitude and practice of community-dwelling adults regarding advance care planning in Malaysia: A cross-sectional study. *BMJ Open* **12**: e048314. DOI: 1136/bmjopen-2020-048314.

23. Lee Y.K., Ng C.J., Lee P.Y., Tong W.T., *et al.* (2022) Shared decision-making in Malaysia: Legislation, patient involvement, implementation and the impact of COVID-19. *ZEFQ* **171**: 89–92. https://doi.org/10.1016/j.zefq.2022.04.020.

24. Jaafar N., Perialathan K., Krishnan M., Juatan N., *et al.* (2021). Malaysian health literacy: Scorecard performance from a national survey. *Int. J. Environ. Res. Public Health* **18**, 5813. https://doi.org/10.3390/ijerph18115813.

25. Martina D., Geerse O.P., Lin C.P., Kristanti M.S., *et al.* (2021). Asian patients' perspectives on advance care planning: A mixed-method systematic review and conceptual framework. *J. Palliative Med.* **35**(10): 1776–1792. https://doi.org/10.1177/02692163211042530.

26. Jimenez G., Tan W.S., Virk A.K., Chan K.L., *et al.* (2018). Overview of systematic reviews of advance care planning: Summary of evidence and global lessons. *J. Pain Symptom Manage.* **56**(3): 436–459.e5. https://doi.org/10.1016/j.jpainsymman.2018.05.016.

Chapter 17

Advance Care Planning in India: Current Status and Future Directions: A Short Narrative Review*

Roop Gursahani[†], Naveen Salins[‡], Sushma Bhatnagar[§],
Savita Butola[¶], Raj K. Mani[‖], Dhvani Mehta[**], and
Srinagesh Simha[††]

[†]*P. D. Hinduja Hospital, Mumbai, India*
[‡]*Department of Palliative Medicine and Supportive Care,
Kasturba Medical College Manipal,
Manipal Academy of Higher Education, Manipal, India*
[§]*National Cancer Institute and Institute Rotary Cancer Hospital,
Department of Onco-Anaesthesia and Palliative Medicine,
All India Institute of Medical Sciences, New Delhi, India*
[¶]*Sector Hospital, Border Security Force, Tripura, India*
[‖]*Critical Care & Pulmonology, Yashoda Hospital,
Kaushambi, Ghaziabad, UP, India*
[**]*Vidhi Centre for Legal Policy, New Delhi, India*
[††]*Karunashraya, Bangalore Hospice Trust, Bengaluru, India*

---

*Re-published with permission from special issue of ZEFQ journal; "Advance Care Planning around the World: Evidence and Experiences, Programmes and Perspectives".

The Indian Healthcare System and Its Challenges

The Indian economy has grown over the past three decades at over 5% annually in real per capita GDP and evolved to lower-middle-income status in 2009.[2] This growth has provided for rapid expansion of the health industry. The public sector has seen significantly higher financial investments and the rapid growth of government-sponsored health insurance schemes. The private sector, which includes both hospitals and insurance has also grown to serve the emerging middle class, especially in smaller cities. Simultaneously this economic transition is largely responsible for the epidemiological transition into 'the age of receding pandemics' with the rise of non-communicable diseases. For instance, stroke was documented to be the leading cause of death in the rural, largely tribal district of Gadchiroli in Maharashtra.[3] The third transition is demographic. Lower birth and death rates have provided a bulge in the working-age population together with an increase in life expectancy and the population of seniors.

India has a mixed health care system with a stated goal of eventually achieving universal health care.[2] The private sector provides the bulk of outpatient encounters (70%), inpatient admissions (58%) and medicine dispensation (90%) with the remainder from the public sector. The public sector is largely responsible for the education and training of healthcare professionals and exclusively responsible for preventive health. The challenges in the public system include (1) fragmented service delivery; (2) inefficient linkages between various components with a patient tendency to bypass primary care for secondary and tertiary levels; (3) inadequacies of personnel, drugs, equipment and infrastructure; (4) lack of public accountability. On the private side, as can be expected, both facilities and workforce are skewed towards locations and specialties based on paying capacity and profits. It has been commented that the public health system is grossly underfunded, and the private sector is inadequately and erratically regulated. The national health policy has an explicit commitment to increasing public spending on health from the current level of 1% of GDP to 2.5% by 2025. It has been estimated that we should be able to achieve universal health care if this figure is doubled to 5% but for reasons somewhat like the United States,[4] that may not be feasible in a country as large and diverse as India. At present, like other low-income countries, healthcare spending in India is predominantly out-of-pocket (about 60–70%) with some community support in the form of not-for-profit (mainly charitable) providers.[5] The average Indian household spends 5–7% of its annual budget on health and in 15–20% of families every year health expenditure crosses the 10% limit that categorizes it as catastrophic. It has been estimated that 55 million Indians descend into poverty annually because of illness. The cost of care continues to grow and is often inappropriate at the end of life,[6] such as when ineffective oncologic treatments are used until death.

ACP: Public Knowledge, Attitude, and Practice

There is very little awareness of advance care planning for serious illness and end of life, either amongst the public or healthcare professionals. A Google Forms survey[7] of graduate internet users showed that less than 30% were aware of Advance Medical Directives. Of note, college graduates constitute less than 7% of the Indian population. Medical professionals fared somewhat better in the same survey: about 63% had heard of ADs. Nevertheless, extrapolating from experiences elsewhere in Asia (Lebanon, Malaysia) and from a large survey in the city of Pune, it can be assumed that most of the adult population have preferences for end-of-life care and would want to have their wishes followed. The Pune population-based survey[8] showed that over 99% were able to express a choice of preferred place of death and in 83% this was at home. The Lebanese study (middle-aged to older adults in primary care) showed that about 90% favored truth-telling and healthcare autonomy while 77% favoured documenting their healthcare values and preferences.[9] The main issue is that Indian concepts of autonomy are relational and not based on the individual. As a filial culture, the reliance on the family structure is seen in two ways: both as a duty to the sick and the expectation of caregiving. Shared decision-making necessarily involves the wider family and collusion to withhold information from the patient is routine.[10] The best insight into our cultural attitudes is from the South Asian diaspora in the West.[11,12] Qualitative studies by Biondo *et al.* (South Asia, Alberta, Canada) and Radhakrishnan *et al.* (South Asian Indians, including physicians, Texas, USA) have reported on focus groups. Issues that were highlighted included (i) the need for educational materials that were tailored for languages and health-literacy levels; (ii) the role of power differentials within families and the scope for involving power figures in the community; (iii) cultural hesitance in discussing death and dying with older family members; (iv) external loci of control with financial limitations and a sense of fatalism. Participants in both studies reported enhanced motivation to participate in ACP after learning about the concepts. This corresponds to the findings of Lim *et al.* (community-dwelling adults, Malaysia) of a positive attitude to and a willingness to participate in ACP after it was explained to them.[13]

ACP: Policy, Legislative and Judicial Aspects in India

Psychiatric advance directives were enabled by federal legislation with the revamp of the Mental Healthcare Act in 2017. A part of this enabled all persons with psychiatric illness to make advance directives for non-voluntary treatment and to nominate representatives for shared decision-making.[14] Mental health reform was driven by India's ratification of the UN convention on the rights of persons with disabilities. We believe it is unrealistic to expect any comparable political or legislative initiative for ACP for serious illness and end of life until and unless there is substantial citizen support for this issue. In fact, a draft bill,[15] which fortunately lapsed, was floated by the Ministry of Health and Family Welfare in 2016, which explicitly declared AMDs and medical power-of-attorney "to be void and not binding on medical practitioners". No politician in power would take the risk of enacting 'death laws' without adequate and universal healthcare. This gap is therefore now being filled in by judicial action in response to litigation initiated by civil society organizations and medical associations.

Enacted in 1950, India has a liberal constitution with strong rights of political and religious liberty. However individual autonomy has never been a major concern for Indians as in other Asian societies. The Indian Supreme Court first began weighing in on the constitutional basis of the right to die with dignity in 1996. In 2017–2018, a triptych of judgments laid the parameters for personal autonomy as regards privacy, sexual choice and health decisions.[16] The absolute right to refuse treatment even at the risk of death was clearly stated in the Common Cause judgment. The judges were however concerned about the misuse of provisions for withholding and withdrawing life support. They have also been traditionally wary of the potential for exploitation of vulnerable individuals through living wills. A judicial functionary (Judicial Magistrate First Class) was thus made the authority both for verifying advance directives (by countersigning them) and their implementation by withholding/withdrawing life support. This became an impossible hurdle and the 2018 judgment effectively remained inoperative.[17] However, initiatives began to evolve guidelines and documents for end-of-life care and most of the current authors were part of these which included a Do-Not-Attempt-Resuscitation policy,[18] draft End-of-life care legislation,[19] a model advance medical directive[20] and institutional guidelines.[21,22] Simultaneously advocacy efforts continued with the government and the courts. This led to a recent review by the Supreme Court in January this year which has significantly eased the situation.[1] This final order allows AMDs to be validated by notarization and the signatures of two witnesses. The JMFC involvement in withholding and withdrawal decision-making has also been removed.

Planning Implementation of ACP with Palliative Care Organizations

As is obvious from the above, ACP implementation currently will have to be a civil society effort while we continue advocacy efforts for government support. Setting up an organization for this is a huge task and efforts are likely to be fragmented and not scalable. In India, we propose the Indian Association of Palliative Care as the nodal agency for ACP until this is determined by legislation or government decision. PC now has a logical role in ACP which has evolved in the past couple of decades. Legacy PC in the 1960s began as a response to the suffering of cancer patients. Even today when PC is provided as a top-down service, the bulk of its services are geared to oncology. Over the past 3 decades, the focus has expanded to non-oncologic diagnoses as exemplified by the emergence of Neuropalliative care as a distinct subspecialty.[23] It has been shown that when PC needs are identified bottom-up by the community, as in the Neighborhood Networks system in Kerala, two neurologic diagnoses (dementia and stroke) have already outstripped cancer.[24] Biologically, in oncology, tumor burden determines when the 'waterfall trajectory' identifies prognosis. In non-oncology, patient/family autonomy and ethical concerns intersect with medical prognosis, making ACP a pillar of shared decision-making. Thus, as PC takes on its responsibility across various illness trajectories at the end of life, it needs to be involved in ACP as much as pediatricians now accept childhood vaccination as part of their brief. In most developed countries, ACP systems (through independent not-for-profits) and PC provision (often through universal health care) have evolved independently but our situation offers an opportunity for experimenting with a middle path. We expect a substantial spin-off benefit in the form of greater visibility and awareness of local PC organizations and services. In addition, since ACP is largely a middle-class concern, facilitation and documentation can also be run as chargeable services.

Suggested Plan for ACP implementation through the IAPC

Pragmatic definitions for ACP and AMD[25–28]:

ACP: This is the process of discussion with an adult subject (and significant others), at any stage of health or illness but often towards the end of life, whereby preferences for future treatment are stated and documented, in preparation for a stage where they can no longer participate in medical decision making. This should preferably include the designation of a proxy/surrogate decision maker/s and preferred place of care/death.

AMD: This is the document containing preferences for future medical care together with underlying values and wishes, meant to be used when the individual is no longer able to comprehend and/or communicate. These can include living wills, healthcare power-of-attorney designation, DNAR orders or physician orders for life-sustaining treatment.

Process

1. Initial public outreach will consist of live webinars in all major Indian languages. The schedule for this will soon be put up on the IAPC website. These recordings will be made available together with appropriate materials on the IAPC or an independent dedicated website. A dedicated response team will be set up for all queries either from laypersons or health professionals.
2. Model advance medical directive: The IAPC will set up a team of experts to review available documents from across the world. One or more of these will be selected, harmonized and validated.
3. Facilitator training and support: The materials for this will be initially developed in English and we request ACP-I for support and collaboration. The IAPC will then set up vernacular language ACP Facilitators training through its state units. Validated materials will undergo

translation and back-translation into the scheduled languages of the Indian Union. Initially, this will be the responsibility of state chapters, but we hope to be able to pass this on to dedicated not-for-profits in the long run. This is especially important in the subsequent phases when community capacity building will likely be the main driver. These materials will also be incorporated into current palliative care training. We will also explore the possibilities of making these available through massive online open courses.

4. Focus groups will be run in major ethno-religious groups to understand if there are significant differences. We will then attempt an outreach to religious power centres to share this responsibility amongst their own congregations.

5. Budgetary support will be required for administrative support and translation since we expect substantial input of voluntary and pro-bono efforts from our members.

Challenges

1. Palliative care capacity in India: Our situation is characterized by both low demand and low supply.[29] Hence it is difficult to imagine IAPC shouldering this effort alone and we hope to be a catalyst for dedicated non-profits to take over.

2. Health and death literacy: Health literacy is the ability to obtain and process information needed for basic health decisions. This information is largely processed through social practices and cultural, community and peer norms help determine the behavior of individuals. Poor health literacy is one of the drivers of potentially inappropriate end-of-life care and low ACP engagement in the USA.[30,31]

3. Religious beliefs: Receptivity to ACP and perspectives on termination of care are probably influenced more by religiosity than by actual religion.[32,33] Perspectives can vary even within the same religion based on the sect and guidance from spiritual leaders. Strategies to promote ACP will need to engage with religious communities.

Conclusions

Advance medical directives were legally and constitutionally validated in India in 2018 but on a practical basis were enabled only in January 2023. This narrative review is an overview of the socio-legal landscape and suggests a road map for the immediate future.

References

1. Common Cause vs. Union of India: Supreme Court of India. Miscellaneous application No. 1699 of 2019 in Writ Petition (Civil) No. 215 of 2005. https://main.sci.gov.in/supremecourt/2019/25360/25360_2019_3_504_41295_Judgement_24-Jan-2023.pdf (Accessed 2023 March 26).
2. Selvaraj S., Karan K.A., Srivastava S., Bhan N., *et al.* (2022). India: Health system review. *Health Syst. Transition* **11**(1). World Health Organization. Regional Office for South-East Asia. https://apps.who.int/iris/handle/10665/352685. License: CC BY-NC-SA 3.0 IGO.
3. Kalkonde Y.V., Deshmukh M.D., Sahane V., Puthran J., Kakarmath S., Agavane V., and Bang A. (2015 July). Stroke is the leading cause of death in Rural Gadchiroli, India: A prospective community-based study. *Stroke* **46**(7): 1764–1768. DOI: 10.1161/STROKEAHA.115.008918.
4. Alesina A., Glaeser E., and Sacerdote B. (2001). Why doesn't the US have a European-style welfare state? Harvard Institute of Economic Research. https://scholar.harvard.edu/files/glaeser/files/why_doesnt_the_u.s._have_a_european-style_welfare_state.pdf (Accessed 2023 April 14).
5. La Forgia G.M. and Nagpal S. (2012). Government-Sponsored Health Insurance in India: Are You Covered? https://openknowledge.worldbank.org/entities/publication/896f4909-aed1-5124-a621-ab68b3db6c24. License: CC BY 3.0 IGO.
6. Das S.K. and Ladusingh L. (2018 September 10). Why is the inpatient cost of dying increasing in India? *PLoS One* **13**(9): e0203454. DOI: 10.1371/journal.pone.0203454.
7. Dhru K.A. and Ghooi R. (2023 February). Advance directives in India: Seeking the individual within the community. In Cheung D. and Dunn M. (Eds.) *Advance Directives across Asia: A Comparative Socio-legal Analysis* (pp. 110–129). Cambridge: Cambridge University Press. ISBN: 9781009152624.
8. Kulkarni P., Kulkarni P., Anavkar V., and Ghooi R. (2014 May). Preference of the place of death among people of pune. *Indian J. Palliative Care* **20**(2): 101–106. DOI: 10.4103/0973-1075.132620.
9. Assaf G., Jawhar S., Wahab K., El Hachem R., Kaur T., Tanielian M., Feghali L., Al Hazzouri A.Z., and Elbejjani M. (2021 October 28). Awareness and attitudes towards advance care planning in primary care: Role of demographic, socioeconomic and religiosity factors in a cross-sectional Lebanese study. *BMJ Open* **11**(10): e052170. DOI: 10.1136/bmjopen-2021-052170.
10. Chaturvedi S.K., Loiselle C.G., and Chandra P.S. (2009 January). Communication with relatives and collusion in palliative care: A cross-cultural perspective. *Indian J. Palliative Care* **15**(1): 2–9. DOI: 10.4103/0973-1075.53485.
11. Biondo P.D., Kalia R., Khan R.A., Asghar N., Banerjee C., Boulton D., Marlett N., Shklarov S., and Simon J.E. (2017 October). Understanding advance care planning within the South Asian community. *Health Expect.* **20**(5): 911–919. DOI: 10.1111/hex.12531.

12. Radhakrishnan K., Saxena S., Jillapalli R., Jang Y., and Kim M. (2017 May). Barriers to and facilitators of South Asian Indian-Americans' engagement in advanced care planning behaviors. *J. Nurs. Scholarsh.* **49**(3): 294–302. DOI: 10.1111/jnu.12293.

13. Lim M.K., Lai P.S.M., Lim P.S., Wong P.S., Othman S., Mydin F.H.M. (2022 February 14). Knowledge, attitude and practice of community-dwelling adults regarding advance care planning in Malaysia: A cross-sectional study. *BMJ Open* **12**(2): e048314. DOI: 10.1136/bmjopen-2020-048314.

14. Philip S., Rangarajan S.K., Moirangthem S., Kumar C.N., Gowda M.R., Gowda G.S., and Math S.B. (2019 April). Advance directives and nominated representatives: A critique. *Indian J. Psychiatry* **61**(Suppl 4): S680–S685. DOI: 10.4103/psychiatry.IndianJPsychiatry_95_19.

15. Ministry of Health and Family Welfare, Government of India (2016). The Medical Treatment of Terminally-ill patients (Protection of Patients and Medical Practitioners) Bill. https://main.mohfw.gov.in/sites/default/files/44374928791462768288.pdf (Accessed 2023 March 27).

16. Gursahani R., Simha S., and Mani R.K. (2020 July–September). Legislation for end-of-life care in India: Reflections on 5 years of the end-of-life care in India taskforce journey. *Indian J. Palliative Care* **26**(3): 269–270. DOI: 10.4103/0973-1075.293879.

17. Mani R.K., Simha S.N., and Gursahani R. (2018 March). The advance directives and foregoing of life support: Where do we stand now? *Indian J. Crit. Care Med.* **22**(3): 135–137. DOI: 10.4103/ijccm.IJCCM_116_18.

18. Mathur R. (2020 April). ICMR consensus guidelines on 'do not attempt resuscitation'. *Indian J. Med. Res.* **151**(4): 303–310. DOI: 10.4103/ijmr.IJMR_395_20.

19. Mehta D. and Agarwal A. (2021). End of life care in India: A model legal framework, 2.0. Vidhi Centre for Legal Policy. https://vidhilegalpolicy.in/research/end-of-life-care-in-india-a-model-legal-framework-2-0/ (Accessed 2023 March 26).

20. Indian Association of Palliative Care: Living Will, 2020. https://www.palliativecare.in/living-will/ (Accessed 2023 March 26).

21. Blue Maple™, 2nd Ed, 2021: Kasturba Hospital Manipal Standard Operating Procedures on Limitation of Life Sustaining treatment and End of life care. https://khmanipal.com/wp-content/uploads/2023/02/Blue-Maple-Second-Edition-2021.pdf (Accessed 2023 March 26).

22. Bhatnagar S., Biswas S., Kumar A., Gupta R., Sarma R., Yadav H.P., Karthik A.R., Agarwal A., Ratre B.K., and Sirohiya P. (2022 February). Institutional end-of-life care policy for inpatients at a tertiary care centre in India: A way forward to provide a system for a dignified death. *Indian J. Med. Res.* **155**(2): 232–242. DOI: 10.4103/ijmr.IJMR_902_21.

23. The Lancet Neurology. (2021 June). New hope for advancing neuropalliative care. *Lancet Neurol.* **20**(6): 409. DOI: 10.1016/S1474-4422(21)00142-3.

24. Philip R.R., Philip S., Tripathy J.P., Manima A., and Venables E. (2018 February 14). Twenty years of home-based palliative care in Malappuram, Kerala, India: A descriptive study of patients and their care-givers. *BMC Palliative Care.* **17**(1): 26. DOI: 10.1186/s12904-018-0278-4.

25. Rietjens J.A.C., Sudore R.L., Connolly M., *et al.* (2017 September). European Association for Palliative Care. Definition and recommendations for advance care planning: an international consensus supported by the European Association for Palliative Care. *Lancet Oncol.* **18**(9): e543–e551. DOI: 10.1016/S1470-2045(17)30582-X.

26. Sudore R.L., Lum H.D., You J.J., *et al.* (2017 May). Defining advance care planning for adults: A consensus definition from a multidisciplinary Delphi panel. *J. Pain Symptom Manage.* **53**(5): 821–832.e1. DOI: 10.1016/j.jpainsymman.2016.12.331.

27. Jimenez G., Tan W.S., Virk A.K., Low C.K., Car J., and Ho A.H.Y. (2018 September). Overview of systematic reviews of advance care planning: Summary of evidence and global lessons. J. Pain Symptom Manage. **56**(3): 436–459.e25. DOI: 10.1016/j.jpainsymman.2018.05.016.

28. Martina D., Lin C.P., Kristanti M.S., *et al.* (2021 February). Advance care planning in Asia: A systematic narrative review of healthcare professionals' knowledge, attitude, and experience. *J. Am. Med. Dir. Assoc.* **22**(2): 349. e1–349.e28. DOI: 10.1016/j.jamda.2020.12.018.

29. Economist Intelligence Unit. The 2015 quality of death index: Ranking palliative care across the world. Commissioned by Lien Foundation, Singapore. https://impact.economist.com/perspectives/sites/default/files/2015%20EIU%20Quality%20of%20Death%20Index%20Oct%2029%20FINAL.pdf (Accessed 2023 March 27).

30. Luo Q., Shi K., Hung P., and Wang S.Y. (2021 June). Associations between health literacy and end-of-life care intensity among medicare beneficiaries. *Am. J. Hosp. Palliative Care.* **38**(6): 626–633.

31. Barker P.C., Holland N.P., Shore O., Cook R.L., Zhang Y., Warring C.D., and Hagen M.G. (2021 January–December). The effect of health literacy on a brief intervention to improve advance directive completion: A randomized controlled study. *J. Primary Care Community Health* **12**: 21501327211000221. DOI: 10.1177/21501327211000221.

32. Chakraborty R., El-Jawahri A.R., Litzow M.R., Syrjala K.L., Parnes A.D., and Hashmi S.K. (2017 October). A systematic review of religious beliefs about major end-of-life issues in the five major world religions. *Palliative Support Care.* **15**(5): 609–622. DOI: 10.1017/S1478951516001061.

33. Pereira-Salgado A., Mader P., O'Callaghan C., Boyd L., and Staples M. (2017 December 28). Religious leaders' perceptions of advance care planning: A secondary analysis of interviews with Buddhist, Christian, Hindu, Islamic, Jewish, Sikh and Bahá'í leaders. *BMC Palliative Care* **16**(1): 79. DOI: 10.1186/s12904-017-0239-3.

Chapter 18

Thailand Experience in Advance Care Planning*

Srivieng Pairojkul[†], Attakorn Raksasataya[†], Chalermsri Sorasit[†],
Duenpen Horatanaruang[‡], and Wanna Jarusomboon[§]

[†]*Karunruk Palliative Care Center, Srinagarind Hospital,
Faculty of Medicine, Khon Kaen University,
Khon Kaen, Thailand*
[‡]*Queen Sirikit National Institute of Child Health,
MOPH, Bangkok, Thailand*
[§]*Peaceful Death Group, Thailand*

Background of Thailand's Health Security System

In the last four decades, Thailand has achieved remarkable social and economic development, moving from a low-income country to an upper-income country in less than a generation.[1] In 2023, the Thai population numbered 70.2 million, with 51.1% in urban areas.[2] Like other developed countries, Thailand's fertility rate is 1.5 live births per woman,[2] which means that Thailand has now entered an aging society with 21.5% of the total population older than 60 years.[3] Regarding accessibility to health

---

*Re-published with permission from special issue of ZEFQ journal: "Advance Care Planning around the World: Evidence and Experiences, Programmes and Perspectives".

services, Thailand has been recognized as having booming development of health services.[4] The Ministry of Public Health (MOPH) is the key health authority responsible for planning, implementing, monitoring, and evaluating health policy and service implementation. There are other autonomous health agencies also established through legislation, notably the Health Systems Research Institute (1992), the Thai Health Promotion Foundation (2001), the National Health Security Office (2002), the National Health Commission Office (2007), and the Healthcare Accreditation Institute (2009).[4] Thailand's policy on universal health coverage has made good progress since implementing the National Health Security Act in 2002.[5] Ninety-nine percent of the population has access to health insurance. The public sector delivers most healthcare services in Thailand, including 1,002 hospitals and 9,765 health stations.

Primary Healthcare System in Thailand

The Thai MOPH tackles health inequality through three core policies: (1) Region-based health services system. This policy aims to facilitate better sharing of resources within each region, including money, human resources, information, medicines/technologies, and to strengthen referral across care levels within the region toward more efficient services. A referral system for healthcare services facilitates referring upstream and downstream between primary health units to community hospitals and higher health facilities at provincial or regional hospitals; (2) Health services development plans or 'Service plans' comprise primary and holistic healthcare as one of 15 service plans that all health facilities under the MOPH will use as their operation plan and implementation. The goals of this primary care and holistic care service plan include providing care by family care teams and establishing long-term community care and health promotion for the elderly, disabled, and vulnerable; and, (3) a District health system that calls for multisectoral collaboration in the community using strategic approaches called "U-CARE": Unity district health team; Community participation; Appreciation; Resource sharing and human development; and, Essential care provision. It is also believed that the district health system could become an active participatory model for harmonizing up- and downstream health services in Thailand.[6]

Cultural Context of Thailand: A Challenge and Barrier to Advance Care Planning

Shared decision-making is a crucial process to facilitate advance care planning. Asian countries are collectivist cultures with strong family values.[7] Thais pay high respect to their parents and forebears. Family is considered the foundation of social life. The Thai family comprises several generations living under the same roof, and their adult children will care for the elderly. A systematic study on advance care planning in Asia[8] found that healthcare professionals recognize the importance of ACP but rarely engage the patient. Instead, they address the family as a unit for fear of conflict with family members and potential litigation. Their lack of knowledge and skills resulted in low engagement and late initiation of ACP.

The culture of East Asia is influenced by the virtue of filial piety, as is Thai culture.[9] It requires a person to honor their parents, elders, and ancestors. Asian societies stigmatize the rejection of these family responsibilities and obligations.[10] This cultural practice reflects the family's participation in shared decision-making and advance care planning; typically, the patient's family makes the final decision. Another obstacle is that Thai healthcare professionals have always encountered a conspiracy of silence[11] and family members who, in an effort to provide the best care possible for their loved ones, choose to prolong life support treatments. This obstacle of family-directed care and the conspiracy of silence must be considered when planning advance care for the elderly in Thai culture.

View of Good Death in Thai and Buddhist Context: Support of Advance Care Planning

The majority of elderly with life-threatening illnesses wish for a peaceful and dignified passing. Most Thai seniors surveyed about their wishes for the end of life wanted to know the truth about their illness and be relieved of uncomfortable symptoms. Seventy-five percent did not desire "life-prolonging" treatments when the likelihood of survival was low.[12] Thai Buddhist family members defined peaceful death as preparing for a peaceful state of mind in the knowledge that one's impending death is neither a time of suffering nor of being alone, but rather a time spent with family members who are not yet in mourning.[13] In palliative care, Thai Buddhist cancer patients undergo three dynamic phases to accept death: participation in suffering, openness to death, and adherence to Buddhist practices to increase death consciousness.[14] A Thai study compares the perspectives of cancer patients and their relatives regarding end-of-life care. Both groups of respondents emphasized the importance of the place of death, the relationship with the family, physical and emotional comfort, and rapport with the medical staff. However, relatives underestimated patients' preferences in three areas: not burdening others, preparation for death, and physical and emotional comfort.[15] Death without suffering (not suffering from life support devices, dying with care), natural death (death with an end-of-life expectancy, death with illness or ailments), and death without worries (preparation for death, spiritual and belief practice toward preparation for death, family and property management before death); death among family members and death in a familiar place are also regarded as good deaths.[16] According to terminal, chronic patients, their caregivers, and the hospital palliative care team in the upper Northern Thai context, the characteristics of a good death are the absence of physical discomfort, psychological and spiritual tranquility, preparation for death, the ability to determine the place of death and the assurance of post-mortem care.[17] The patient's involvement in treatment decisions was the only difference between the end-of-life care preferences of the adult and older adult groups. According to a population-based study conducted in southern Thailand, receiving the truth about their illness, being free of distressing symptoms, having loved ones nearby, and living a meaningful life were essential preferences for end-of-life care for both adult and older adult groups.[18] Relief suffering, preparation for death, being with family, and the place of death were consistently mentioned in these studies, and these elements can be interpreted as the Buddhist definition of a good death. In advance care planning, the concept of a good death has always been used to comprehend values and preferences. The definition of advance care planning is the process of assisting adults of any age or health status in understanding and communicating their values, life goals, and care preferences for the future.[19] In this circumstance, a good death could be attained by organizing one's advance care plan.

Thailand's Experience with the Advance Directive

Thailand issued The National Health Act in 2007. Section 12 states that a person shall have the right to make a living will in writing to refuse the public health service provided merely to prolong his/her terminal stage of life or to make a living will to refuse the service to cease severe suffering from illness. Section 12 also allows a person to nominate an authorized substitute decision-maker for health decisions. In the early period of implementation of Section 12 of the National Health Act, doctors firmly rejected it. In Thailand, withholding or withdrawing life support remains a contentious issue, so doctors were concerned about the degree of confidence in the diagnosis of dying. The conspiracy of silence is quite strong in Thai culture, and patients have less opportunity to share in decision-making and less opportunity to prepare for future healthcare plans.[11] The patient and family feel reluctant to sign the advance directive, fearing the healthcare team will neglect them. Automatically the family will take the position of decision-maker, sometimes without any patient's consent. When Section 12 was enacted, the development of palliative care in Thailand was still in the early stages.[20] In 2014, Thailand announced the Palliative Care Policy. The inclusion of Palliative Care in the 2016 health service plan is the most crucial factor that has prepared the system to provide palliative care.[21]

Palliative Care Development in Thailand

Palliative care was recognized during the AIDS epidemic, but the care provided was mainly psychosocial and spiritual. After the epidemic had ended, palliative care was confined to advanced cancer patients. In 2012, Thailand's palliative care service was classified in Group 3a, which is localized palliative care provision, so it had not yet reached a measure for use by main service providers.[20] Since palliative care services were not integrated into the MOPH service plan, there was no career path, funding support, or time allocation for personnel. The services were run on a voluntary basis. The lack of doctor education perpetuated and exacerbated the situation. As a result, the development of palliative care policies went very slowly. In 2006, the Healthcare Accreditation Institute included several palliative care indicators in hospital accreditation. The indicators included pain management and psychosocial/spiritual care. In 2009, the

National Health Security Office supported hospitals in developing a palliative care network. It was in 2016 when palliative care was finally integrated into the MOPH Service plans,[21] a giant leap in palliative care development.

The National Health Security Office has endorsed palliative home care since 2016 by providing e-claim for palliative home care, which has had a tremendous impact on palliative home care service. The 2019 Service Plan Inspection report shows that 97.3% of regional and general hospitals and 96.1% of community hospitals have a palliative care program.[21] The management of the National Palliative Care Program is supervised, monitored, and evaluated by the MOPH through health inspection. The next step is to implement quality improvement. The Karunruk Palliative Care Center and the Thai Palliative Care Network developed Quality Standard for Palliative Care in 2019, and the MOPH adopted it as a guideline for hospital palliative care units to be used for quality assessment and improvement.[22] As a result, by 2017, palliative care in Thailand was classified as Category 4a: Palliative care services in the preliminary stage of integration into mainstream healthcare services.[23]

Difference between Advance Care Planning and the Advance Directive

Advance care plans are fundamentally different from advance directives (referred to as living wills). The basis of advance care planning is ongoing communication with health providers, family members, and potential surrogate decision-makers; they are not focused exclusively on end-of-life or life-threatening conditions. Advance care plans ensure patient-centred care by allowing healthcare providers and patients to identify their values, preferences, and the care they prefer in a medical crisis if they cannot communicate the care they want.[24]

Thailand Moving Forward to Advance Care Planning

Section 12 of the National Health Act in 2007 was enacted for nearly 16 years, but progress has been slow. A public awareness survey on attitudes toward palliative care in Thailand using a questionnaire that interviewed 2,394 participants from all regions of Thailand in 2018 found that 21%

had heard of a living will. The rate was higher in women aged 40–59 and 44% in Bangkok. Only 14% had a living will, but after receiving information, 72% planned to make a living will, and 13% insisted that they did not want such planning ahead of death.[25] Advance care planning conversation is conducted primarily in palliative care patients. A point prevalence survey from 14 hospitals in Thailand found that 18.9% of patients met the criteria for palliative patients, but only 17.3% had access to palliative care consultation.[26] In the group that received palliative care consultation, 88.8% had ACP recorded in their medical document, compared to 15.7% in the nonconsult group.

There was awareness of ACP, and continuous movement has occurred. For example, in 2019, the Karunruk Palliative Care Center invited Dr. Raymond Ng Han Lip and his team from Singapore to conduct an ACP communication workshop in Bangkok. After that, 14 hospitals all over Thailand started ACP clinics in their hospitals. Karunruk also hosted the ACP conference in 2019 and co-hosted with other significant organizations, including the MOPH, the National Health Commission Office, the Thai Heath Promotion Foundation, the National Health Security Office, the Thai Palliative Care Society, and the Thai Palliative Care Network. Thereafter, there has been a significant coordinated development in the ACP.

In 2019, the Thai Palliative Care Network and the Karunruk Palliative Care Center worked together to establish Thai Quality Standards for PC, an essential tool for quality assessment and improvement, with the goal of best practice and benchmarking. ACP is one of the 11 quality standards. ACP KPIs include accessibility to ACP communication; ACP documentation; accessibility of healthcare team to patients' ACP; and percentage of preferences honored.[22] A pilot project used this quality standard to audit the quality of hospital palliative care units in 2021. Ninety-nine regional and general hospitals throughout Thailand (83.19%) were included in the study. The results revealed: accessibility to ACP at 3.8 ± 0.9 (out of 5); ACP documentation at 4.0 ± 0.9; accessibility of healthcare team to patients' ACP at 3.4 ± 1.1; and, preferences honored at 3.4 ± 1.3.[27] Advance care planning is a significant component of palliative care. The management of the National Palliative Care Program is supervised, monitored, and evaluated by the Ministry of Public Health through health inspection. By 2020, ACP had been included as one of the 3 other significant KPIs for health inspection, but still, ACP was conducted primarily in palliative patients. Most palliative patients were provided palliative care at their primary doctors' requests, and rarely that the patients request palliative care and request for advance care planning by themselves.

Scaling Up Movement of Advance Care Planning Implementation

In 2021, the National Health Commission Office brought ACP into a national-level action.[28] First, a committee created a common national ACP form and standard operating procedure. The ACP form consisted of values, preferences, and the degree of medical treatment according to the person's wishes. It also includes an advance directive and proxy appointment at the end of the form. Next, a referendum was conducted among health and social professionals, including a public hearing, which the National Health Commission committee affirmed. The form and procedures were then distributed to the government and the public sector to be implemented. The National Health Commission office has since appointed a steering committee to move forward with the nationwide implementation of ACP, which is to integrate ACP into various stages and care settings, including:

- Healthy adults
  Primary/community care
  Public awareness
- Chronic disease patients
  Specialist OPD
  Hospital in-patient
- High-needs/frail patients
  LTC and nursing home
  Geriatric and Palliative services

Thailand's Government Movement of Advance Care Planning Implementation

The Office of the National Health Commission, the major player in implementing ACPs, has established strategies for implementing ACPs by coordinating/facilitating with other organizations.

1. Set up a National Steering Committee to move ACP into a national-level movement.

2. Integration of ACP into all other related national policies: National Plan for the Elderly; National Service Plan for Palliative Care.
3. Implementation of the ACP form: Implementation and monitoring in all 13 Health Areas through the Palliative Care Service Plan set ACP ≥ 60% as a Palliative Care KPI.
4. Work with the National Health Security Office on possible hospital reimbursement for ACP.
5. Coordination with the Thai Palliative Care Society developed curricula for Palliative Care and ACP E-learning for professionals and the public.
6. Implement public awareness of the ACP through regional conferences.
7. Building champions in Health Areas 5, 9, and 12.

Institutional and Community Implementation Programs

Integrating ACP into Chronic Kidney Disease

The Karunruk Palliative Care Center has coordinated with the Thai Nephrology Society, the National Service Plan for Palliative Care, and the National Service Plan for Kidney Health, MOPH. A prototype of the Kidney Supportive Care Program of Srinagarind Hospital has been used to integrate palliative care into nephrology. A "Palliative Care in End-Stage Kidney Disease" conference was held in January 2023 to provide palliative and nephrology professionals with knowledge and skills. In addition, a plan to increase skills in sharing decision-making and communicating ACP will be provided through hands-on workshops for palliative and nephrology personnel in all service areas in Thailand.

Integrating ACP into the Long-term Care Program

The National Health Security Office piloted the Long-Term Care (LTC) program in 2016 to encourage multisectoral collaboration for community eldercare that targets dependent older adults, people with disabilities, and people with chronic diseases. The National Health Security Office receives an annual budget from the government and distributes funds to local administrative organizations. The LTC program covers 80% of the area and will soon expand to 100%. A nurse from the primary care unit manages the program and provides patient care through trained caregivers. The majority of program participants are elderly people with ADL

$\geq$11. The care manager conducts the evaluation and develops the care plan. One caregiver will be responsible for 10–20 clients and make regular visits per the care plan. The Department of Health requires care managers for the LTC program to complete a 70-hour training program. The care manager training curriculum is reviewed regularly. Still, palliative care was not integrated into the curriculum, and ACP was not made mandatory when recruiting clients for the program until 2023.

Advance Care Planning Education

The palliative care team conducts the majority of ACP communications with palliative patients. Therefore, training other health professionals in the knowledge and skills required for ACP is necessary. Healthcare professionals and the general public are offered workshops regarding education and training on ACP knowledge and skills.

- Karunruk Palliative Care Center has designed a program called "Training for the Trainers for Serious Illness Conversation and Advance Care Planning Communication" and has conducted several workshops to train a group of facilitators for further training for palliative care and nephrology professionals in the National Service Plan of the MOPH. Thereafter this workshop could be conducted regularly for other health professionals.
- The Peaceful Death Group has created a group of facilitators to help conduct regular workshops called the "Bao Jai classroom" for the public and volunteers.

Many public and non-public organizations have crafted articles, materials, e-learning, and videos to promote ACP and palliative care.

Role of NGOs on Public Awareness

Several NGOs have actively promoted the issue of public awareness of palliative care and advance care planning (namely, Budnet Foundation, Peaceful Death Group, and Cheewamitr Social Enterprise). Together, they coordinate and also work with healthcare sectors.

The Budnet Foundation's founder, Phra Phaisan Visalo, distributed a workshop on "Preparation for a Peaceful Death" in 2003, which teaches about end-of-life spiritual care and preparing the mind for a good and peaceful death. Palliative care education has been incorporated into the workshop. Planning for a good death is inextricably linked to advance care planning. This workshop is held several times a year, and health professionals and members of the general public have responded positively.

The Peaceful Death Group is a non-profit organization founded in 2018 to promote death with dignity. The group has created the "Bao Jai booklet",[29] which aids in the development of its advance directive. The promotion of advance care planning and living through this program, as well as the regular schedule of the Bao Jai classroom, will be ongoing in the community. The group also used validated card games to facilitate discussion on sensitive topics. The activity was designed to be a small group discussion in person. Using Zoom[30] during the COVID-19 pandemic, they develop an innovative practice of teaching participants about ACP and Palliative care using a card game. One can also learn about advance care planning and palliative care on their website. To promote ACP, the group collaborated with numerous influencers and journalists.

Future of Advance Care Planning in Thailand

Thailand is rapidly improving national palliative care services and implementing ACP on a large scale. There are still many challenges and barriers to overcome, but close coordination between government and nongovernmental organizations is critical. Furthermore, lessons from other countries and our experiences may help improve the program.

Acknowledgments

The authors thank Mr. Bryan Roderick Hamman, under the aegis of the KKU Publication Clinic, for assistance with the English-language presentation of the manuscript.

References

1. World Bank. The World Bank in Thailand. https://www.worldbank.org/en/country/thailand/overview. (Access 2023 March 30).
2. Thailand population. https://www.worldometers.info/world-population/thailand-population/ (Access 2023 March 30).
3. Thailand — Demographic change. https://www.population-trends-asiapacific.org/data/THA. (Access 2023 March 30).

4. Asia Pacific Observatory on Health Systems and Policies. (2015). The Kingdom of Thailand health system review. *Health Syst. Transition* **5**: 153–5.

5. Tangcharoensathien V., Prakongsai P., Lim-wattananon S., Patcharanarumol W., Jongudomsuk P. (2009). From targeting to universality: Lessons from the health system in Thailand. In Townsend P. (Ed.) *Building Decent Societies: Rethinking the Role of Social Security in Development.* Palgrave Macmillan, Hampshire, pp. 310–22.

6. World Health Organization. (2017). *Primary Health Care Systems (PRIMASYS): Case Study from Thailand, Abridged Version.* World Health Organization, Geneva. Licence: CC BY-NY-SA 3.0 IGO.

7. Marcia Carteret M.E. (October 21, 2010). https://www.dimensionsofculture. com/2010/10/cultural-values-of-asian-patients-and-families/   (Accessed 2023 March 7).

8. Martina D., Lin C.L., Kristani M.S., Bramer W.M., Mori M., *et al.* (2021). Advance care planning in Asia: A systematic narrative review of professionals' attitude, knowledge and experience. *JAMDA.* **22**: 349.e1–349.e28.

9. Filial Piety. https://en.wikipedia.org/wiki/Filial_piety (Accessed 2023 March 30).

10. Zhan H.G., Feng Z., Chen Z., and Feng X. (2011). The role of the family in institutional long-term care: Cultural management of filial piety in China. *Int. J. Soc. Welfare* **20**: S121–S134. DOI: 10.1111/j.1468-2397.2011.00808.x.

11. Saimmai P., Hathirat S., and Nagaviroj K. (2022 March 31). What challenges do Thai general practitioners and family physicians confront when discussing advance care planning with palliative care patients and families?: A qualitative study. *J. Dept. Med. Ser.* **47**(1): 94–102. [cited 2023 March 31]. https://he02.tci-thaijo.org/index.php/JDMS/article/view/252203.

12. Srinonprasert V., Kajornkijaroen A., Na Bangchang P., Wangtrakuldee G., Wongboonsin J., *et al.* (2014). A survey of opinions regarding wishes toward the end-of-life among Thai elderly. *J. Med. Assoc. Thai* **97**(Suppl. 3): S216–S222. Full text. e-Journal. http://www.jmatonline.com.

13. Kongsuwan W., ChaipetchO., and Matchim Y. (2012). Thai Buddhist families' perspective of a peaceful death in ICUs. *Nur. Crit. Care* **17**(3): 151–159. DOI: 10.1111/j.1478-5153.2012.00495.x. Epub 2012 February 15.

14. Upasen R., Thanasilp S., Akkayagorn L., Chimluang L., Tantitrakul W., *et al.* (2022). Death acceptance process in Thai Buddhist patients with life-limiting cancer: A grounded theory. *Global Qual. Nur. Res.* **9**: 1–10.

15. Chindaprasirt J., Wongtirawit N., Limpawattana P., Srinonprasert V., Manjavong, M., *et al.* (2019). Perception of a "good death" in Thai patients with cancer and their relatives. *Heliyon* **5**: e02067.

16. Tipwong A., Ruamsook T., Hongkittiyanon T., Kgowsiri K. (2020). The perceptions on good death of the older adults in the semi-urban community: A qualitative study. *Int. J. Nur. Sci.* **9**: 389–396.

17. Panuthai S., Srirat S., and Wonghongkul T. (2020). Characteristics of a good death as perceived by related people in the upper northern Thai context. *Thai J. Nur. Council* **35**(4): 35–53.

18. Jiraphan A. and Pitanupong J. (2022). General population-based study on preferences towards end-of-life care in Southern Thailand: A cross-sectional survey. *BMC Palliative Care* **21**: 36: 1–11. https://dci.org/10.1186/s12904-022-00926-3.

19. Sudore R.L., Lum H.D., You J.J., Hanson L.C., Meier D.E., *et al.* (2017). Defining advance care planning for adults: A consensus definition from multidisciplinary Dephi Panel. *J. Pain Symptom Manage.* **53**: 821–832. DOI: 10.1016/j.jpainsymman.2016.12.331.

20. Worldwide Palliative Care Alliance. Global atlas of palliative care at the end of life. https://www.who.int/nmh/Global_Atlas_of_Palliative_Care.pdf (Accessed 2020 March).

21. Ministry of Public Health. Inspection guideline: Service plan — Palliative care. 2019 report.

22. Pairojkul S. (2019). *Quality Standard for Palliative Care.* Klung Nanathum Publishing, Khon Kaen. https://www.karunruk.org/quality-standard/.

23. Clark D., Baur N., Clelland D., *et al.* Mapping levels of palliative care development in 198 countries: 616 The situation in 2017. https://doi.org/10.1016/j.jpainsymman.2019.11.009.

24. MyHomecareBiz.com. The difference between advance care planning and advance directive. https://go.myhomecarebiz.com/blog/train-home-health-nurses-on-oasis-c2-advance-directives. (Accessed 2023 March 30).

25. Kunakornvong W. and Naosri K. (2020). Public awareness and attitude toward palliative care in Thailand. *Siriraj Med. J.* **5**: 424–430.

26. Pairojkul S., Thongkhumcharoen R., Raksasattaya A., *et al.* (2021). Integration of specialist palliative care into tertiary hospitals: A multicenter point prevalence survey from Thailand. *Palliative Med. Rep.* **2**(1). DOI: 10.1089/pmr.2021.0003.

27. Pairojkul S. Report project "Situational analysis and developing of quality hospital palliative care services". Supported by National Research Council of Thailand. N0. SUNN65001.

28. National Health Commission Office. Advance care planning. https://www.nationalhealth.or.th/th/standard-operation-procedures-sop (Accessed 2023 March 30).

29. Peaceful Death Group. Bao Jai Booklet. https://peacefuldeath.co/activities/baojai/ (Access 2023 March 30).

30. Phenwan T., Peerawong T, Jarusomboon W., Sittiwantana E., Satian C., and Supanichwatana S. (2021 July 18). Using Zoom and card game to conduct advance care planning classes: An innovative practice. *J. Death Dying.* OnlineFirst. https://doi.org/10.1177/00302228211032735.

Chapter 19

Advance Care Planning in South Korea*

Yu Jung Kim[†] and Sun-Hyun Kim[‡]

[†]*Division of Hematology and Medical Oncology,
Department of Internal Medicine, Seoul National University
Bundang Hospital, Seoul National University College of Medicine,
Seongnam, Republic of Korea*
[‡]*Department of Family Medicine, International St. Mary's Hospital,
College of Medicine, Catholic Kwandong University,
Incheon, Republic of Korea*

Introduction

As of 2023, South Korea is an aging society that is rapidly entering a super-aged society with an elderly population accounting for 18.4% of the total population of about 52 million. The total number of deaths in 2022 is 372,800, and the most common cause of death is cancer.[1] Half of the decedents are over the age of 80,[1] and due to this increase in the elderly population, interest in end-of-life (EOL) care and the quality of death is increasing. However, South Korea is one of the Asian countries that traditionally avoids discussing death openly.[2] Particularly, even when a person is suffering from an incurable disease and is about to die, it is customary for the family members to make surrogate decisions without directly informing

---

*Re-published with permission from special issue of ZEFQ journal; "Advance Care Planning around the World: Evidence and Experiences, Programmes and Perspectives".

the patient of the disease status or discussing life-sustaining treatment (LST).[2,3] However, due to a series of social events such as the Boramae case[4] and the Grandma Kim case,[5] a social consensus was sought on the importance of individual autonomy, good death, discontinuation of futile LST, and advance care planning (ACP), and eventually the Life-Sustaining Treatment Decisions Act was enforced in 2018. In this article, we summarized the current situation of ACP and decisions on LST in South Korea.

Background — Culture and Landmark Medical-Legal Cases

Traditionally, South Korea is one of those countries where family consensus is more important than individual autonomy. In the case of an elderly patient, family members often thought that the best filial piety is to perform LST until death without informing the patient of the diagnosis or prognosis so as not to discourage their parents. It was also considered a cultural practice to withhold cardiopulmonary resuscitation (CPR) just before death according to the family's decision rather than the patient's self-determination.[6–11] In addition, society was not accustomed to openly discussing death.[2]

However, two historical events occurred. One was the "Boramae Hospital case" in 1997 when an inebriated older man fell and received emergency surgery for intracerebral hemorrhage. The wife, who could not afford the cost of the intensive care unit, strongly demanded the withdrawal of LST, and the patient died immediately after being discharged. Later, the patient's brother sued the patient's wife and the doctors, and the doctors were convicted of aiding and abetting murder. After this incident, doctors would not stop LST fearing legal responsibility even for patients with no possibility of recovery, and this led to frequent conflicts between family members and doctors.[4] The second was the "Grandma Kim case", in which the family members requested to withdraw mechanical ventilation, but the hospital refused and the family filed a lawsuit to discontinue futile LST. Grandma Kim was in a vegetative state following complications of a lung biopsy in February 2008. The family demanded to withdraw the mechanical ventilation because Grandma Kim had previously told them she would not want futile LST. After a lengthy lawsuit, in May 2009, the Supreme Court ruled that Grandma Kim's LST was meaningless, and the LST was discontinued.[5] These events sparked social controversy, and a full-fledged discussion began to achieve a social consensus on the discontinuation of meaningless LST. Based on these social discussions and the growing awareness of the importance of EOL care, the Life-Sustaining Treatment Decisions Act was legislated in 2016 by merging with the existing hospice-related laws and was fully implemented on February 4, 2018.[12]

In addition, the National Health Insurance Service began to partially apply insurance fees for counseling and paperwork related to LST decisions for terminally ill patients. South Korea has had National Health Insurance Service for all citizens since July 1989.[13] In July 2015, inpatient hospice services were incorporated into the National Health Insurance Service after several years of demonstration projects. Since then, home care hospice and consultation hospice services have been added, and the use of hospice services is gradually increasing.[14,15]

There is still a reluctance to tell patients directly about hospice or terminal diagnoses, so family members often make surrogate decisions and do not always respect patients' wishes.[8,16] However, South Korean studies show patients want to know the prognosis of their disease and want to discuss ACP directly.[17,18] Failure to consider patient's own values and wishes may increase unnecessary medical use, increase medical costs,[17,19,20] and reduce the quality of life of patients and caregivers.[21,22]

Policy or Legislative Efforts/Milestones to Foster ACP Implementation into the National Health Care System (From AD to ACP)

Before the enactment of Life-Sustaining Treatment Decisions Act, most hospitals were able to discontinue LST without the consent of the patient if the family members made a surrogate decision and signed the do-not-resuscitate (DNR) form of the institution, and these decisions were usually made just before death.[6–8,10,11] After the case of Grandma Kim, some private organizations or associations created their own advance directive (AD) forms, but they were not widely used because they were not common forms and had no legal effect.

After the Boramae hospital case in 1997, there were social attempts to discuss the discontinuation of LST, but discussions faded without changes made to health policy. It was after the case of Grandma Kim that the need for legislation related to the discontinuation of LST came to the fore. In 2013, the National Bioethics Committee prepared a recommendation on futile LST decisions, and after continuous discussions, it was integrated with the existing hospice-related laws in 2016 to enact the Life-Sustaining

Treatment Decisions Act, which was fully implemented on February 4, 2018.[12] According to the Life-Sustaining Treatment Decisions Act, the National Agency for Management of Life-Sustaining Treatment under the supervision of the Ministry of Health and Welfare plays a central role in the overall management of medical institutions and registry agencies, including supervision, education, system establishment and operation. The Ministry of Health and Welfare is supposed to establish a comprehensive plan for hospice and LST every five years, based on reviews by the National Committee for Hospice Care and Life-Sustaining Treatment. This committee is a social consultative body composed of a total of 15 members, including members from the medical, religious, ethical, legal, and patient groups, with the Vice Minister of Health and Welfare as the chairperson. The National Agency for Management of Life-Sustaining Treatment is currently performing its functions under the mandate of the Korea National Institute for Bioethics Policy (Figure 1).[23]

The purpose of the Life-Sustaining Treatment Decisions Act is to protect the dignity and value of human beings by ensuring the best interests of the patients at the end stage of disease by respecting their self-determination. Patients can express their preferences by completing the legal forms including an AD or a Life-Sustaining Treatment Plan which is a type of a Physician Orders for LST (POLST). Whether it is because of the legal background of the Boramae case or the Grandma Kim case, or

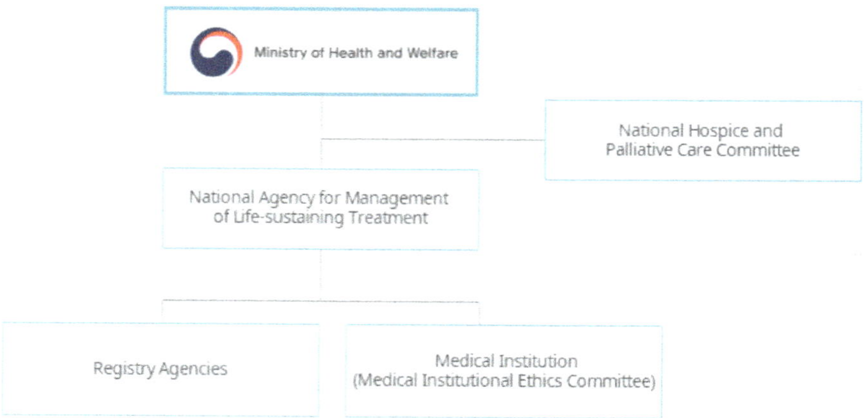

Figure 1. System of the National Agency for Management of Life Sustaining Treatment.[23]

Source: Figure from National Agency for Management of Life-sustaining Treatment.

because of the penalties for violations, currently there is a tendency to focus on completing the relevant legal forms rather than focusing on in-depth ACP discussions between patients, their families, and medical team. Before the enactment of this law, most hospitals left their own DNR documents without legal effect on medical records. The content of these DNR forms was limited to whether or not CPR was performed and were usually completed by the family members at the time of imminent death.[6,7] After the enactment of the law, documents related to LST were unified into above mentioned legal forms.[24] These documents are not only legal forms, but are reimbursed by National Health Insurance once they are completed and registered in the national system.

Definitions and Models of ACP in South Korea

Many aspects of the Life-Sustaining Treatment Decisions Act mirror the process of ACP, but the word "ACP" is not specified anywhere in the law.[12] However, the purpose of protecting human dignity and respecting patient autonomy is the same as that of the ACP, and the legal forms related to LST can be regarded as a documented result of the ACP.

To reduce the confusion that may arise after the implementation of the law in 2018, the Korean Medical Association published a consensus guideline clarifying the definitions of "the end stage of disease" and "the last days of life" after analyzing reports and laws of other countries.[25–27] In this guideline, ACP was defined as "a process in which patients and medical team discuss the goals of care and specific methods of future treatment so that the patient's autonomy and best interests can be realized".[28] According to the guideline, ACP can be performed at any time of the disease trajectory and is often initiated at the request of the patient or at the recommendation of the doctor while the disease is worsening. The doctor participating in the ACP provides the patient with information about the pros and cons of the medical treatment that can be selected in the future to help the patient make a decision and documents the contents of ACP as a medical record. Medical records may include discussions of legal forms such as AD or discussions about hospice and palliative care.

The appropriate time to discuss ACP is not limited to the end stage of the disease and is preferred to be done early in a healthy state. Therefore, not only terminally ill patients but also patients with chronic disease and even healthy people can perform ACP at any time.[28]

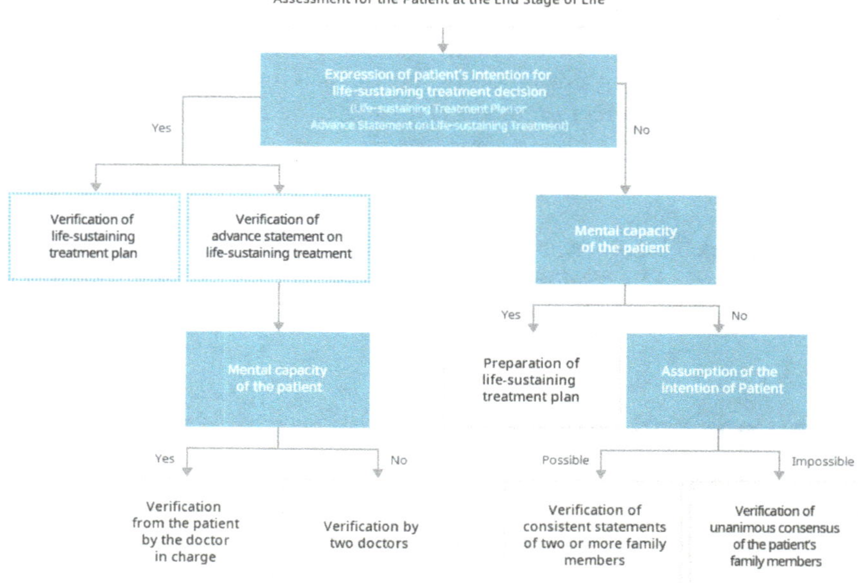

Figure 2.   Procedure diagram.[29]

Source: Figure from National Agency for Management of Life-sustaining Treatment.

To withhold or withdraw life-sustaining treatment (LST), three steps are required. First, two physicians (the primary physician and one medical specialist) must confirm that a patient is in the end-of-life process (Form 9). Second, a patient should express his or her intention in person with an advance statement regarding LST or Form 1 (Life-Sustaining Treatment Plan). When the patient lacks "decision-making capacity", family members take on this role and must provide two or more identical statements regarding patient's intent to withhold or withdraw LST (Form 11). When it is impossible to verify a patient's intent, "all" members of patient's family should show unanimous consensus on withholding or withdrawing LST (Form 12). The "patient's family" herein refers to all immediate family members who are 19 years of age or older. Finally, the primary physician should fill out an execution form (Form 13), clarifying which LSTs will be withheld or withdrawn, and take the necessary action.

According to the Life-Sustaining Treatment Decisions Act, all adults can complete an AD at national registry agencies whenever they want. Patients at the end stage of the disease and in their last days of life can complete a Life-Sustaining Treatment Plan with their doctors. If the patient is under the age of 19, the patient's parental authority completes the documents on behalf of the patient. When a patient does not have a decision-making capacity, an AD or Life-Sustaining Treatment Plan cannot be completed (Figure 2).[12,29] When the patient had a consistent intention for LST decisions, 2 or more legal immediate family members can complete a legal form to verify the patient's wishes. If the patient's intentions are unknown, all immediate family members should draw up a unanimous consensus regarding LST decisions.

Education/Training of Health Care Professionals and Non-health Care Professionals in ACP

Formal education is provided by the National Agency for Management of Life-Sustaining Treatment.[30] The subjects of education are divided into workers at registry agencies, medical teams at medical institutions, the general public, and general medical institutions. The contents of education differ according to the role of the target of education and are divided into a basic course and an advanced course.

Information Materials Used, Documentation and Digitalization of ACP Processes in the Health Care Sector and Beyond

All legal forms should be uploaded to the Life-Sustaining Treatment Information Processing System (https://intra.lst.go.kr/login/pkiLogin.do), managed by the National Agency for Management of Life-Sustaining Treatment. If it is not possible to fill out the documents, audio or video files can also be registered. Since the system is highly secure, only authorized institutions and individuals can access it. Once registered in this system, institutions registered at the National Agency for Management of Life-Sustaining Treatment can check the patient's LST decision status by linking it to the electronic medical records of each institution. In 2019, AD registration cards were issued for individuals who completed ADs, and in 2020, voice barcodes for the visually impaired were introduced.[31]

Examples of Institutional and Community Implementation

Since the implementation of the Life-Sustaining Treatment Decisions Act, as of March 7, 2023, there are 602 registry agencies that can prepare and register AD, and 375 medical institutions that can prepare documents and carry out procedures for LST decisions.[32] The number of AD registered so far is 1,655,507, and Life-Sustaining Treatment Plan is 107,902. Local health institutions such as public health centres, medical institutions, non-profit organizations, public institutions, and senior welfare centres can assist with AD preparation and registration, if they are designated by the Ministry of Health and Welfare. These institutions are commonly located in each region and are easily accessible. Medical institutions can carry out procedures for discontinuing life-sustaining treatment according to the law only when an institutional ethics committee is established. Before the law was enacted, the rate of patients making decisions about LST by self-determination, was very insignificant.[6,7] However, it gradually increased to 32.4% immediately after the implementation of the law and 40.9% in 2021.[31,33]

ACP Research and Quality Improvement

In order to firmly establish this law, the law stipulates that the Ministry of Health and Welfare should announce a comprehensive plan related to promotion direction, education, operation, manpower, institution, research, and investigation every 5 years.[12] About 100 million won of the budget allocated to the National Agency for Management of Life-Sustaining Treatment is allocated for research every year. After the law was enacted, the National Agency for Management of Life-Sustaining Treatment continuously conducted public surveys on LST decisions, research to improve policies, and research to establish publicity strategies. However, these researches focused on systems and laws, rather than ACP or counseling. Recently, papers on difficulties in communication related to LST decisions have been published,[34] and we think that policy support and research on counseling and communication in ACP are also needed. In addition to research activities, symposiums, press conferences, and various events related to LST decisions are held.[31]

Patient and Public Involvement (Patient Movement) in Research and Development of ACP

Right after the case of Grandma Kim, people from all walks of life suggested the need for social consensus and a system for LST decisions, and currently the National Committee for Hospice Care and Life-Sustaining Treatment under the Ministry of Health and Welfare is composed of 15 members from the medical, religious, ethical, legal, and patient groups. The committee is designed to reflect the opinions of patients or the public and deliberate on important matters related to hospice and LST (Figure 1).[23] In addition, the National Agency for Management of Life-Sustaining Treatment is conducting essay contests on LST-related experiences and publishing casebooks to promote publicity, and to introduce public participation.[31]

Addressing Diversity and Vulnerabilities (Cultural Social) Regarding ACP Access and Use

To raise awareness among the public and the medical society, the National Agency for Management of Life-Sustaining Treatment operates a website and conducts education and consultation. They use a Social Network Service (SNS) for promotion and also produced promotional videos that were submitted for national broadcasting. Recently, senior welfare centres were included in registry agencies, and an MOU was signed with Korea Blind Union for the activation of AD.[31]

Main Challenges and Barriers

Since the discussion and legislation on LST decisions were triggered by legal disputes, the medical society tended to focus on completing legal documents to avoid legal responsibility rather than performing an ideal ACP after the enforcement of the Life-Sustaining Treatment Decisions Act. Therefore, although concepts such as LST decision, communication, autonomy, AD, and Life-Sustaining Treatment Plan are all included in the broad concept of ACP, the term "ACP" itself is still unfamiliar to medical staff in South Korea. The ACP itself lacks publicity and education, and legal and systematic support is still insignificant. As in Taiwan, it may be a good solution to provide national support for ACP consultation clinics, so that patients, families, and medical teams can have ongoing discussions about ACP together at an early stage.[35]

Because the Life-Sustaining Treatment Plan can be completed only after the patient is determined to be at the end stage of the disease by two doctors, ACP counseling is often conducted too late.[20,24,36] In addition, patients cannot designate a proxy in advance, and many family members choose to make surrogate LST decisions after the patient loses their decision-making capacities. Thus, unlike the purpose of the law, patients' right to self-determination is not well protected yet. However, Korean society is changing quite rapidly in the direction of respecting individual autonomy, and the law was enacted in this atmosphere. Therefore, we believe that through more publicity and education, ACP in South Korea will move toward respecting individual autonomy as much as possible.

Finally, although ACP should be based on in-depth communication between patients and the medical team, spending time on ACP counseling is not rewarded, and doctors often cannot afford additional time to communicate due to heavy clinical loads.

Collaborations with Other Countries/Programs Regarding ACP

Officially, there is no international collaboration program at the national level yet, but there is physician-led international research collaboration. For example, an ACP Delphi research study in five East Asian countries (South Korea, Japan, Taiwan, Singapore, and Hong Kong) is in progress and is expected to be published soon.

Conclusion

Since the implementation of the Life-Sustaining Treatment Decisions Act in 2018 in South Korea, many people have started to think and decide about future medical treatment, but the ratio is still unsatisfactory. Additionally, LST discussions and decisions tend to focus on the legal process and completion of legal forms, while the concept of ACP is unfamiliar to many people and not widely accepted. There are still many areas to be improved in order to establish an optimal environment for ACP, and we believe that the current situation could be improved through systematic support, research, and education based on social consensus.

References

1. Korea S. (2023). Statistical Database Korea: Statistic Korea [population projections, number of deaths, total fertility rate, etc]. Available from: https://kosis.kr/index/index.do. Accessed March 14, 2023.

2. Shin D.W., Lee J.E., Cho B., *et al.* (2016). End-of-life communication in Korean older adults: With focus on advance care planning and advance directives. *Geriatr. Gerontol. Int.* **16**(4): 407–15. doi: 10.1111/ggi.12603 [published Online First: 20151013].

3. Yamaguchi T., Maeda I., Hatano Y., *et al.* (2021). Communication and behavior of palliative care physicians of patients with cancer near end of life in three East Asian countries. *J. Pain Symptom Manage.* **61**(2): 315–322 e1. doi: 10.1016/j.jpainsymman.2020.07.031 [published Online First: 20200807].

4. Court S. (2004). 2004.6.24 sentence 2002 Do 995 Korea: Korean Law Information Center, Ministry of Goverment legislation [Boramae hospital case Judgment]. Available from: https://www.law.go.kr/%ED%8C% 90%EB%A1%80/(2002%EB%8F%84995). Accessed March 14, 2023.

5. Court S. (2009). 2009.5.21 Sentence 2009 Da 17417 Korea: Korean Law Information Center, Ministry of Goverment legislation [Grandmother Kim's case judgment]. Available from: https://www.law.go.kr/%ED%8C%90% EB%A1%80/(2009%EB%8B%A417417). Accessed March 14, 2023.

6. Oh D.Y., Kim J.H., Kim D.W., *et al.* (2006). CPR or DNR? End-of-life decision in Korean cancer patients: A single center's experience. *Support. Care Cancer* **14**(2): 103–108. doi: 10.1007/s00520-005-0885-5 [published Online First: 20050908].

7. Kim D.Y., Lee K.E., Nam E.M., *et al.* (2007). Do-not-resuscitate orders for terminal patients with cancer in teaching hospitals of Korea. *J. Palliat. Med.* **10**(5): 1153–1158. doi: 10.1089/jpm.2006.0264.

8. Lee J.K., Keam B., An A.R., *et al.* (2013). Surrogate decision-making in Korean patients with advanced cancer: A longitudinal study. *Support Care Cancer* **21**(1): 183–190. doi: 10.1007/s00520-012-1509-5 [published Online First: 20120531].

9. Jho H.J., Nam E.J., Shin I.W., *et al.* (2020). Changes of end of life practices for cancer patients and their association with hospice palliative care referral over 2009–2014: A single institution study. *Cancer Res. Treat.* **52**(2): 419–425. doi: 10.4143/crt.2018.648 [published Online First: 20190903].

10. Shim B.Y., Hong S.I., Park J.M., *et al.* (2004). DNR (do-not-resuscitate) order for terminal cancer patients at hospice ward. *J. Hosp Palliat. Nurs.* **7**(2): 232–237.

11. Baek S.K., Chang H.J., Byun J.M., *et al.* (2017). The association between end-of-life care and the time interval between provision of a do-not-resuscitate consent and death in cancer patients in Korea. *Cancer Res. Treat.* **49**: 502–508.

12. Welfare MoHa. (2016). Act on Decisions on Life-Sustaining Treatment for Patients in Hospice and Palliative Care or at the End of Life (Act No.14013) Korea: The Korean Law Information Center. Available from: https://law. go.kr/LSW/lsInfoP.do?lsiSeq=180823&viewCls=engLsInfoR&urlMode=en gLsInfoR#0000. Accessed March 14, 2023.

13. Service HIRaA. (2023). History of Universal Health Coverage: Health Insurance Review and Assessment Service. Available from: https://www.hira.or.kr/dummy.do?pgmid=HIRAJ010000003000. Accessed March 14, 2023.

14. Kim K.W., Park B.H., Gu B.J., *et al.* (2022). The national hospice and palliative care registry in Korea. *Epidemiol. Health* **44**. doi: https://doi.org/10.4178/epih.e2022079 [published Online First: 21 September 2022]

15. National Hospice Center. (2022). 2021 National Hospice and Palliative Care Annual Report. National Hospice Center, National Cancer Center, Korea.

16. Mo H.N., Shin D.W., Woo J.H., *et al.* (2012). Is patient autonomy a critical determinant of quality of life in Korea? End-of-life decision making from the perspective of the patient. *Palliat. Med.* **26**(3): 222–231. doi: 10.1177/0269216311405089 [published Online First: 20110511].

17. Yun Y.H., Kwon Y.C., Lee M.K., *et al.* (2010). Experiences and attitudes of patients with terminal cancer and their family caregivers toward the disclosure of terminal illness. *J. Clin. Oncol.* **28**(11): 1950–1957. doi: 10.1200/JCO.2009.22.9658 [published Online First: 20100308].

18. Park H.Y., Kim Y.A., Sim J.A., *et al.* (2019). Attitudes of the general public, cancer patients, family caregivers, and physicians toward advance care planning: A nationwide survey before the enforcement of the life-sustaining treatment decision-making act. *J. Pain Symptom Manage.* **57**(4): 774–782. doi: 10.1016/j.jpainsymman.2018.12.332 [published Online First: 20181227].

19. Kim J.S., Yoo S.H., Choi W., *et al.* (2020). Implication of the life-sustaining treatment decisions act on end-of-life care for Korean terminal patients. *Cancer Res. Treat.* **52**(3): 917–924. doi: 10.4143/crt.2019.740 [published Online First: 20200323].

20. Kim D., Yoo S.H., Seo S., *et al.* (2022). Analysis of cancer patient decision-making and health service utilization after enforcement of the life-sustaining treatment decision-making act in Korea. *Cancer Res. Treat.* **54**(1):20–29. doi: 10.4143/crt.2021.131 [published Online First: 20210412].

21. Farber S.J., Egnew T.R., Herman-Bertsch J.L., *et al.* (2003). Issues in end-of-life care: Patient, caregiver, and clinician perceptions. *J. Palliat. Med.* **6**(1): 19–31. doi: 10.1089/109662103605510082.

22. Grunfeld E., Coyle D., Whelan T., *et al.* (2004). Family caregiver burden: Results of a longitudinal study of breast cancer patients and their principal caregivers. *CMAJ* **170**(12): 1795–1801. doi: 10.1503/cmaj.1031205.

23. Treatment NAfMoL-s. System overview Korea: Korea National Institute for Bioethics Policy [System]. Available from: https://www.lst.go.kr/eng/decn/management.do. Accessed March 14 2023.

24. Baek S.K., Kim H.J., Kwon J.H., *et al.* (2021). Preparation and practice of the necessary documents in hospital for the "act on decision of

life-sustaining treatment for patients at the end-of-life". *Cancer Res. Treat.* **53**(4): 926–934. doi: 10.4143/crt.2021.326 [published Online First: 20210602].

25. Prevention CfDCa. (2012). CDC Healthy Aging Program. Advance care planning: Ensuring your wishes are known and honored if you are unable to speak for yourself. In: Prevention CfDCa, USA.

26. National Medical Ethics Committee. (2010). Guide for healthcare professionals on the ethical handling of communication in advance care planning.

27. National Health Service. (2013). More care, less pathway: A review of the liverpool care pathway. London: GOV.UK.

28. Lee S.M., Kim S.J., Choi Y.S., *et al.* (2018). Consensus guidelines for the definition of the end stage of disease and last days of life and criteria for medical judgment. *J. Korean Med. Assoc.* **61**(8): 509–521. doi: https://doi.org/10.5124/jkma.2018.61.8.509.

29. Treatment NAfMoL-s. (2023). Procedure diagram Korea: Korea National Institute for Bioethics Policy; [Available from: https://www.lst.go.kr/eng/half/procedure.do. Accessed March 14, 2023.

30. Treatment NAfMoL-s. Education Portal for Life-sustaining treatment decision system Korea: Korea National Institute for Bioethics Policy [Education Portal online site]. Available from: https://www.lst.go.kr/edu/. Accessed March 14, 2023.

31. Treatment NAfMoL-s. (2022). 2021 Yearbook of life-sustaining treatment decision system. National Agency for Management of Life-sustaining Treatment, Korea.

32. Treatment NAfMoL-s. (2023). Homepage of National Agency for Management of Life-sustaining Treatment Korea: Korea National Institute for Bioethics Policy; [Registration number of AD and PCLST]. Available from: https://www.lst.go.kr/main/main.do. Accessed March 14, 2023.

33. Park S.Y., Lee B., Seon J.Y., *et al.* (2021). A national study of life-sustaining treatments in South Korea: What factors affect decision-making? *Cancer Res. Treat.* **53**(2): 593–600. doi: 10.4143/crt.2020.803 [published Online First: 20201121].

34. Yoo S.H., Choi W., Kim Y., *et al.* (2021). Difficulties doctors experience during life-sustaining treatment discussion after enactment of the life-sustaining treatment decisions act: A cross-sectional study. *Cancer Res. Treat.* **53**(2): 584–592. doi: 10.4143/crt.2020.735 [published Online First: 20201119].

35. Cheng S.Y., Lin C.P., Chan H.Y., *et al.* (2020). Advance care planning in Asian culture. *Jpn. J. Clin. Oncol.* **50**(9): 976–989. doi: 10.1093/jjco/hyaa131.

36. Kim M. (2018). The problems and the improvement plan of the hospice/palliative care and dying patient's decisions on life-sustaining treatment act. *Korean J. Hosp. Palliat. Care* **21**(1): 1–8. doi: https://doi.org/10.14475/kjhpc.2018.21.1.1.

Chapter 20

Advance Care Planning in Singapore: The Genesis and Evolution of a National Programme*

Raymond Ng[†,‡], Koh Lip Hoe[‡,§], Jane Lim[¶],
and Liao Weifen[¶]

[†]*Palliative and Supportive Care, Woodlands Health, Singapore*
[‡]*National Advance Care Planning Steering Committee, Singapore*
[§]*Palliative Care Service, Changi General Hospital, Singapore*
[¶]*Agency for Integrated Care, Singapore*

Introduction

Singapore is an island country in Southeast Asia with a population of approximately 5.6 million people. It has an efficient healthcare system with one of the highest life expectancies in the world at 83.5 years.[1] Singapore's healthcare system works to ensure that quality and affordable medical services are available for all through a mixed financing system known as the 3Ms; Medishield Life, a universal basic health care insurance, Medisave, a national medical savings scheme and Medifund, the government's safety net for needy Singaporeans.

---

*Re-published with permission from special issue of ZEFQ journal; "Advance Care Planning around the World: Evidence and Experiences, Programmes and Perspectives".

The Need for an ACP Programme

Singapore's population is also aging rapidly. It is estimated that by 2030, one in four will be aged over 65 years old.[2] The number of elderly with more complex care needs as well as chronic sick living in longer years of disability will likewise rise. Over the decades, advance care planning (ACP) has become especially important. Technological and medical advances prolong life expectancies but may sometimes result in poor quality of life as well as missed opportunities to engage patients in discussions to understand what really matters to them. Such person-centred conversations with individuals typically happen late in a patient's illness trajectory or not at all. In a retrospective chart review of 683 adult patients who passed away in a tertiary hospital in Singapore in 2007, orders to limit life-sustaining therapies as well as discussions with patients on end-of-life decisions were infrequent and excessive burdensome interventions at the end-of-life were observed. Multiple factors conspire in this state of affairs including low awareness of ACP,[3] cultural taboo in talking about potential serious illness scenarios and end-of-life matters, a lack of systematic training of healthcare professionals as well as the lack of a system and culture of preemptive conversations and documentation.[4]

The Advance Medical Directive and Mental Capacity Acts

The earliest and only known statute that directly governs advance decision-making process in healthcare in Singapore is the Advance Medical Directive or AMD. Enacted in 1996, the AMD is a legal document that an individual signs in advance, to inform treating doctors that one does not want extraordinary life-sustaining treatment to prolong one's life in the event one is terminally ill and unconscious.[5] There has been poor uptake of the AMD by the public and up till 2015, less than 25,000 people signed the AMD.[6]

The AMD applies only to a very narrowly defined scenario when one is terminally ill and death is imminent and when life-sustaining measures serve to only prolong the dying process. It does not adequately address the broader spectrum of ACP and goals of care conversations as well as the values and personhood of individuals that underlie these discussions.

Unlike ACP and goals of care conversations that explore individuals' goals, preferences, values and personhood, the AMD does not adequately address the broader spectrum of scenarios when one loses mental capacity nor does it enhance the physician-patient relationship which is paramount in healthcare decision making.

The Mental Capacity Act (MCA) was passed in 2008 allowing individuals (called "donors") to plan ahead and appoint a "donee" in a Lasting Power of Attorney (LPA) to make financial and healthcare-related decisions for them if they lose mental capacity. This Act precludes the donee from making decisions regarding potentially life-sustaining treatment on behalf of the donor. It also stipulates that when making best interests decisions for an individual, one must consider, so far as is reasonably ascertainable, the person's past and present wishes and feelings (including any relevant written statement made by the person when the person had capacity) as well as the beliefs and values that would likely influence his/her decision if the person had capacity.

The provision of MCA highlighted the importance of respecting the autonomous right of persons with capacity and protecting the welfare of those who have lost mental capacity. Advance care planning is an important enabler in helping care teams make best interests decisions for patients who have lost mental capacity. While making best-interest decisions may be viewed as paternalistic in some settings in the world, Singapore's system of substitute decision-making is similar to the system in the United Kingdom, in which the best-interests approach incorporates having regard to the person's wishes as far as possible.

However, Singapore lacked a national programme and roadmap in ACP implementation.

Genesis of the Living Matters Programme

In 2009, on the invitation of the National Healthcare Group in Singapore, the faculty of Respecting Choices (RC) from Gunderson Health System, USA, came to Singapore to train healthcare professionals in RC's paradigm of ACP. RC taught that ACP is a staged conversation, suitable for individuals in any state of health or illness. A healthy individual can be engaged regarding his/her personhood as well as to articulate values that would influence future healthcare decisions, nominate a healthcare spokesperson, and to articulate what he/she would have wanted in the unfortunate event of a sudden, catastrophic and permanent neurological injury. This is known as General ACP. (First Steps in RC's current model) An individual with a chronic progressive illness such as heart, lung or renal disease may also be engaged regarding scenarios related to his/her underlying disease and his/her choices should these complications take place. This is known as Disease Specific ACP in Singapore. (Next Steps in RC's current model) Finally, an individual with an advanced serious illness and advanced frailty may be engaged regarding more specific treatment choices related to resuscitation, type of medical care as well as preferred places of care and death. This is known as Preferred Plan of Care in Singapore. (Advanced Steps in RC's current model) All such discussions are always person-centred in approach, contextualized, step-wise, and built upon elicitation and shared understanding of what matters to each individual.

Subsequently, small pilot projects were attempted by various hospitals in disciplines such as Cardiology, Respiratory Medicine, Geriatric Medicine and Neurology. However, these fledgling efforts were hindered by the lack of clinician time to facilitate ACP as well as the perspective that ACP is secondary to clinical treatment. The greatest pushback was from clinicians, who were concerned about what patients and caregivers would think should such topics be raised or were generally apathetic. Though a developed country with a multi-cultural society, Singapore's culture is largely conservative and traditional taboos exist. Over the last decade or so, attitudes amongst healthcare providers started to change as policies and programmes were implemented at a national level.

In 2010, the Ministry of Health in Singapore commissioned the Lien Centre for Palliative Care to formulate a National Strategy for Palliative Care that delineated ten key goals for palliative care in Singapore, including that all patients at the end of life have access to ACP.

In 2011, the Ministry of Health of Health appointed the Agency for Integrated Care (AIC) to helm the national ACP programme. The programme was aptly named "Living Matters", drawing focus to ACP as conversations about what living well means and not about death and dying.

Each public hospital is funded for efforts in ACP and to employ a small team of full-time ACP facilitators supported by 1–2 administrators. A national steering committee on advance care planning was concurrently set up, to advise on policies and implementation plans on ACP as well as engage healthcare partners and foster an ecosystem of ACP stakeholders in Singapore. The steering committee comprised of senior clinicians in geriatric, internal, family and palliative medicine as well as senior social workers, a lawyer and ethicists. AIC served as the programme manager; overseeing the alignment of ACP forms and certification of ACP facilitators. Various sub-committees were set up to assist the ACP steering committee in ACP work. These include the training and curriculum sub-committee, the ACP research and development sub-committee, the children and young persons sub-committee and the nursing home sub-committee. RC taught that the four pillars of any successful ACP programme are (1) engagement of the community, (2) training in ACP facilitation, (3) building a system to capture and honour preferences and (4) implementing audit checks, tracking and quality improvement measures.

Engagement of Healthcare Professionals and the Community

Engagement proved to be a key step in winning hearts and minds in "ACP naïve" units and organisations. Key leaders and change-makers were engaged with regards to the benefits of ACP in fostering person centred care, to understand ground constraints and to tailor interventions that may enhance adoption of ACP within the unit. Hospitals organised forums to educate about ACP, including talks by ethicists and lawyers to clear misconceptions and explain nuances of the ethical implementation of ACP. Healthcare professionals were encouraged to embrace ACP through fun and games such as conversation cards, photo competition on what living well means and "death cafes". In some departments, passionate individuals were identified as clinical champions to oversee ACP efforts in the units. The engagement efforts reached a tipping point in some units where ACP became a core activity that is viewed as part of routine patient care. Engagement efforts also began in the heartlands of the community. Various advocacy groups such as the Singapore Hospice Council and ACP teams in hospitals held outreach activities to educate the public about the importance of ACP as part of future care or life planning. Various other organisations partnered with physicians in some of these engagements. They include the Law Society of Singapore which featured ACP together with legal literacy webinars about wills and estate planning, the National Library of Singapore which launched outreach within libraries and over Zoom webinars as well as the Artswok collaborative which sought to harness the power of arts to create more "die-logues". The momentum built up by various organisations has culminated in consensus to organize an

ACP Week every year in May, in Singapore. The media was also engaged and ACP was featured in mainstream print media, social media, YouTube videos, radio talk shows, news channels and television talk shows.

Training Healthcare Professionals

Training of healthcare professionals in ACP facilitation and advocacy has picked up over the years. In Singapore, a nationally standardized training curriculum and certification process is implemented in regular workshops run by ACP trainers in each public hospital. Healthcare professionals deemed to be most likely to facilitate ACP in their primary roles volunteer for the courses or are nominated by their departments. These may be a mix of physicians, nurses, medical social workers and other vocations such as community workers. As of today, more than 5000 ACP facilitators are trained in various healthcare settings from the community to the hospitals. However, only approximately 50–60% of those trained go on to facilitate one ACP. It was realized that training alone is insufficient to sustain the implementation effort and some organisations have put in place mentoring processes for newly trained facilitators to build confidence and be shown the ropes. Nevertheless, each organization may have some "super-facilitators", who were either full-time ACP facilitators or ardent advocates who enjoy ACP work and see ACP facilitation as part of routine patient care.

Building an "ACP System"

Early on in the national ACP programme, efforts were made to contextualize and align discussion worksheets and forms for General ACP, Disease Specific ACP and Preferred Plan of Care in Singapore, so that they are standardized and recognizable across all healthcare settings. As part of building the "ACP infrastructure", ACP work processes were drawn up; such as how to identify suitable patients for the appropriate type of ACP as well as how to sign and pass copies of the forms to patients and their caregivers. An ACP information technology system was built and refined over the years to capture ACP information and to transmit the latest advance care plans to the National Electronic Health Record (NEHR) system. ACP alerts were built into native electronic medical systems of different healthcare systems which alert frontline clinicians to the existence of ACP in NEHR, which then can be viewed by 1 or 2 clicks in the system.

Quality Improvement and Audit

The fourth pillar of ACP implementation taught by RC was quality improvement, tracking and audit. These were implemented at both the grassroots level as well as by AIC, the manager of the national ACP programme. Number of advance care plans lodged in the national ACP IT system are routinely tracked. While it is known that simply tracking the numbers of ACPs is not ideal, there is no international gold standard or set of consensus criteria to evaluate an ACP programme, including the quality of conversations held and quality of care delivered. Currently, there are ongoing engagement efforts by AIC and the Ministry of Health with various stakeholders regarding consensus indicators to evaluate ACP programmes. While research in ACP will be relevant in this fourth pillar, it is not routinely funded on a continual basis as part of the national ACP programme. Rather, research bodies in Singapore are tasked to evaluate the national ACP programme in the last two phases of funding of ACP, namely in ACP 1.0 and ACP 2.0. Various other independent researchers have contributed research in ACP that add to current knowledge of ACP in Singapore.

Challenges Remain in Implementing ACP

Since 2009 when Respecting Choices visited, ACP has become part of the vernacular in many medical units in Singapore. More than 30,000 advance care plans have been lodged in the national ACP IT system since the inception of the system almost 10 years ago.

However, challenges persist. These include misconceptions that conflate ACP with palliative care, an overt focus by some clinicians on ACP forms as utilitarian tools for CPR decisions and a perceived lack of time by clinicians for ACP facilitation. There was also wide variation in the implementation of ACP between organisations, dissonance with family's expectations as well as gaps in public awareness, physician engagement and in the ACP training framework.

ACP is commonly viewed by clinicians as secondary to other more pressing clinical tasks and the implementation of ACP is not uniform across all levels of the healthcare system and in all departments. As ACP first started from within hospitals and is mostly initiated with patients with advanced illness, it is an upstream effort to bring ACP conversations to outpatient and general practice clinics. Disease-specific and General ACP types of conversations are less frequently practised as compared to Preferred Plans of Care conversations. Primary care doctors in Singapore do not routinely facilitate ACP with their patients and people are generally apathetic towards ACP when healthier.

Research in ACP and Implementation Science

Local research has also highlighted that the end-of-life preferences of patients with heart failure are not stable suggesting that ACP documents should be regularly re-evaluated. Systematic reviews of the international literature on outcomes in ACP showed mixed results and low quality of available evidence. A recent systematic review showed more consistent evidence of the efficacy of ACP in the improvement of proximal patient outcomes such as decisional conflict as compared with distal outcomes such as goal concordant care.[7] This research highlights the complex and multi-dimensional nature of any ACP programme implementation. It is not a one size fits all approach and will need to be contextualised to each setting.

The Geriatric Education and Research Institute (GERI) has recently partnered with AIC and other stakeholders in forming an ACP Quality Implementation workgroup.

This workgroup will use the knowledge-to-action framework in implementation science to co-create a consensus framework on quality ACP implementation in Singapore, including definitions and scope of ACP in Singapore, best practice recommendations and consensus quality indicators.

Healthier SG and Future Opportunities in ACP

Singapore is currently undergoing a period of healthcare reform known as Healthier SG (SG is a common short form for Singapore). Taking a life course approach, it aims to promote wellbeing, improve physical and mental health outcomes as well as reduce inequalities across the entire population. Core components of this government-led programme include the mobilization of Singapore's network of family physicians, community partnerships to support better health as well as enhancements of policy, training and financial structures supporting the scheme. A key step in this approach is to encourage each resident to enrol with one family physician and for physicians to proactively discuss care plans with patients. ACP will eventually form an integral part of such care plans. This announcement augurs well for the ACP movement in Singapore. The Minister of Health has openly spoken about the need "to normalize death and dying as a topic".[8]

Plans are underway to roll out a public campaign to encourage residents about future care planning, including nominating their lasting power of attorney. There are also plans for ACP to come on board the digital revolution in Singapore. The My Legacy portal serves to make accessible information and tools related to the end of life, including an ability for the layperson to plan, store and share one's legal, healthcare and estate matters safely with people whom he/she trusts in a digital vault.[9]

Apart from all these efforts at raising awareness and self-ownership of the ACP process, there are also endeavours at encouraging ACP conversations as an iterative process of engagement between physicians and patients. To ensure ACP is uniformly accessible in various populations, special workgroups have been set up to promote ACP in children and young persons with serious illnesses as well as within the long-term care sector. Renewed efforts are underway to engage clinicians from cardiology, respiratory medicine, geriatric medicine, renal medicine, dementia care and primary care to both customize and align ACP forms that would best suit the various settings and disciplines.

Conclusion

Being a globally connected city, Singapore is at the cusp of change on many fronts, including in ACP. In May 2023, Singapore hosted the 8th international conference in advance care planning, where the latest trends, research and innovations in ACP and person-centred care were shared.

There is still much that is to be done in fostering better quality ACP in Singapore and it is hoped that every effort will help us to better answer the question "What matters to you?" as well as to promote the dignity of every individual when he/she is most vulnerable.

References

1. www.singstat.gov.sg. Accessed 11/04/2023.
2. https://www.channelnewsasia.com/commentary/singapore-ageing-population-grow-old-care-burden-3321546. Accessed 11/04/2023.
3. Ng Q.X., Kuah, T., Loo, G., *et al.* (2017). Awareness and attitudes of community-dwelling individuals in Singapore towards participating in advance care planning. *Ann. Acad. Med. Singap.* **46**(3): 84–90. March 2017. https://doi.org/10.47102/annals-acadmedsg.V46N3p84.
4. Phua J., Kee A., Tan A., *et al.* (2011). End-of-life care in the general wards of a Singaporean hospital: An Asian perspective. *J. Palliat. Med.* **14**(12): 1296–1301. December 2011. https://doi:10.1089/jpm.2011.0215.
5. https://www.moh.gov.sg/policies-and-legislation/advance-medical-directive. Accessed 11/04/2023.
6. https://www.straitstimes.com/opinion/lets-talk-about-advance-care-planning-to-die-with-dignity. Accessed 11/04/2023.
7. Maholtra C., Shafiq M., and Batcagan-Abueg A. P. M. (2022). What is the evidence for efficacy of advance care planning in improving patient outcomes? A systematic review of randomized controlled trials. *BMJ Open* **12**: e060201. doi:10.1136/bmjopen-2021-060201.
8. https://www.straitstimes.com/singapore/health/palliative-care-services-to-be-boosted-topic-of-death-needs-open-discussion-ong-ye. Accessed 11/04/2023.
9. www.mylegacy.life.gov.sg. Accessed 11/04/2023.

Chapter 21

Advance Care Planning in Japan*

Jun Miyashita[†] and Megumi Kishino[‡]

*†Department of General Medicine, Shirakawa Satellite for Teaching and
Research, Fukushima Medical University, Fukushima, Japan*
‡Cicely Saunders Institute, King's College London, London, UK

Introduction

Japan has one of the most rapidly aging societies in the world. In terms of the speed of aging, defined as the doubling time of the proportion of the aged population from 7% to 14%, East Asian countries, including Japan, are aging faster than the United States and European countries. Therefore, Japan is expected to retain its status as having the highest proportion of the aged population over the next 30 years.[1] The year 2025 will represent a milestone in Japan because the so-called baby-boomer generation will reach the age of 75 years and over, making the proportion of the aged population exceed 30% for the first time in the world. As a result, in Japan, 1.5 million deaths annually are expected by 2025.[2] How to handle the mounting financial and social burdens of end-of-life care for older adults has been of great concern in Japan.[3] The Japanese government has promoted a shift from "family care" to the "socialization of care," which means that social security benefits will cover the labor and costs of care

---

*Re-published with permission from special issue of ZEFQ journal; "Advance Care Planning around the World: Evidence and Experiences, Programmes and Perspectives".

that have traditionally been left to the family, and further to "care in the community," which means adapting socialization of care not only to long-term care but to the care of all residents in the community. For this purpose, the Japanese government has been developing a community-based integrated care system that aims to enable older adults to continue living in their community by securing comprehensive medical care, long-term care, care prevention, and support for housing and independence in daily life.[4] Needless to say, older adults' wishes regarding medical treatment and care should be respected. Healthcare providers involved in care for older adults should be engaged as a team in advance care planning (ACP) to protect their dignity.[5] Therefore, promoting ACP in the super-aged society of Japan is essential to ensure an effective community-based integrated care system and support older adults in continuing to live in the community until the end of life. In considering how to promote ACP in Japan, the cultural and historical backgrounds of medical decision-making need to be taken into account. Therefore, in this paper, we first describe the environment and historical backgrounds surrounding ACP in Japan, and based on the results, introduce research and education programs regarding its implementation.

Cultural and Historical Backgrounds Surrounding ACP in Japan

Japan has a long tradition of family-centred decision-making.[6] Illness has long been considered a family matter instead of an individual one. Japanese family-centred decision-making has been based on a tradition of high collectivism and a high-context culture, in which people are deeply involved in each other's lives, and most information exchange depends on situations and internalized personal experiences.[7] The Japanese agree tacitly based on implicit cues rather than explicit verbal communication.[6] This family-centred decision-making based on high collectivism and a high-context culture greatly influences the care of older adults by their family members. The cultural values at the core of family caregiving include strong family ties and a sense of empathy.[8] This sense of empathy, *omoiyari*, is defined as the ability and willingness to feel what others are feeling and is an important value in Japanese culture.[9] Through this, Japanese people try to infer what their family potentially wants.[10] In this context, there has often been discordance between the wants of Japanese older adults at the end of life, and what they felt compelled to do for their family members.[11] This discordance has been considered important in the process of Japanese older adults' discussions about ACP.

It is also true that there have been significant changes in Japanese perceptions of end-of-life care over the past 30 years within the context of its family-centred decision-making culture. Until the 1990s, it was considered taboo to talk about death and end of life. At that time, most patients with cancer were not informed of their diagnosis. The proportion of patients with cancer who knew their diagnosis before death was about 25%,[12] and the proportion of physicians who informed patients with cancer of their disease was only about 13%.[13] However, as the aged population in Japan has increased rapidly, Japanese people have become increasingly interested in expressing and enhancing their autonomy in medical decisions made at the end of life.[14,15] In this social context, in 2002, the Supreme Court of Japan changed its view on disease notification from "Disease notification is within the physician's discretion" to "Considering disease notification is the physicians' duty". In addition, some cases were seen in which physicians who were suspected of murder after withdrawing patients' life-sustaining treatments were referred to the Public Prosecutor's Office.[16] These cases started to raise public opinion about end-of-life care. In 2007, triggered by a case involving the removal of a ventilator at Imizu Municipal Hospital in Imizu City, guidelines regarding the decision-making process for end-of-life medical treatment and care were formulated for the first time.[16] Subsequently, many organizations and academic societies developed guidelines about end-of-life care. By 2016, the proportion of patients with cancer who knew their diagnosis exceeded over 95%.[17] The prevalence of ACP discussions doubled from about 20% in 2006[18] to about 40% in 2017.[19] However, as of March 2023, Japan has yet to establish either mandatory advance directives or legislation supporting ACP. In 2018, the Japanese government revised the guidelines regarding the decision-making process for end-of-life medical treatment and care.[20] In these 2018 guidelines, the general direction of the ACP process in Japan was set forth for the first time.

Research on ACP in Japan

Recently, the momentum for widespread ACP discussions in Japan has been building. At the same time, evidence of ACP in Japan has been accumulating. Previous qualitative and quantitative studies have revealed that experience as a family caregiver could be a catalyst for ACP discussions in Japan.[21,22] This experience acts as a trigger for positive attitudes toward ACP discussions. Moreover, Japanese adults with an equal relationship with a spouse or relative in the same generation tend to discuss ACP among themselves.[21,23] As described above, there has often been discordance between the wants of Japanese older adults at the end of life and what they feel compelled to do for their family members. In this context, Japanese older adults have come to understand that failing to make their own future healthcare decisions made would burden their children. However, at the same time, they are afraid that having strong opinions on what they want at the end of life could also burden their children. Therefore, ACP discussions between Japanese older adults and their spouses and relatives in the same generation are important for reaching a consensus about end-of-life treatment and care that their children can use as a reference to make final decisions without experiencing the sense of an emotional burden.[21] Another issue is that Japanese healthcare providers, especially physicians, tend to be unaware of patients' desires for more information about end-of-life care before they become incapacitated. Previous studies have pointed out discordance between physicians' and patients' preferred timing of initial ACP.[24,25] More than 70% of patients in Japan are willing to begin ACP discussions while they are still healthy, and 90% before being incapacitated.[24] However, only 50% of physicians in Japan are willing to begin ACP discussions while their patients are still healthy, and more than half tend to postpone such discussions until their patients' imminent end of life.[25] Therefore, to promote timely ACP discussions, it is essential to bridge this perception gap between physicians and patients.

Japan's Advance Care Planning

In 2022, a culturally adapted consensus definition and action guideline, "Japan's Advance Care Planning," was developed to facilitate the implementation of ACP in the context of Japanese society.[26] This definition and action guideline was based on previous evidence and expert opinions and developed using a multidisciplinary modified Delphi method. In seven rounds, 56 experts evaluated sentences delineating the definition, scope, subjects, and action guidelines for ACP in Japan. As a result, the 29-item set reached the target consensus level. ACP was defined as "an individual's thinking about and discussing with their family and other people close to them, with the support as necessary of health-care providers who have established a trusting relationship with them, preparations for the future, including the way of life and medical treatment and care that they wish to have in the future." One of the significant features of this definition and action guideline is that it incorporates the concept of *relational autonomy*. ACP based on an individualistic interpretation of autonomy emphasizing self-determination may be difficult to implement in Japan because of its family-centred decision-making and high-context culture. From the viewpoint of relational autonomy, social relationships can both promote and compromise autonomy. Therefore, this definition emphasizes the support and enhancement of autonomous decision-making of people reluctant to express their wishes to their family members because of the burden it would impose (Figures 1–4).

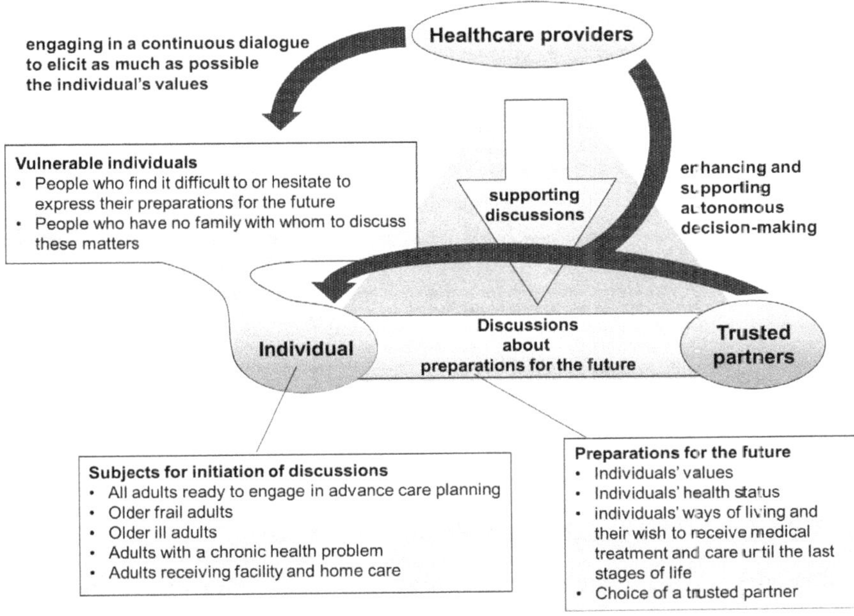

Figure 1.   Conceptual framework of Japan's advance care planning.

Source: Reprinted from Miyashita *et al.* (2022) with permission from Elsevier.

1. Definition

Brief definition. Advance care planning is an individual's thinking and discussing with his or her family and other people close to them[(1)] with the support as necessary of healthcare providers[(2)] who have established a trusting relationship with the individual concerning preparations for the future: his or her current state of health and future way of life and medical treatment and care that the individual wishes to receive in the future.

Consideration for vulnerable individuals. In particular, for people who are finding it increasingly difficult or who hesitate to express in words their preparations for the future, or who have no family or other parties with whom to discuss these matters, healthcare providers should engage in a continuous dialogue to elicit as much as possible the individual's values and provide suitable support.

Purpose of advance care planning. When individuals find it difficult to make decisions by themselves, their family and the healthcare providers engage in discussions based on statements the individual has made in the past regarding preparations for the future, with the aim of respecting the individual's values and providing medical treatment and care that reflects the individual's intentions.

[(1)]Hereinafter "the family"; [(2)]The medical, nursing, and welfare services staff in charge of the individual's medical treatment and care.

2. Scope: "preparations for the future"

To prepare for the future means the following things:

> ***Individuals' values.*** It means for individuals to imagine, looking back on their life thus far, what kind of person they would like to be and what kind of life they would like to lead henceforth. It means for them to consider, in order to achieve these aspirations, what their preoccupations and anxieties are and what they regard as lastingly important.
>
> ***Individuals' health status.*** It means to be aware of and accept one's present and expected future state of health and one's prospects in regard to illness, injury, and ensuing disabilities.
>
> ***Individuals' ways of living and their wish to receive medical treatment and care until the last stages of life.*** It means imagining where, with whom, and how one wishes to live in the last stages of life. It means thinking about what types of medical treatment and care one wishes to have and what types one wishes not to have, in order to realize, to the greatest possible degree until the last moments of one's life, the kind of life one wants to lead — including the conditions under which one wishes or not to receive those medical treatments and care.
>
> ***Choice of a trusted partner.*** It means to take into consideration the choice of a trusted partner[(3)] who, when it has become too difficult to decide one's intention(s) oneself, will act on one's behalf to ensure that one's intention(s) will be reflected in discussions with healthcare providers. One's chosen trusted partners will attempt to represent one's intentions, and only when one's intentions are unclear will they make inferences and discuss one's intentions with healthcare providers to make medical treatment and care choices based on one's values.

[(3)]Trusted partners are normally chosen from among family members. Here the term "trusted partner" is used, although elsewhere other terms such as "spokesperson" and "substitute decision maker" are used by specialists or organizations.

3. Subjects

All adults ready to engage in advace care planning. Any adult who is ready and willing to undergo advance care planning is the subject of advance care planning.

In particular, advance care planning is recommended for people with existing or potential physical or mental status changes or changes in their living environment, as in the following cases:

> ***Older frail adults.*** Anyone of advanced age who feels the effects of aging more markedly than they did before (for example, if they feel that they are losing weight, getting tired more easily, becoming weaker, walking more slowly, or becoming less active);
>
> ***Older ill adults.*** Anyone of advanced age who goes regularly to see a doctor or who is under treatment in a hospital for an illness or injury;
>
> ***Adults with a chronic health problem.*** Anyone with a physical, intellectual, or psychiatric disability as a result of illness or injury who may suffer deterioration in their physical functions or capacity to make decisions with worsening of their disability;
>
> ***Adults receiving facility and home care.*** Anyone who will be admitted to a nursing care facility or receive home medical or nursing care or who is already receiving such services.

Consideration for individuals reluctant to discuss advance care planning. For people who are reluctant to discuss advance care planning, the healthcare providers need first to build a trusting relationship and, on that basis, to probe the reasons for their reluctance, and then to sit down to talk with them about when is the most appropriate time to begin discussions and what to discuss.

Figure 2.   Definition, scope, and subjects of Japan's advance care planning (Items 1–3).

Source: Reprinted from Miyashita *et al.* (2022) with permission from Elsevier.

Education Programs for ACP in Japan

In this context of Japanese society, several programs for promoting ACP in Japan have been developed and implemented. In March 2014, the Ministry of Health, Labour and Welfare of Japan (MHLW) issued an opinion survey report on end-of-life medical treatment and care.[14] It stated the

4. Preparations for the future: developing ideas
It is recommended that individuals make preparations for the future upon accepting the state of their health and thinking about how they would like to live henceforth and until the last stages of their life, and about the medical treatment and care they desire. People who have experience caregiving for family members or keeping company with a dying family member until the end, by recalling this experience and preemptively imagining themselves in the same position, hold the key to preparations for their own future.

5. Discussing preparations with others: sharing ideas
It is recommended that individuals decide to discuss their preparations for the future with their family. People who have experienced family caregiving or being with a dying family member until the end will share their thoughts with others based on their direct experience. However, when individuals are conscious of the need to communicate these things but fail to find someone with whom to talk, it is recommended that they seek advice about with whom and how to discuss preparations for the future from their primary-care physician or the nursing and welfare facility staff they regularly see

6. Choosing trusted partners
How to choose a trusted partner. To prepare for a time when it will become too difficult for individuals to make decisions, they are advised to choose in advance from among their family a trusted partner with whom they have discussed these matters and who will speak on their behalf with the healthcare providers. If they wish to delegate to the trusted partner the power to make decisions on their behalf, it is recommended that they communicate this intention to the trusted partner in advance.
Roles of a trusted partner when intentions cannot be realized. It sometimes turns out to be too difficult actually to put into practice previously established preparations for the future. This happens, for example, when one can no longer live at home as one hoped to do. In this case, healthcare providers and one's trusted partners try to offer the second-best treatment and care that respects the individual's wishes to the maximum feasible degree. Individuals and their trusted partners ought to discuss beforehand the possibility of this occurrence.

7. Healthcare providers' support for others' preparations
It is recommended that healthcare providers harness their respective areas of expertise and their ties with each other to comprehend from different standpoints the individual's personal values. On this basis healthcare providers will assist in preparations for the future both by providing information about available medical treatments and care and by helping individuals to consider how to live in the future and to imagine concretely the final stages of their life.

8. Healthcare providers' support for discussions
Supporting discussions with individuals. It is recommended that healthcare providers establish a trusting relationship with individuals and create opportunities for discussions with those individuals and their family about preparing for the future. They will help the family to understand well and accept the individual's preparations for the future.
Supporting discussions with solitary individuals. In the case of individuals who have no family with whom to discuss preparations for the future, if the individual so desires, trusted healthcare providers will serve as interlocutors in discussions regarding preparations for the future.
Supporting discussions with hesitant individuals. In the case of individuals who hesitate to put their preparations for the future into words, the family and the healthcare providers will try to grasp through persistent dialogue with the individual his or her reasons for hesitation and, with the individual's consent, help them to express their feelings and personal values in words.

Figure 3.   Action guidelines regarding Japan's advance care planning (Items 4–8).

Source: Reprinted from Miyashita *et al.* (2022) with permission from Elsevier.

importance of (1) securing opportunities for the general public to consider end-of-life medical treatment and care, (2) developing training programs to support decision-making in accordance with guidelines on end-of-life medical treatment and care, and (3) the need to educate health-care providers. In response, in 2016, after a 2-year pilot phase, an education program for health-care providers regarding decision-making support for end-of-life treatment and care and ACP discussions, titled "Education For Implementing End-of-Life Discussion (E-FIELD)," was launched.[27] In addition to the program, leaflets and websites were created and released to raise awareness of ACP among the general public, and these have been used by local authorities and institutions throughout Japan. The program and materials developed are described as follows.

9. Continuity of discussions and flexible case-by-case response
Discussing repeatedly. The outcome of any discussion is the individual's will at that point in time; it may change. It is recommended that all parties (i.e., individuals, their family, and healthcare providers) have repeated discussions at every opportunity and revise their joint understanding of what has been confirmed in accordance with changes in the individual's feelings and thoughts.
Discussing more details with end-of-life approaching. With changes in disease status or as the end of the individual's life approaches and medical treatment and care become necessary, all parties will discuss increasingly specifically, if the individual so desires, the details of medical treatment and care.
Response when individuals' cognitive capacity is declining. Should the individual's condition worsen suddenly and cognitive capacity markedly decline, the healthcare providers and the individual's trusted partners will make efforts to infer the individual's will at that moment based on the tenor of previous discussions.

10. Response to a sudden emergency in the absence of prior discussion
There are cases when individuals who are suddenly found to be in critical condition or to have markedly impaired cognitive function before discussions about preparations for the future take place. It is recommended that healthcare providers make efforts together with the family, or in some cases with neighbors or municipal staff providing livelihood support, to provide medical treatment and care that respects those individuals' personal values by extrapolating those values from their way of life and their previous conversations.
Note: Though the contents of this section 10 are not included in the definition of Japan's advance care planning, they are listed here among the action guidelines because such situations are often faced in decision making in the medical and nursing care setting.

11. Record-keeping
General approach to record-keeping. It is recommended that records be kept as necessary of discussions regarding preparations for the future. It is recommended that records regarding specific items related to medical treatment and care be maintained, if possible, in a special written format[4]. The drafting of these documents is not obligatory, nor do these documents have legally binding power; they may be revised at any time. One approach is to use forms prepared by a regularly visited medical institution or by a municipality or by an organization promoting living wills.
Purpose of records. When individuals become unable to communicate their wishes, the records and documents drafted based on previous discussions become the keystone enabling healthcare providers, in collaboration with the trusted partner, to deliver medical treatment and care reflecting the individual's wishes.
Record-keeping for solitary individuals. For individuals who have no family with whom to discuss preparations for the future, healthcare providers can, if the individuals so desire, become interlocutors; it is best to take minutes of discussions.
Record-sharing among healthcare providers. It is recommended that healthcare providers keep in mind to describe the individual's preparations for the future in the medical record, share them among staff members, and transmit them to any new person in charge.
[4]Special written format: e.g., advance directives such as "living wills" in which individuals record their future plans, or other medical forms in which medical practitioners record principally the life-support treatments to be provided to individuals who have life-threatening illnesses.

Figure 4.   Action guidelines regarding Japan's advance care planning (Items 9–11).

Source: Reprinted from Miyashita *et al.* (2022) with permission from Elsevier.

Education Program for Health-Care Providers: Education for Implementing End-of-Life Discussion (E-FIELD) Workshop

E-FIELD is a 1- to 2-day training program that includes lectures regarding the basics of laws and ethics related to end-of-life care and guidelines on decision-making for end-of-life treatment and care, as well as group work and role-play sessions for practical methods to support decision-making among individuals at the end of life and their family members and discussions on ACP. The target audience for E-FIELD is all healthcare providers who assist in making-decision for end-of-life treatment and care. In 2020, the training program was revised to be held continuously, even during the quarantine stage of the COVID-19 pandemic (see Tables 1 and 2 for learning objectives and program structure, respectively).

Table 1.   E-FIELD learning objectives.

Learning objectives
• To understand and adopt the practice in line with the current guideline for the decision-making process for end-of-life medical treatment and care;
• To obtain the legal and ethical knowledge necessary for decision-making regarding end-of-life medical treatment and care;
• To be able to make decisions after having sufficient discussions with individuals;
• To be able to provide decision-making support for family members so that they can make decisions about treatment and care that reflect an individual's values; and
• To be able to assess an individual's readiness for initiating ACP discussions.

Table 2.   E-FIELD program structure.

Six Contents of E-FIELD
1. Basic legal and ethical knowledge and outlines of the current guideline (on-demand video pre-learning).
2. How healthcare providers should evaluate an individual's decision-making capacity (lecture and group discussion)
3. How healthcare providers should support decision-making in cases where individuals still have a capacity for decision-making (lecture and group discussion).
4. How healthcare providers should support decision-making in cases where individuals have lost their capacity for decision-making, but their wishes can be inferred by their family members (lecture and group discussion).
5. How healthcare providers should determine the best interests of individuals in cases where they have lost their capacity for decision-making and have neither family members nor others close to them who can infer their wishes (lecture and group discussion).
6. How healthcare providers should discuss and share individuals' values, goals, and preferences with their families so that their wishes are respected, even when they lose their capacity for decision-making (lecture and role-play).

The participants learn the six parts through work groups and role-play sessions using several health stages in a scenario of a case whose health condition declines. In this training program, participants can obtain the essential knowledge and skills necessary for goal-concordant care by learning different types of decision-making processes that include "in-the-moment decision-making with individuals who still have a capacity for decision-making" and "surrogate decision-making in case that individuals lose their capacity for decision-making". Especially, the experience of learning how difficult it is to support surrogate decision-making through group discussions can help participants realize that ACP is essential for goal-concordant care for individuals who have lost their capacity for decision-making.

Outcomes of the E-FIELD Workshop and Future Prospects

The MHLW rolled out this program by developing local champions in each prefecture throughout Japan, so they would continuously hold the program on their own in the long run. As of 2023, neighboring prefectures collaborate to hold the program every year under the Ministry's support, and more than 8500 healthcare providers have completed this program since it began in 2016. An evaluation of the program found that the participants' confidence in the knowledge and practice of ACP significantly increased compared with before the training, and their confidence was maintained for 6 months. In addition, the number of ACP discussions significantly increased 6 months after compared with before the training, and a trend toward a decrease in difficulties related to ACP practice was observed.[28,29] The original government-commissioned program will be revised for delivery by prefectures and local authorities. In addition, a training program for instructors will be held continuously to realize this.

Materials for the General Public

It is important to promote public awareness of ACP through websites and leaflets, as these materials can facilitate people's exploring and identifying what they regard as important in their lives and sharing their values with their family members.

Website: Let's Have Jinsei Kaigi, (Literally Life Meeting in Japanese)[30]

The MHLW gave ACP the appellation *Jinsei Kaigi*. Kobe University, which implemented a project for promoting an ACP education program commissioned by the MHLW, has published a website that explains *Jinsei Kaigi* to the general public using texts and videos. The website provides links to related information to help individuals comprehend ACP, including "Who knows your thoughts and values well?", "What should I talk about at *Jinsei Kaigi*?", and "What happens when you call an ambulance for patients at the end of life?" Based on the results of a nationwide survey in 2018 revealing that only 3% of the participants thoroughly discussed their values and preferences with their family, and that although 66% agreed to ACP documentation, only 8% actually documented, the website points out that few people take action in relation to ACP, even though the majority agree that individuals should be able to receive the medical treatment and care that aligns with their wishes through ACP.

The following three steps are introduced for individuals to proceed with ACP: (1) Thinking about their values, their way of living at the end of life, and their preferences for treatment and care at the end of life, (2) Selecting a surrogate decision-maker, and (3) Sharing their values and preferences with their surrogate decision-maker. There are also webpages in which advance directives can be easily made and printed out by selecting responses from multiple-choice question items and describing ideas in detail in the free-description field.

Leaflet: Discussions on Future Treatment and Care[31]

Kobe University also created a leaflet promoting ACP, the outline of which is almost the same as that of the website. However, the leaflet incorporates additional steps (e.g., asking individuals' physicians about their medical condition and prognosis, discussing their values and preferences with their physician) to help patients with serious illnesses think thoroughly and concretely about the way to live their end of life and what kind of treatment and care they want or wish to refuse. This is because, unlike the website, which can be accessed by the general public, the leaflet is assumed to be primarily for patients under the guidance of a healthcare provider.

Conclusion

In Japanese society, family-centred decision-making and a high-context culture still strongly influence end-of-life care. In this context, it is necessary to create an environment where autonomous decision-making among adults reluctant to express their opinions about their end-of-life treatment and care are supported and enhanced by their family members and the trusted healthcare providers involved in their treatment and care. To that end, culturally adapted ACP should be familiarized, spread, and implemented. At the same time, it is also true that Japanese people have become increasingly interested in expressing and enhancing their autonomy in medical decisions. Most Japanese adults want to consider and obtain more information about their end-of-life treatment and care before their health declines. Healthcare providers should consider Japanese adults' demands and provide adequate support at an appropriate time for ACP implementation. To achieve this, effective programs for educating healthcare providers about how to support ACP implementation in Japan, such as E-FIELD, should be continuously provided.

References

1. Cabinet Office. (2018). Annual Report on the Aging Society: 2018 (Summary). Available at: https://www8.cao.go.jp/kourei/english/annualreport/2018/2018pdf_e.html. Accessed April 1, 2023.
2. National Institute of Population and Social Research. (2017). Population Projections for Japan: 2016 to 2065 (Appendix: Auxiliary Projections 2066 to 2115). Available at: https://www.ipss.go.jp/pp-zenkoku/e/zenkoku_e2017/pp_zenkoku2017e.asp. Accessed April 1, 2023.
3. Hirakawa Y. (2017). Towards structuring community-based integrated care systems in Japan: Research and practice. *Med. Res. Arch.* **5**(4): 1–8.
4. Asakura K. (2022). The "community-based integrated care system" and discourse ethics — from the viewpoint of autonomy and solidarity. *Jpn. Soc. Cult.* **4**(6): 80–92.
5. The Japan Geriatrics Society Subcommittee on End-of-Life Issues, Kuzuya M., Aita K., *et al.* (2020). Japan Geriatrics Society "Recommendations for the promotion of advance care planning": End-of-life issues subcommittee consensus statement. *Geriatr. Gerontol. Int.* **20**(11): 1024–1028.
6. Matsumura S., Bito S., Liu H., *et al.* (2002). Acculturation of attitudes toward end-of-life care: A cross-cultural survey of Japanese Americans and Japanese. *J. Gen. Intern. Med.* **17**(7): 531–539.
7. Hall E.T. (1989). *Beyond Culture.* Anchor Books, New York, NY.
8. Yamaguchi S., Cohen S.R., and Uza M. (2016). Family caregiving in Japan: The influence of cultural constructs in the care of adults with cancer. *J. Fam. Nurs.* **22**(3): 392–418.
9. Lebra T.S. (1976). *Japanese Patterns of Behavior.* University of Hawaii Press, Honolulu, Hawaii 96822.
10. Fukushima S. (2011). A cross-generational and cross-cultural study on demonstration of attentiveness. *Pragmatics* 21549–21571.

11. Bito S., Matsumura S., Singer M.K., *et al.* (2007). Acculturation and end-of-life decision making: Comparison of Japanese and Japanese-American focus groups. *Bioethics* **21**(5): 251–262.

12. Seo Y. (1997). A preliminary study on the emotional distress of patients with terminal-stage cancer: A questionnaire survey of 1380 bereaved families over a 12-year period. *Jpn. J. Clin. Oncol.* **27**(2): 80–83.

13. Tanida N. (1994). Japanese attitudes towards truth disclosure in cancer. *Scand. J. Soc. Med.* **22**(1): 50–57.

14. Ministry of Health Labour and Welfare. (2014). Shuumatsuki iryou nikansuru ishikichousatou kentoukai houkokusho 2014. Available at: https://www.mhlw.go.jp/file/04-Houdouhappyou-10802000-Iseikyoku-Shidouka/0000042774.pdf. Accessed April 1, 2023.

15. Akabayashi A., and Slingsby B.T. (2003). Biomedical ethics in Japan: The second stage. *Camb. Q. Healthc. Ethics: CQ: Int. J. Healthc. Ethics Comm.* **12**(3): 261–264.

16. Tanaka M., Kodama S., Lee I., Huxtable R., and Chung Y. (2020). Forgoing life-sustaining treatment — a comparative analysis of regulations in Japan, Korea, Taiwan, and England. *BMC Med. Ethics* **21**(1): 99.

17. Higashi T., and Okuyama A. (2018). Hospital Based Cancer Registry 2016 Nationwide Report: National Cancer Center for Cancer Control and Information Services. Available at: https://ganjoho.jp/public/qa_links/report/hosp_c/pdf/2016_report.pdf. Accessed April 1, 2023.

18. Miyata H., Shiraishi H., and Kai I. (2006). Survey of the general public's attitudes toward advance directives in Japan: How to respect patients' preferences. *BMC Med. Ethics* 7E11.

19. Ministry of Health Labour and Welfare. (2017). The attitude survey for end-of-life care, Summary of the report 2017. Available at: https://www.mhlw.go.jp/toukei/list/dl/saisyuiryo_a_h29.pdf. Accessed April 1, 2023.

20. Ministry of Health Labour and Welfare. (2018). Jinsei no saishudankai niokeru iryo kea no ketteipurosesu nikansuru gaidorain 2018. Available at: https://www.mhlw.go.jp/file/06-Seisakujouhou-10800000-Iseikyoku/0000197721.pdf. Accessed April 1, 2023.

21. Miyashita J., Kohno A., Yamamoto Y., *et al.* (2021). How psychosocial factors contribute to Japanese older adults' initiation of advance care planning discussions: A qualitative study. *J. Appl. Gerontol. Off. J. Southern Gerontol. Soc.* **40**(10): 1180–1188.

22. Miyashita J., Shimizu S., Azuma T., *et al.* (2021). Experience as an informal caregiver and discussions regarding advance care planning in Japan. *J. Pain Symptom Manage.* **61**(1): 63–70.

23. Miyashita J., Yamamoto Y., Shimizu S., *et al.* (2019). Association between social networks and discussions regarding advance care planning among Japanese older adults. *PLoS One* **14**(3): e0213894.

24. Miyashita J., Kohno A., Cheng S.Y., *et al.* (2020). Patients' preferences and factors influencing initial advance care planning discussions' timing: A cross-cultural mixed-methods study. *Palliat. Med.* **34**(7): 906–916.
25. Miyashita J., Kohno A., Shimizu S., *et al.* (2021). Healthcare providers' perceptions on the timing of initial advance care planning discussions in Japan: A mixed-methods study. *J. Gen. Intern. Med.* **36**(10): 2935–2942.
26. Miyashita J., Shimizu S., Shiraishi R., *et al.* (2022). Culturally adapted consensus definition and action guideline: Japan's advance care planning. *J. Pain Symptom Manage.* **64**(6): 602–613.
27. Ministry of Health Labour and Welfare. (2021). Reiwa 3 nendo jinsei no saishudankai niokeru Iryo kea taisei seibi jigyou 2021. Available at: https://www.mhlw.go.jp/stf/newpage_25608.html. Accessed April 1, 2023.
28. Miura H., Kizawa Y., Bito S., *et al.* (2017). Benefits of the Japanese version of the advance care planning facilitators education program. *Geriatr. Gerontol. Int.* **17**(2): 350–352.
29. Okada H., Morita T., Kiuchi T., Okuhara T., and Kizawa Y. (2021). Health care providers' knowledge, confidence, difficulties, and practices after completing a communication skills training program for advance care planning discussion in Japan. *Ann. Palliat. Med.* **10**(7): 7225–7235.
30. Kobe University. Zero Kara Hajimeru Jinsei Kaigi. Available at: https://www.med.kobe-u.ac.jp/jinsei/index.html. Accessed April 1, 2023.
31. Kobe University. Adobansukeapuranningu (Jinsei Kaigi), Ippantekina ACP. Available at: https://www.med.kobe-u.ac.jp/jinsei/acp_kobe-u/acp_kobe-u/acp01/index.html. Accessed April 1, 2023.

Chapter 22

Advance Care Planning in Taiwan[*]

Yingwei Wang

*Center for Palliative Care, Hualien Tzu Chi Hospital,
Hualien, Taiwan R.O.C*

Background of the Health Care System

As of approximately 2023, the population of Taiwan stands at around 23.33 million. The healthcare services available encompass medical centres, regional hospitals, local hospitals, and primary health care. While these healthcare facilities are established by both the government and private sector, they are all included under the universal health insurance system. Taiwan's universal health coverage has achieved an impressive coverage rate of 99%. In the case of major illnesses such as cancer, individuals are not required to bear any medical expenses.

The development of palliative care in Taiwan can be divided into three waves.[1] The first wave occurred prior to 1995. Starting in 1983, civil organizations in Taiwan began promoting the concept of palliative care, actively advocating for the idea of compassionate care. Starting in 1983, civil groups began advocating for the concept of palliative care, with a focus on end-stage cancer. At that time, palliative care was provided through hospice wards and home care services. The first hospice ward was established in 1990. In 1995, the government began promoting palliative

---

[*] Re-published with permission from special issue of ZEFQ journal; "Advance Care Planning around the World: Evidence and Experiences, Programmes and Perspectives".

care services. In 1996, the trial program of palliative home care was included in the National Health Insurance system. In 2000, palliative care in hospital settings was covered by National Health Insurance, and at the same time, the Hospice Palliative Care Act was passed. In 2003, the Cancer Control Act was also established, which mandated the provision of palliative care for cancer patients in the terminal stage. At the same time, various professional palliative care groups began certification processes to ensure the quality of care for end-stage patients.

The second wave of palliative care development occurred between 2006 and 2015. During this time, non-cancer patients became eligible for health insurance coverage for palliative care, and civil society groups began promoting the concept of advance care planning. The government also promoted shared decision-making between patients and healthcare providers, and palliative care was extended to include intensive care units for critically ill patients.

The third wave of palliative care development began after 2016 and included palliative care for newborns, children, frail elderly individuals, and community-based care in long-term care facilities. Compassionate communities were also established, and the Patient Right to Autonomy Act was passed during this period to protect the rights of patients.

Policy or Legislative Efforts/Milestones to Foster Advance Care Planning Implementation into the National Health Care System

In Taiwan, the legislation concerning advance care planning can be divided into two phases. The first phase was the passage of the Hospice Palliative Care Act (HPCA) in 2000. The second stage occurred in 2016 with the enactment of the Patient Right to Autonomy Act (PRAA). These two laws coexist, and there is some overlap in their concepts. This differs from the development process in many other countries.

In 2000, the Taiwanese government announced the Hospice Palliative Care Act.[2] According to the act, if two specialist physicians determined that a patient was in the terminal stage of an illness, life-sustaining measures could be withheld in certain situations. However, if life-sustaining medical treatment or cardiopulmonary resuscitation had already begun, they could not be withdrawn. The implementation of this law faced challenges as it did not align with the ethical principle of withholding or withdrawing treatment in equal importance. In 2002, the law was amended for the first time to allow the withholding or withdrawal of life-sustaining medical treatment for patients who had signed HPCA and were in a terminal condition. In 2011, further amendments were made to allow patients' preferences to be noted on their health insurance cards and stored in a cloud-based system for easy access during emergency situations, ensuring that healthcare providers are aware of the patient's wishes.[3]

In 2013, the Hospice Palliative Care Act underwent its third amendment to redefine concepts such as "palliative care," "do not cardiopulmonary resuscitation (DNR)," and "life-sustaining medical treatment." The purpose was to prevent misunderstandings and avoid the perception that hospice palliative care equates to "giving up". The amendments aimed to provide greater flexibility and multiple options for end-of-life medical choices. In other words, the decision between hospice palliative care and life-sustaining medical treatment can be made separately as diverse options for terminally ill patients.

When a terminally ill patient has not signed the letter of intent of HPCA or designated a medical proxy, decisions regarding the implementation, withdrawal, or termination of CPR or life-sustaining medical treatment should be made based on the patient's best interests, following consultation with hospice palliative care professionals.

In the second phase, the "Patient Right to Autonomy Act" was passed in 2015,[4] which differs from the "Hospice Palliative Care Act" that specifically targets end-of-life patients with the concept of "life-sustaining treatment," referring only to "medical measures that can prolong the dying process." At this stage, "life-sustaining therapy" encompasses "any necessary medical treatment that has the potential to prolong a patient's life" and has a broader scope. The traditional concept and practice of "informed consent" was relatively paternalistic and centred on the physician, with the patient expected to assent to the physician's recommendations. This law emphasizes patient autonomy, with recognition of the patient's right to informed choice and decision-making. While the Medical Care Act and Physician Act have already stipulated the obligation of medical institutions and physicians to provide information, the target of information disclosure is not prioritized on the patient. Therefore, this law specifies that informed consent is a patient's right and that medical institutions or physicians should disclose information to the patient as a principle. At the same time, if the patient has not expressed objection, medical institutions or physicians may also disclose relevant information to their relatives.

Patients who have undergone consultation and signed an advance medical decision under the PRAA may have the option to withdraw or withhold life-sustaining treatments, artificial nutrition, and hydration if they meet the diagnoses confirmed by two relevant specialists and if the palliative care team has conducted at least two consultations to confirm specific clinical conditions. These clinical conditions may include the following circumstances:

1. The patient is in a terminal stage of illness.
2. The patient is in an irreversible coma.
3. The patient is in a permanent vegetative state.
4. The patient is suffering from severe dementia.
5. Other disease conditions, as determined by the central competent authority, meet the following requirements: the conditions or sufferings are unbearable, the disease is incurable, and there are no other appropriate treatment options available according to the prevailing medical standards at the time of the disease's occurrence.

Definition and Model of Advance Care Planning Used

According to the principles of Advance Care Planning (ACP), patients have the fundamental right to receive information about their disease diagnosis, available treatment options, and the potential benefits and risks associated with each option. Additionally, patients hold the autonomy to make decisions and choose among the treatment options provided by their physicians. It is imperative that the patient's legal representative, spouse, relatives, health care agents, and other closely related individuals do not impede the medical institution or physician from adhering to the patient's treatment decisions. When seeking medical care, the medical institution or physician must promptly and appropriately provide the patient with information regarding their disease diagnosis, treatment plan, proposed procedures, medications, prognosis, potential adverse reactions, and other pertinent matters, as deemed suitable by the medical institution or physician.

In order to establish an advance decision, the declarant must fulfill the following requirements:

1. The declarant must have received advance care planning consultation from a medical institution and have the institution's seal affixed to their advance decision.

2. The advance decision must be notarized by a notary public or witnessed by two or more individuals with full legal capacity.
3. The advance decision must be registered in the declarant's National Health Insurance IC card.

The terms used in this Act are defined as follows:

1. Life-sustaining treatment: necessary medical measures that can prolong the lives of patients, such as cardiopulmonary resuscitation, mechanical life-support system, blood products, special treatments for specific diseases, and antibiotics against severe infections etc.
2. Artificial nutrition and hydration: Provision of food or fluids via tubes or other invasive means.
3. Advance decision: A prior written and signed statement expressing the willingness of a person to accept or refuse life-sustaining treatment, artificial nutrition and hydration, or other types of medical care and a good death when he/she is in specific clinical conditions.
4. Declarant: A person who makes an advance decision in writing.
5. Health care agent: A person who has received written authorization from a declarant to express his or her wishes on his or her behalf when he or she is unconscious or unable to clearly express his or her wishes
6. Advance care planning: The process of communication between the patient and medical service providers, relatives, and other related parties regarding the proper care that shall be offered to the patient and the options he or she has to receive or refuse life-preserving treatments and artificial nutrition and hydration when the patient is in specific clinical conditions, unconscious or unable to clearly express his or her wishes.
7. Palliative care: Relieving and supportive medical treatment provided to alleviate or eliminate the patient's physical, psychological, and spiritual suffering to improve his or her life quality.

Education/Training of Health Care Professionals and Non-health Care Professionals in Advance Care Planning

In Taiwan, professionals who provide ACP counselling are required to complete proper training. Physicians are required to attend a 4-hour workshop, while nurses and social workers or clinical psychologists must attend a 6-hour and 8-hour workshop, respectively. The training program was offered by the Hospice Foundation of Taiwan, which is an officially authorized training centre sanctioned by the government. The Patient Autonomy Research Center is another institution commissioned by the government to provide continuing education. It also offers online learning courses through which physicians and nursing staff can obtain certification. The centre plays a vital role in educating healthcare professionals about patient autonomy and supporting them in facilitating patient-centred decision-making processes.

Over the course of five years (2018–2022), a total of 7328 individuals have participated in the training program, consisting of 1806 physicians, 6717 nurses, 1169 social workers, and 482 clinical psychologists. Out of all the participants, 2853 of them enrolled in the onsite workshop.

Information Materials Used, Documentation and Digitalization of Advance Care Planning Processes in the Health Care Sector and Beyond

Taiwan has placed great emphasis on the promotion of the Hospice and Palliative Care Act and Advance Care Planning. The central government has shown significant commitment by establishing an information system on the website of the Ministry of Health and Welfare.[3] This allows individuals to sign HPCA online and provides real-time updates on the progress of ACP implementation in different regions. The Hospice Foundation of Taiwan and the Patient Autonomy Research Center play a major role in promoting ACP within the civil sector. Various advocacy materials, including brochures and videos, are produced by both the government and private organizations. Local hospitals that offer ACP services can also be searched on the government's website.

People can sign or revoke HPCA online, but Advance Decision must go through a legal consultation process before it can be legally recorded in the cloud-based system. Both HPCA and AD can be digitally linked to an individual's national health insurance card after signing, enabling healthcare institutions to access people's preferences in real time.

Examples of Institutional and Community Implementation

After the implementation of HPCA, the Health Promotion Administration provides funding, and private organizations are responsible for advocacy. Due to the requirements of hospital accreditation, various hospitals have started internal promotion and assistance to help people sign HPCA.

In 2019, with the passage of ACP, to encourage its implementation, the indicators in hospital accreditation were adjusted to include the promotion outcomes of ACP. Local health authorities, under the policy promotion of the Ministry of Health and Welfare, also promote ACP at the local government level.

Research Agenda on Advance Care Planning

In Taiwan, there have been several studies conducted on HPCA. Although the concept of HPCA is closely related to ACP, there has been limited international collaboration primarily due to variations in terminology. However, with the formal promotion of ACP, research teams in Taiwan have engaged in collaborations with several countries in the Asia-Pacific region to study ACP and gain insights into its implementation across diverse cultural contexts.[5,6]

Regarding research funding, there has been a focus on practical research in the initial stages. The National Science and Technology Council has played a role in providing research grants, and many researchers have submitted applications to secure funding for conducting ACP-related research.

Addressing Diversity and Sociocultural Vulnerabilities Regarding ACP Access and Use

The government in Taiwan provides subsidies to non-governmental organizations (NGOs) for the development of promotional materials in various languages for both HPCA and ACP. Given the significant number of foreign spouses and foreign caregivers from Southeast Asia, promotional videos in languages such as Indonesian and Vietnamese have been developed to cater to their needs. Regular outreach efforts are also conducted in indigenous communities, where information is shared in their native languages to ensure better understanding. The emphasis is primarily on explaining the core concepts of HPCA and ACP. As each indigenous tribe has unique perspectives on death, local healthcare professionals within the communities play a vital role in driving the promotion and implementation of these initiatives.

Main Challenges and Barriers

It is generally believed that discussing death is a taboo topic among the Taiwanese population. However, after years of advocacy and promotion, there has been a more accepting attitude towards Advance Care Planning (ACP). In addition, government and civil society collaboration has resulted in life education being taught in elementary school curricula and regular promotion in senior community centres, leading to a significant shift in mindset.

The main challenge faced is that healthcare professionals often have differing views on the timing of initiating High-Performance CPR and ACP.[7] Many are still in the mindset of only providing CPR or implementing a do-not-resuscitate (DNR) order and are unfamiliar with the patient's choices and the use of time-limited trials of care.

Regarding the ACP consultation process, strict requirements are in place, including a one-hour explanation of the various options by three types of professionals. However, some people may sign without fully understanding, leading to difficulties in execution later.

Although ACP discussions began earlier, many studies have shown that people cannot truly understand future scenarios. Therefore, their choices may cause problems in the future. In practical terms, the provision of end-of-life care is a more urgent and critical issue compared to the other four conditions, namely irreversible coma, permanent vegetative state, severe dementia, and other diseases determined by the central authority. However, the government's focus on promoting the PRAA has impeded the progress of the much-needed HPCA. In the end, both efforts have reached a bottleneck in terms of implementation.

Upon reviewing the official data from the Ministry of Health and Welfare R.O.C. between 2013 and 2022, it was observed that a total of 852,754 individuals had signed the HPCA agreement, while 43,466 individuals had signed Advance Decision (AD) between 2019 and 2022. There was an increasing trend in HPCA signatories prior to the implementation of the ACP/AD program in 2019. The turning point in this trend can be attributed to the Coronavirus disease 2019 pandemic and the introduction of the ACP Act. However, it appears that the promotion of ACP/AD not only slowed down the growth of HPCA but also did not achieve the desired outcomes for those who made declarations.

Collaborations with Other Countries/Programs Regarding Advance Care Planning

Advance Care Planning (ACP) is based on the universal value of respecting patients' choices, but different cultural contexts in different countries may prioritize different aspects. In Chinese society, for example, individual autonomy often takes into account the opinions of family members. Therefore, in cross-national collaborations, experiences from different countries can be referenced and adapted to local immigrant communities in order to achieve the spirit of ACP. In Taiwan, due to the presence of many foreign spouses and migrant workers, culturally based ACP explanatory brochures in multiple languages have been established, and can also serve as a reference for other countries.

Conclusion

Taiwan has made significant progress in the development of end-of-life care, from the enactment of the Hospice Palliative Care Act over 20 years ago to the recent implementation of the Patient Autonomy Act. However, there is still room for improvement in terms of execution, including how to ensure that both the public and healthcare professionals have a thorough understanding of the content of ACP and when it is appropriate to execute it. By referring to the implementation models of other countries, Taiwan can further advance the promotion of ACP and enable more individuals to participate in making their own healthcare decisions.

References

1.   National Health Research Institutes. (2019). White Paper on Palliative and Hospice Care Policy in Taiwan. (in Chinese).

2. Ke L.S. (2012). Advance care planning in Taiwan. *Patient Educ. Couns.* **89**(1): 213.

3. Welfare M.o.H.a. *Hospice Palliative Care Act.* 2021 [cited 2023 May 10]. Available from: https://law.moj.gov.tw/ENG/LawClass/LawAll.aspx?pcode= L0020066.

4. Welfare M.o.H.a. *Patient Right to Autonomy Act.* 2021 [cited 2023 May 10]. Available from: https://law.moj.gov.tw/ENG/LawClass/LawAll.aspx?pcode= L0020189.

5. Lin C.P., *et al.* (2019). 2019 Taipei declaration on advance care planning: A cultural adaptation of end-of-life care discussion. *J. Palliat. Med.* **22**(10): 1175–1177.

6. Cheng S.Y., *et al.* (2020). Advance care planning in Asian culture. *Jpn. J. Clin. Oncol.* **50**(9): 976–989.

7. Martina D., *et al.* (2021). Advance care planning in Asia: A systematic narrative review of healthcare professionals' knowledge, attitude, and experience. *J. Am. Med. Dir. Assoc.* **22**(2): 349 e1–349 e28.

Chapter 23

Advance Care Planning in the Philippines: A Continuing Narrative of Advocacy[*]

Rumalie Alparaque-Corvera[†], Djhoanna Aguirre-Pedro[†],
Erwin Phillip E. Francisco[‡], and Andrew E. Ang[§]

[†]*The Ruth Foundation, Unit 2719 Entrata Tower 1, Filinvest Corporate
City, Alabang, Muntinlupa, Philippines*
[‡]*Asian Hospital and Medical Center, 2205 Civic Dr., Alabang,
Muntinlupa, 1780 Metro Manila, Philippines*
[§]*Department of Family and Community Medicine, Philippine General
Hospital, Taft Ave, Ermita, Manila, 1000 Metro Manila, Philippines*

The Philippine Backdrop for Healthcare Decisions

In the 2017–2022 National Objectives for Health, the Philippine health system was described as operating within a "fragmented environment", a mixture of private and public provision.[1] The majority of which is the private sector, mainly self-paying and out of pocket from the patients. This is further demonstrated in the Local Government Code of 1991 that led to a dual governance of health, with the Department of Health (DOH) governing the national level and the Local Government Units (LGU) at the subnational level. Though this system defined and perhaps

---

[*]Re-published with permission from special issue of ZEFQ journal; "Advance Care Planning around the World: Evidence and Experiences, Programmes and Perspectives".

strengthened the role of the DOH as the overall steward and technical authority on health being the national health policy-maker and regulatory institution, it was dependent on the LGU for the actual rollout of existing and future policies and standards. Such fragmentation poses probable risks for more gaps between orders and implementations, most especially for new and emerging ethical health standards such as Advance Care Planning (ACP).

To date, there is no standard form that is being used for ACP in the Philippines. Hospitals, medical institutions and private providers that may have such forms, base them on international templates. There are also no specific legislations that foster ACP implementation into the Philippine national health care system. Perhaps the nearest attempt ever made was the Senate Bill 1887 filed in 2013 by the late Senator Miriam Defensor-Santiago.[2] This was entitled appropriately as the "Natural Death Act". The bill defined and outlined how any person of legal age and sound mind may execute a written instruction *directing the withholding or withdrawal of life-sustaining treatment in a terminal condition or permanent uncon-scious condition.* The proposed legislation even provided the template for a "Health Care Directive" that should be honored by the patient's family and health care providers as the final expression of their legal right to refuse medical or surgical treatment given the qualified conditions. That Senate Bill was brought to many levels of scrutiny by Bioethics and Legal communities alike. Unfortunately, it was not passed and to date nothing quite similar to it has been brought to the priority table of lawmakers.

Patient autonomy, as cited by Cheng *et al.* in the article "Advance care planning in Asian culture", is consequently subordinate to family values and physician authority within the Southeast Asian culture.[3] This is very much descriptive of the Filipino attitude towards health decision-making, thus making the mere suggestion of preparing for death most often taboo in any conversation. Lanaban *et al.* in a local study done in the Southern Philippines about their perspective on death and dying, viewed that it was important for a person to have a sense of *"readiness"* in order to achieve a good death. With these contrasting views, Advance Care Planning is the ideal tool to be used for the Filipino patient and family to be equipped to deal with end of life issues and further options for further palliative care.[4]

Difficult Decision-Making throughout the Pandemic

In 2020, the world experienced COVID-19. The pandemic ruthlessly challenged the norms of the global healthcare force irrespective of systems, resources and culture. Actual accounts to demonstrate this reality were that of an older Filipino patient who began with respiratory distress from the dreaded virus and was advised by the Pulmonologist if he would consent to endotracheal intubation as indicated. He unhesitatingly answered, "Why should I, when I know I will die anyway?" Then there is that of another elderly patient who was brought to one of the most congested emergency rooms in the country. He had rapidly escalating respiratory distress and was quickly brought by his son to the emergency room physician. Little did the son know that it would be the last time he would see his father alive. No questions were asked as the hospital was too overwhelmed and would promptly give the required medical treatment. It was during this critical time in the history of our country, and of the whole world, that everyone had to collectively confront the sinister nature of death head-on. No one was spared from the exposure to death as the number of fatalities increased worldwide.

In the hospital wards and emergency rooms, the role of Palliative Medicine specialists was largely in the area of care in the final hours and bereavement support. The members of the Philippine Society of Hospice and Palliative Medicine (PSHPM) assumed not only "front-liner" duties but also took on an even stronger role in the battle lines against the deluge of health-related suffering that the pandemic has brought with it. Difficult conversations, decision-making and ACP discussions were more common following a shared-decision making strategy model during family conferences and individual counselling. Palliative Care consultants also volunteered in the "back-room" with the crafting of COVID-19 guidelines and process flows.

They worked side by side with other medical and ethical specialists for policies and unified algorithms, which also included one for Advance Care Planning.[5] An electronic publication by the University of the Philippines Manila COVID-19 Ethics Study group also included a guideline on Advance Care Planning under the section of "Communication of Care".[6] Along with these, there were institutional initiatives and documents that tentatively embraced the value of Advance Care Planning.

Organizational and National Movements for Advance Care Planning

Prior to the pandemic, PSHPM alongside the National Council for Hospice and Palliative Care in the Philippines (Hospice Philippines) played a significant role in promoting and supporting Advance Care

Planning (ACP) in the country. As the Philippine government-recognized national organization, composed of physicians, nurses, and other allied health professionals and advocates with a special interest in hospice and palliative care, Hospice Philippines had been working to improve the quality of life for patients with life-limiting illnesses and their families since it's foundation back in 2003. The organization's involvement in ACP can be seen through several key activities:

1. *Education and Training* through programs aimed at enhancing the knowledge and skills of healthcare professionals in managing patients with life-limiting illnesses. These would include addressing their physical, emotional, and spiritual needs, and facilitating ACP discussions with patients and their families.
2. *Advocacy* for the integration of both Palliative care and ACP into the Philippine health care system. The organization works closely with government agencies, educational institutions, and other stakeholders to promote awareness and understanding of ACP and its importance in providing comprehensive, patient-centred care.
3. *Research and Development* with the support of research initiatives in hospice and palliative care, including ACP. Through research, the organizations seek to generate evidence-based knowledge that can inform and improve the practice of ACP in the Philippines.
4. *Networking and Collaboration* among health care professionals, government agencies, non-governmental organizations, and other stakeholders involved in ACP. Hospice Philippines and PSHPM actively organize and participate in national and international conferences, workshops, and meetings to exchange ideas, experiences, and best practices in hospice and palliative care, as well as ACP skills.
5. *Policy Development and Support* in contributing to the development of policies and guidelines related to hospice and palliative care, with special interest in ACP. Both PSHPM and Hospice Philippines work together with the DOH and other relevant agencies in ensuring that these policies are consistent with international standards and best practices.

Learning from the Past and Marching Forward

Throughout the years 2020–2021 the DOH has also strengthened the capacity of healthcare professionals in Palliative care and consequently in the areas of ACP discussions. This led to the crafting and publishing of the National Training Manuals for Palliative Care.[7] It was from this reference that the recognized definition of Advance Care Planning is "a process which entails planning for future medical care if the person can no longer retain the capacity to decide on his own". Further to this definition, they described the ACP process as allowing a competent individual and his or her family to participate in future medical decisions even before a medical crisis happens.

Though we are now currently at a far better point of ACP orientation than we were pre-pandemic, actual implementation and integration into patient care remain unfledged and sparse. The Philippines still has a great shortage of healthcare professionals trained in ACP and palliative care, leading to inadequate support for patients and their families. Additionally, the lack of dedicated hospice and palliative care facilities limits the accessibility of ACP services. With these barriers, the ongoing challenges for ACP in the Philippines are as follows:

A. Prevailing cultural barriers

Filipino culture places a strong emphasis on family values and interdependence, which sometimes leads to reluctance in discussing end-of-life issues. Moreover, there is a prevailing belief in "bahala na," or leaving things to fate, making it difficult for some individuals to engage in ACP. Religiosity is also a huge part of Filipino culture and letting things be out of faith to the higher being is commonplace even if it meant prolonged suffering and emotional distress to those involved.

B. Continuing lack of awareness and understanding of ACP

Many Filipinos are unaware of the concept of ACP or do not fully understand its importance. This lack of awareness extends to healthcare professionals, who may not be well-equipped to initiate ACP discussions with patients and their families.

C. Limited resources and infrastructure

The Philippines faces a shortage of healthcare professionals trained in ACP and palliative care, leading to inadequate support for patients and their families. Furthermore, the lack of dedicated hospice and palliative care facilities limits the accessibility of ACP services.

In order to overcome these challenges, there must be a willingness for all stakeholders to be aware and be active in the training of healthcare professionals to do ACP. The capacity building of non-healthcare professionals is also crucial. These can be carried out through the following recommendations:

A. Community-based education

Local government initiatives can play a crucial role in promoting ACP awareness by organizing community-based education programs. These programs may include seminars, workshops, and support groups that educate the public about the importance of ACP. Non-government organizations (NGOs) and advocacy groups can also help increase public awareness of ACP by conducting educational campaigns and providing resources for patients and their families. These organizations can also collaborate with healthcare professionals to ensure a holistic approach to ACP.

B. Faith-based organizations

Spirituality is an essential component of ACP, as it addresses the emotional and spiritual needs of patients and their families. Training programs should equip faith leaders and pastoral care providers with the necessary skills to support individuals during the ACP process.

C. Public information campaigns

Traditional, digital, and social media platforms can play a significant role in promoting ACP awareness. By featuring stories, interviews, and expert opinions on ACP, media outlets can help educate the public about its importance and benefits. Key individuals and influencers may help bring awareness to more reach, especially to the Filipino public.

An area of importance that must be tackled is lobbying for stronger and more intentional legal and policy frameworks that support ACP in the Philippines. The Expanded Senior Citizens Act of 2010 is able to provide for the rights and privileges of senior citizens in the Philippines, including access to quality healthcare services.[8] In turn, the Republic Act No. 11215 otherwise known as the National Integrated Cancer Control Act (NICCA) of 2019 and Republic Act No. 11223, also known as the Universal Health Care Act,[9] both include Palliative health services in their declarations of principles and policies. While not directly addressing ACP, these legislations highlight the need for comprehensive care for those with advanced age and illness, together with end-of-life care planning. As the DOH issued Administrative Order No. 2015-0052 has provided the primary policy framework for palliative and hospice care in the Philippines,[10] it consequently emphasizes the importance of ACP in providing patient-centred care and calls for the integration of ACP services within the Philippine health care system. Even more so there is a need to advocate for proposed legislations that aim to further support ACP in the Philippines. These would include legislative bills concerning patients' rights to make end-of-life decisions and those that would strengthen the eventual rollout of the national hospice and palliative care program. These proposed laws have the potential to create a more supportive environment for ACP implementation and practice.

Conclusion

ACP awareness and practice is still in its infancy and is a continually evolving practice in the Philippines, as it is around the world. It is essential to monitor the progress and outcomes of existing initiatives. Continuous research, evaluation, and feedback can help identify areas for improvement and guide future strategies for promoting ACP among healthcare professionals and the general public. Moreover, further investment in resources and infrastructure, as well as the development of a comprehensive legal and policy framework, is crucial for ensuring the long-term success of ACP initiatives in our country.

The Filipino people have long been known for resilience, and it is with such strong cultural traits that we move forward towards the goal of equitable attention to health-related suffering. This will allow each of our citizens the basic human right of participating in their future medical decisions, well before any health crisis happens.

References

1. Department of Health. (2018). National Objectives for Health Philippines 2017–2022. Department of Health, Manila, Philippines.
2. Santiago M. (2013). *Senate Bill No. 1887;* An Act Recognizing the Fundamental Right of Adult Persons to Decide Their Own Health Care, Including the Decision to Have Life-Sustaining Treatment Withheld or Withdrawn in Instances of a Terminal Condition or Permanent Unconscious Condition . Retrieved April 14, 2023, from https://legacy.senate.gov.ph/lis-data/1812315368!.pdf. October 24, 2013.

3. Cheng S. Y., Lin C. P., Chan H. Y., Martina D., Mori M., Kim S. H., and Ng R. (2020). Advance care planning in Asian culture. *Jpn. J. Clin. Oncol.* **50**(9): 976–989. doi: 10.1093/jjco/hyaa131. PMID: 32761078.

4. Lanaban A. R., Sorrosa R., and Concha M. E. (2016). Perspectives of good death and dying among patients with cancer, their caregivers, and health care providers. *SPMC J. Health Care Ser.* **2**(1): 8. http://N2T.NET/ARK:/76951/JHCA4JT8Z4.

5. Unified COVID-19 Algorithms. (2021). Unified COVID-19 Algorithms. https://www.psmid.org/unified-covid-19-algorithms-5/. October 1, 2021.

6. University of the Philippines COVID-19 Ethics Study Group. (2020). *Ethics Guidelines on COVID-19 Crisis-Level Hospital Care.* University of the Philippines Manila. Retrieved April 14, 2023, from https://www.upm.edu.ph/node/3549.

7. Department of Health. (2021). *Palliative and Hospice Care Basic Training Course for Primary Care Providers Participant's Manual* (1st edn.). Department of Health.

8. Republic Act No. 11215; An Act Institutionalizing a National Integrated Cancer Control Program and Appropriating funds therefor; Retrieved April 14, 2023, from https://www.officialgazette.gov.ph/2019/02/14/republic-act-no-11215/.

9. Republic Act No. 11223; An Act Instituting Universal Health Care for all Filipinos, prescribing reforms in the health care system and appropriating funds therefor; Retrieved April 14, 2023, from https://www.officialgazette.gov.ph/downloads/2019/02feb/20190220-RA-1223-RRD.pdf.

10. Administrative Order No. 2015-0052; National Policy on Palliative and Hospice Care in the Philippines; Retrieved April 14, 2023, from https://doh.gov.ph/sites/default/files/health_programs/AO%202015-0052%20National%20Policy%20on%20Palliative%20and%20Hospice%20Care%20in%20the%20Philippines.pdf.

Chapter 24

Advance Care Planning in Indonesia: Current State and Future Prospects*

Diah Martina[†,‡], Maria Astheria Witjaksono[§], and
Rudi Putranto[†,‡]

[†]*Division of Psychosomatic and Palliative Medicine, Department of
Internal Medicine, Universitas Indonesia, Jakarta, Indonesia*
[‡]*Cipto Mangunkusumo National Center Hospital, Jakarta, Indonesia*
[§]*Dharmais National Cancer Center, Jakarta, Indonesia*

Palliative Care Landscape in Indonesia

Indonesia is undergoing an epidemiological transition toward an ageing society and a high rate of advanced cancer. With over 275 million inhabitants, Indonesia is the fourth most populated nation in the world.[1] Its average life expectancy at birth is 74 years, a significant increase from 45 years in 1970 and 64 years in 1990.[1,2] Due to this situation, the population has begun to age, with the elderly population growing from 22 million in 2017 to a projected 61 million in 2050, or 19% of the overall population.[2] More than one-fourth of people in this age range reported having a disability of some kind. Over the past five years, the prevalence of cancer in this nation has increased to 29%, with more than 70% of cases being

---

*Re-published with permission from special issue of ZEFQ journal; "Advance Care Planning around the World: Evidence and Experiences, Programmes and Perspectives".

diagnosed at an advanced stage. These changes highlighted the critical need for high-quality palliative and end-of-life care.

Indonesia is a lower-middle-income country where palliative care is still underdeveloped.[3] Since palliative care was introduced in Indonesia in 1989, it has been scarcely available, disproportionally dispersed, and inadequately funded.[4] The majority of palliative care services are self-funded or supported by charitable donations. According to a recent study undertaken by Comprehensive Cancer Care of Cipto Mangunkusumo Hospital (PKaT), WHO Indonesia, and the Indonesian Ministry of Health, it was known that, apart from initiatives led by several non-profit organizations, the bulk of palliative care services in Indonesia are centred in the hospital settings.[5] Palliative care has not been formally integrated into the national health system or mentioned in national policies, with the exception of a small number of the Ministry of Health's policies and several guidelines linked to cancer and HIV, as well as a small number of regional policies.

Based on the Institute for Health Metrics & Evaluation Global Burden of Disease 2017 data[6] and the calculation method of the Lancet Commission Report on Palliative Care and Pain Relief,[7] it is estimated that approximately 1,451,100 persons in Indonesia need palliative care annually. This figure is a conservative estimate; thus, it is vital to assume that the actual need is higher. Only 1% of cancer patients in Indonesia who were experiencing pain could obtain morphine, according to an unpublished study that was conducted as part of a collaboration project between the Indonesian National Cancer Control Committee (KPKN), International Atomic Energy Agency (IAEA), World Health Organization-International Agency for Research in Cancer (WHO-IARC).[8] A comparative study revealed that cancer patients in Indonesia had a disproportionately high degree of unmet palliative care needs in all areas (physical, psychological, spiritual, and social).[9]

The cornerstone of patient-centred care is delivering care that is in line with patients' values, wishes, and preferences, even under incapacitating conditions.[10] However, such values, wishes, and preferences are not always known by healthcare professionals and family members.[11,12] Additionally, the advancement of medical technologies often enables care options that may not be in accordance with patients' values, wishes, and preferences.[13] Advance care planning (ACP) is a process that enables medical practitioners better understand patients' values, wishes and preferences for future care and treatment in order to make sure that the care they receive is in accordance with those aspects. Up to 70% of Indonesian patients with cancer were already in advanced stages upon admission to healthcare facilities,[14] when rapid deterioration and unexpected deaths frequently occur.[15] To ensure that care and treatment are provided in accordance with patients' values, it is, therefore, crucial to communicate wishes and preferences about future care and treatment in a timely manner.

Policies or Legislative Achievements Fostering ACP Implementation

Advance care planning has yet to be explicitly mentioned in the national legislative documents. However, in 2007 — 15 years after palliative care was first introduced in Indonesia — the Minister of Health of Indonesia issued a decree on palliative care, including some elements of advance care planning.[3,16,17] In this decree, it was mentioned that when the patient is competent to make a decision for his/her future medical treatment, the palliative care team should endeavour to obtain statements or declarations from him/her regarding what should or should not be done to him/her if his/her competence deteriorates in a written document (advance directive). This statement can specify exactly what actions should or should not be taken, and/or name someone who will subsequently represent the patient in making decisions on his/her behalf if he/she is unable to do so. This written statement should act as the primary guide for the palliative care team in making a final decision.[17]

This decree also regulates code status, in which a competent patient has the right to determine whether he/she wants to be resuscitated as long as he/she has received the information needed to make an informed decision. This decision should be written in advance (advance directive or informed consent). This discussion should begin as soon as the patient meets with the palliative care team. In general, unless specified in an advance directive, the next of kin may not make a DNR decision. However, in certain circumstances and with suitable considerations, all immediate family members may petition the court to grant their request for DNR. Finally, the palliative care team is allowed to make a DNR decision if a patient is believed to be terminal and resuscitation would not save the patient or improve the quality of life based on scientific evidence at the moment.

Another, national legislative document governing advance care planning is the Regulation of the Minister of Health Number 37, 2014, concerning the "Determination of Death and Utilization of Donor Organs," specifically Chapter 3 about "Withholding and withdrawal of life-sustaining treatment," clauses.[14–15,18] It was suggested that if life-sustaining treatment was deemed futile in the incurable, terminal stage, it might be withheld or withdrawn. The hospital director determines what constitutes a terminal illness and a futile treatment.

After conferring with an ethical or medical committee, the teams of treating physicians should decide whether to withhold or withdraw life-sustaining treatment. This decision should be communicated to and approved by the patient's family or surrogate. Among life-sustaining treatments that can be withheld or withdrawn are intensive care unit, cardiopulmonary resuscitation, dysrhythmia control, tracheal intubation, mechanical ventilation, vasoactive drugs, parenteral nutrition, artificial organs, transplant, blood transfusion, invasive monitoring, antibiotic, and other medical interventions specified in the standard medical care. However, life-sustaining treatments such as oxygen, enteral feeding, and crystalloid infusion fell under the treatments that should not be withdrawn or withheld.

In addition, clause 15 states that if a patient is incapable of making decisions, their family may request that life-sustaining care be withheld or withdrawn, or that patient's condition be evaluated to determine whether to do so. In the case that there is a disagreement between the family's request and the recommendation of the team chosen by the medical committee or ethical committee, and the family still seeks the termination or postponement of life support therapy, the family bears legal responsibility.

Despite the fact that there is no clear definition of advance care planning in Indonesia, it is mentioned in the national guideline for cancer palliative care program and is translated as "living will" or "last will" and focuses on the withdrawal or withholding of life-sustaining treatment and resuscitation.[19] The most recent draft of Health Law in Indonesia has finally included palliative care along with promotion, prevention, curation, and rehabilitation.[20] Revision of the Minister of Health Regulation on Palliative Care is needed "advance care planning" as one of the palliative care services the newest among other services such as symptom management, psycho-socio-spiritual support, bereavement support, and end-of-life care. Nonetheless, more recommendations on how advance care planning could be applied in Indonesia have yet to be developed.

All existing documents on advance care planning have mainly focused on patients with terminal illnesses and have not addressed advance care planning as a continuous process of values exploration regarding future care and treatment among healthy populations or other specific conditions such as dementia, psychiatric conditions, or paediatric patients. Furthermore, aside from the do-not-resuscitate (DNR) order form and the informed consent form, no specific form is recognized and commonly used to document advance care planning conversations.[21]

The Implementation of Advance Care Planning in Indonesia

Indonesia is the largest archipelagic country in the world with an estimated 17,504 islands in a land area of 1,811,570 km^2, extending 5,120 km from east to west and 1,760 km from north to south.[22] This geographical landscape poses significant challenges in delivering equitable healthcare and education. Furthermore, Indonesia is home to 1,340 ethnic groups who speak over 800 different languages and dialects and are mostly collectivist — where one's health and illness are considered as a collective matter and care for an individual is primarily viewed as a family responsibility.[23-25] Finally, with over 87% of its population being Muslim, Indonesia has the largest Islamic population in the world.[26] A global survey showed that Indonesia is one of the most religious countries in the world, where faith drives many aspects of life, including healthcare decision-making.[27-29] Indonesian geographical and cultural landscapes, including the religious devoutness of its people, are known to influence advance care planning implementation in Indonesia.[30-32]

According to a survey of 1,030 Indonesian cancer survivors, 46–69% wished to discuss different topics of advance care planning (end-of-life treatments, resuscitation, health care proxies, and what matters at the end of life); however only 21–42% had done so.[30] Nearly 70% of cancer survivors who had considered those topics but had never discussed them with others were willing to do so. This study suggests the lack of advance care planning implementation and that healthcare professionals have failed to address patients' needs for advance care planning. Furthermore, 36–79% of individuals who wished to discuss these topics preferred to do so with family members. This study demonstrates the significance of family members in Indonesian advance care planning. Other studies among Indonesian cancer patients, their family members, and cancer care providers have validated the relevance of family involvement in advance care planning.[31,32]

Different circumstances may bring practical challenges to advance care planning in Indonesia. The first one is system-related barriers. In most of the nation, palliative care services are yet to be integrated. This, combined with healthcare professionals' low awareness of advance care planning, results in patients being referred to palliative care after they have become cognitively impaired, further impeding patients' chances of timely engagement in advance care planning.[31] Due to healthcare professionals' poor knowledge and skills in advance care planning, they often feel anxious about discussing death and dying with patients and family members. Healthcare professionals argued that patients' health literacy would influence their ability to understand and appreciate the aim of advance care planning. Other challenges encountered by Indonesian healthcare professionals are their workload and time constraints. Furthermore, the majority of Indonesian healthcare facilities' paper-based medical record systems restricted the accessibility and accountability of advance care planning-related documents. The lack of institutional and legal support has also been identified as significant impediments to advance care planning.[31,32] Healthcare professionals expressed a need for a written statute to protect them from the legal consequences of engaging in advance care planning. They also indicated that integrating advance care planning into financial platforms would be critical to ensuring patients' access to it. Finally, Indonesian healthcare professionals require clear recommendations and guidelines for advance care planning, specifically regarding who should be in charge of delivering it, when and how to initiate the conversations, what elements should be discussed, and how to deal with family members.[31]

Aside from all of those system barriers, there are also cultural challenges. Firstly, in Indonesian collectivist culture, family plays an important role in healthcare decision-making, even more among the elderly.[31–33] Being ill is a family concern, and telling the patients they are dying is frowned upon.[31,32,34] Patients could especially be deprived of meaningful opportunities to participate in advance care planning if their families took the lead in decision-making. For instance, families' unwillingness to inform patients of their poor prognosis contributed to missed opportunities for patients to timely participate in advance care planning. Certain family structures and dynamics, particularly those involving hierarchy, were observed to possibly hinder advance care planning, sometimes preventing patients' desires from being carried out. Secondly, despite the fact that both patients and doctors are seeking mutual understanding, paternalistic way of communication still frequently occurs between doctors and patients.[31,32,35] In addition to that, patients sometimes viewed the use of direct language to be rude and preferred more euphemistic communication.[31,32] Finally, studies among Indonesian cancer survivors showed that only one-third of them preferred to be informed about their estimated life expectancy, less than half of them would discuss resuscitation and would document their wish in an advance directive.[30] Finally, Indonesian healthcare professionals stated that patients' religious views influence their participation in advance care planning.[31,32] Patients who believe in God's control over their lives may find the concept of future planning contradictory. Patients who believed that life is a sacred gift from God and it should be protected at all costs would often avoid conversations about limiting aggressive interventions. The most important reasons for not being willing to engage in advance care planning were the desire to surrender to God's will and to focus on the here and now.[30] All of these cultural barriers, combined with system barriers, have made advance care planning implementation in Indonesia exceedingly complex.[31,32,36]

Education and Research on Advance Care Planning in Indonesia

One of the main barriers to advance care planning in Indonesia, as mentioned above, is a lack of knowledge, skills, and confidence among healthcare professionals.[31] Due to no nationally systematic training on advance care planning, unsurprisingly, Indonesian healthcare professionals are largely unfamiliar with the complex concept of advance care planning as a continuous process of value identification, even though it may have been practiced to some extent without being formally recognized as advance care planning.

Since 2015, a series of palliative care training of trainer (ToT) programs targeting health-care professionals in referral and regional hospitals have been held in Jakarta and West Java as part of a joint collaboration between local and international non-governmental organizations (e.g., Indonesian Cancer Foundation, Rachel House Foundation, Indonesian Palliative Society and Singapore International Foundation).[21] Additionally, the Indonesian Ministry of Health has been conducting palliative care training for internists and pediatrics in provincial hospitals, general practitioners, and nurses in primary care clinics throughout Indonesia's 34 provinces. Both of these trainings covered serious illness communication, including advance care planning. However, except in a few institutions, such as the Internal Medicine sub-specialty of Psychosomatic and Palliative Medicine at Universitas Indonesia, advance care planning has not been included in the national curricula of formal education for health-care professionals in Indonesia. Finally, public education on advance care planning has been limited to initiatives by several civic societies or patient support groups.

Several international collaborative efforts in education have been conducted in the past as a result of a collaboration between Indonesian professional organizations and international organizations (e.g., International Palliative Care Workshop in 2017 as a collaboration between the Indonesian Association of Psychosomatic Medicine and the American Society of Clinical Oncology).[37]

In Indonesia, research on advance care planning has primarily focused on exploring patients', family members', and healthcare professionals' experiences and perspectives on advance care planning in order to better understand how advance care planning can be implemented in the local context, including potential barriers and facilitators.[30–32] In addition, an Indonesian representative has participated in numerous regional collaborative research projects supported by the Asia Pacific Hospice Palliative Care Network (APHN) and grants from certain collaborating countries. This work has resulted in several advocacy papers in Asia[21,38,39] and nurtured cross-learning between respective countries.

Future Directions for Advance Care Planning in Indonesia

Studies on advance care planning in Indonesia suggested that patients, family members, and healthcare professionals were willing to engage in advance care planning, but also considered that cultural sensitivity mattered to their engagement in it.[30–32] Culturally sensitive advance care planning in Indonesia should consider the importance of respecting the cultural aspects of collectivism (e.g., by facilitating open communication between patients and their families), communication norms (implicit versus explicit), the diverse perspectives on information provision and religious beliefs. Rather than focusing on writing treatment plans in advance,

advance care planning should focus on the continuous effort of exploring individuals' values, wishes, and preferences through their trajectory of illness.

Future directions for advance care planning implementation in this nation should include capacity building for advance care planning through establishing awareness through systematic education, both formal and informal. At a national level, the government in collaboration with professional organizations should establish systematic training programs on advance care planning, including its culturally sensitive approach, for all healthcare professionals. Civil society organizations and media should engage and raise public awareness through public education and campaign about advance care planning. To enable advance care planning implementation, national health policy should acknowledge the importance of respecting patients' autonomy and right to be involved in decision-making for their care at the end of life. Policymakers should integrate advance care planning into the national healthcare system and establish a financing platform. The government should develop national practice guidelines for advance care planning for various conditions (oncology and non-oncology, including dementia, pediatrics, etc.). Healthcare institutions should develop protocols for advance care planning and establish a documentation system for advance care planning.

Future research should focus on how advance care planning is implemented and evaluated in diverse settings and populations. Moreover, more studies are needed to understand how different communication styles (such as implicit communication, euphemism, metaphor, etc.) and religious views affect participation in advance care planning. International and regional research and education collaboration should be maintained, with an emphasis on how to assist and learn from one another.

References

1. National Statistic Bureau. (2022). *Statistical Yearbook of Indonesia 2022* [cited 25 April 2023]; Available from: https://www.bps.go.id/indicator/12/1975/1/jumlah-penduduk-pertengahan-tahun.html.
2. Mboi N., *et al.* (2018). On the road to universal health care in Indonesia, 1990–2016: A systematic analysis for the Global Burden of Disease Study 2016. *Lancet,* **392**(10147): 581–591.
3. Putranto R., *et al.* (2017). Development and challenges of palliative care in Indonesia: role of psychosomatic medicine. *BioPsychoSoc. Med.* **11**(1): 29.

4. Connor S. (2020). *Global Atlas of Palliative Care* (2nd edn.). Worldwide Palliative Care Alliance, London, UK.
5. Comprehensive Cancer Care of Cipto Mangunkusumo Hospital. (2023). Assessment of Palliative Care Integration into the Primary Healthcare System in Indonesia [unpublished study].
6. Institute for Health Metrics and Evaluation (IHME). *GBD Compare: Indonesia.* 2019 [cited 26 April 2023]. Available from: https://www.health-data.org/indonesia.
7. Knaul F. M., *et al.* (2018). Alleviating the access abyss in palliative care and pain relief-an imperative of universal health coverage: The Lancet Commission report. *Lancet,* **391**(10128): 1391–1454.
8. Gondhowiardjo S. (2019). Integrated Missions of the Programme of Action for Cancer Therapy (imPACT Reviews) in Indonesia [unpublished study].
9. Effendy C., *et al.* (2015). Comparison of problems and unmet needs of patients with advanced cancer in a European country and an Asian country. *Pain Pract.* **15**(5): 433–440.
10. Barry M.J., and Edgman-Levitan, S. (2012). Shared decision making — The pinnacle of patient-centered care. *N. Engl. J. Med.* **366**(9): 780–781.
11. Shalowitz, D. I., Garrett-Mayer, E., and Wendler, D. (2006). The accuracy of surrogate decision makers: A systematic review. *Arch. Intern. Med.* **166**(5): 493–497.
12. Coppola K.M., *et al.* (2001). Accuracy of primary care and hospital-based physicians' predictions of elderly outpatients' treatment preferences with and without advance directives. *Arch. Intern. Med.* **161**(3): 431–440.
13. Sabatino C. P. (2010). The evolution of health care advance planning law and policy. *Milbank Q,* **88**(2): 211–239.
14. Soerjomataram I., and Bray, F. (2021). Planning for tomorrow: Global cancer incidence and the role of prevention 2020–2070. *Nat. Rev. Clin. Oncol.* **18**(10): 663–672.
15. Hui D. (2015). Unexpected death in palliative care: What to expect when you are not expecting. *Curr. Opin. Support. Palliat. Care,* **9**(4): 369–374.
16. Witjaksono M.A., Sutandiyo N., and Suardi D. (2014). Regional support for palliative care in Indonesia [cited 21 February 2019]; Available from: https://ehospice.com/international_posts/regional-support-for-palliative-care-in-indonesia/.
17. Minister of Health of the Republic of Indonesia. (2007). Decree of the Minister of Health of the Republic of Indonesia No 812/Menkes/SK/VII/207 about Palliative Care Policy. M.o.H.o.t.R.o. Indonesia.
18. Ministry of Health of the Republic of Indonesia. (2014). Regulation of the Minister of Health Number 37 about the Determination of Death and Utilization of Donor Organs. Ministry of Health of the Republic of Indonesia, Jakarta.

19. Ministry of Health of the Republic of Indonesia. (2015). Pedoman Nasional Program Paliatif Kanker. The Ministry of Health of the Republic of Indonesia, Jakarta.
20. President of the Republic of Indonesia. (2023). Draft of Law of the Republic of Indonesia about Health. T.M.o.S. Secretary, Jakarta.
21. Cheng S.Y., *et al.* (2020). Advance care planning in Asian culture. *Jpn. J. Clin. Oncol.* **50**(9): 976–989.
22. Mahendradhata Y., *et al.* (2017). *The Republic of Indonesia Health System Review*. World Health Organization, Regional Office for South-East Asia, India.
23. Mori M., and Morita, T. (2020). End-of-life decision-making in Asia: A need for in-depth cultural consideration. *Palliat. Med.* 02692163198896932.
24. Effendy C., *et al.* (2015). Dealing with symptoms and issues of hospitalized patients with cancer in indonesia: The role of families, nurses, and physicians. *Pain Pract.* **15**(5): 441–446.
25. Kristanti M. S., *et al.* (2019). The experience of family caregivers of patients with cancer in an Asian country: A grounded theory approach. *Palliat. Med.* **33**(6): 676–684.
26. Claramita M., *et al.* (2013). Doctor-patient communication in Southeast Asia: A different culture? *Adv. Health Sci. Educ. Theory Pract.* **18**(1): 15–31.
27. Rochmawati E., Wiechula, R., and Cameron, K. (2018). Centrality of spirituality/religion in the culture of palliative care service in Indonesia: An ethnographic study. *Nurs. Health Sci.* **20**(2): 231–237.
28. Pew Research Center. (2020). The global God divide [cited 22 November 2021]. Available from: https://www.pewresearch.org/global/2020/07/20/the-global-god-divide/.
29. Garrido M.M., *et al.* (2013). Pathways from religion to advance care planning: Beliefs about control over length of life and end-of-life values. *Gerontologist*, **53**(5): 801–816.
30. Martina D., *et al.* (2023). Cancer survivors' experiences with and preferences for medical information disclosure and advance care planning: An online survey among Indonesian cancer support groups. *JCO Glob. Oncol.* (9): e2300003.
31. Martina D., *et al.* (2022). Opportunities and challenges for advance care planning in strongly religious family-centric societies: A focus group study of Indonesian cancer-care professionals. *BMC Palliat. Care*, **21**(1): 110.
32. Martina D., *et al.* (2022). Advance care planning for patients with cancer and family caregivers in Indonesia: A qualitative study. *BMC Palliat. Care*, **21**(1): 204.
33. Pradnyani N., and Suariyani, N. (2016). Family role in decision making of health seeking behavior on elderly in Tabanan Regency, Bali, Indonesia. *Epidemiology* (sunnyvale) **6**(218): 1–5.

34. Iskandarsyah A., *et al.* (2014). Psychosocial and cultural reasons for delay in seeking help and nonadherence to treatment in Indonesian women with breast cancer: A qualitative study. *Health Psychol.* **33**(3): 214–221.
35. Claramita M., *et al.* (2011). Doctor-patient communication in a Southeast Asian setting: The conflict between ideal and reality. *Adv. Health Sci. Educ. Theory Pract.* **16**(1): 69–80.
36. Wessner P. (2018). Last chance to care: An autoethnography of end-of-life care in Indonesia. *Qual. Rep.* **23**(9): 2238–2250.
37. American Society of Clinical Oncology. (2017). Interview with IPCW Indonesia Faculty. 3 July 2017 [cited 27 April 2023]. Available from: https://connection.asco.org/magazine/asco-international/interview-ipcw-indonesia-faculty-video.
38. Lin C. P., *et al.* (2023). Letter to the editor: Improving access to advance care planning in current and future public health emergencies: International challenges and recommendations. *J. Palliat. Med.* **26**(4): 462–463.
39. Lin C.-P., *et al.* (2019). 2019 Taipei declaration on advance care planning: A cultural adaptation of end-of-life care discussion. *J. Palliat. Med.* **22**(10): 1175–1177.

Chapter 25

Advance Care Planning in Australia: Progress in Research and Implementation*

Craig Sinclair[†,‡], Jill Mann[§], Liz Reymond[¶,‖],
and Xanthe Sansome[**]

†School of Psychology, University of New South Wales, Sydney, Australia
‡Neuroscience Research Australia (NeuRA), Sydney, Australia
§Barwon Health Advance Care Planning Program, Geelong, Australia
*¶Statewide Office of Advance Care Planning, Brisbane South Palliative
Care Collaborative, Metro South Health, Brisbane, Australia*
*‖Griffith University School of Medicine
and Dentistry, Brisbane, Australia*
***Advance Care Planning Australia, Austin Health,
Melbourne, Australia*

Advance care planning (ACP) has developed steadily in Australia during the past two decades, following the establishment of the Respecting Patient Choices program in one Australian state. The foundational work of the Respecting Patient Choices program employed specialists, non-medical health professional facilitators, to assist patients, clients, family members and health professionals in initiating ACP discussions and

---

*Re-published with permission from special issue of ZEFQ journal; "Advance Care Planning around the World: Evidence and Experiences, Programmes and Perspectives".

documenting patient preferences. This work has since been developed by Advance Care Planning Australia, state and territory agencies, and non-government organisations. During this period, the six state and two territory jurisdictions in Australia have developed policy and practice in ACP, in accordance with their local resources, legislation and populations. These initiatives have contributed to some progress in embedding ACP as part of routine care in Australia, a goal identified by the Royal Australian College of General Practitioners.[1] While the international COVID-19 pandemic stimulated public discussion and brought issues of ACP to the fore,[2] there are a number of ongoing challenges. These include discomfort with ACP discussion, a lack of consistency in legislation and ACP documentation across jurisdictions, poor accessibility and quality control of completed ACP documents, difficulties accessing ACP documents at the point of care and broader challenges in coordinating implementation for a diverse, ageing and geographically dispersed population. This chapter presents the historical and legal foundations of ACP in Australia and provides an update on recent implementation work across different settings.

Background of the Australian Health and Social Care System

The Australian healthcare system is considered to be advanced in a number of respects, including well-developed primary, secondary and tertiary sectors, and infrastructure to support digital health and clinical research. The Australian healthcare system also provides services to a population across vast geographic distances, and island communities outside of the mainland part of the continent. The rural and remote health system providing these services is mostly coordinated by primary care professionals (e.g., general practitioners and community-based nurses along with some rurally-based specialists), as well as locum specialists and support staff, and infrastructure for emergency transfers to tertiary hospitals in metropolitan centres. While the healthcare system is funded and administered by state and territory governments, aged care services[a] (provided to older adults who meet assessed

---

[a]Aged care services provide: (i) home- or centre-based supports, to meet person-centred needs for cleaning, social support, clinical support and palliative care in the person's home or the organisation's centre; or (ii) long-term care, where a person moves into a room in a residential aged care home. An aged care home resident shares the facility with 10–400 other residents and has access to 24-hour care, inclusive of meals, personal care, activities of interest, clinical care and end-of-life care.

criteria) are delivered through approved providers of community-based or residential aged care services, which are funded and regulated at a national level by the Australian government. The Australian population is rapidly ageing, with a projected increase in the older adult population (people 65 years of age or older) from 4.31 million to 6.66 million between 2021 and 2041, an increase of 54%.[3] The older adult population in Australia is also culturally and linguistically diverse, with 37% of the older adult (65 years and over) population being born overseas.[4] Aboriginal and Torres Strait Islander peoples are the First Nations people of Australia, representing over 250 unique language groups and 3.3% of the Australian population. These unique geographic and population characteristics have influenced the focus of ACP policy and practice in Australia.

Policy and Legislative Frameworks

Australia has a federated system of state and territory governments, with primary responsibility for legislation and service delivery relating to healthcare. There are legal frameworks in place across all states and territories for recognising substitute decision-makers (SDMs) nominated by a person, to make health or lifestyle decisions. Advance care directives (ACDs) are also recognised in all jurisdictions, either under statutory legislation or common law precedent.[5] In all cases individuals who are over 18 and who have full legal capacity for decision-making may complete formal ACP documents, as well as revising or revoking their existing ACP documents at any time.

While these legal frameworks are in place across Australia, there are inconsistencies between the states and territories in their laws, terminology for ACP documents, circumstances under which ACDs can be overridden and local policy initiatives.[6] These inconsistencies make it challenging to coordinate a national approach to ACP implementation, as well as generating confusion and anxiety among health professionals and community members.

At a national level, quality standards for hospitals and aged care providers require provision of information about ACP and maintenance of systems for storing and accessing ACP documents.[7,8] However as these health and aged care services are typically organised and delivered at a regional or district level, or by non-government organisations, there is no overarching system for measuring the frequency or quality of ACP discussions or documentation across these settings. These policy and legislative inconsistencies, divide between state and federal level regulation, along with the diversity of the relevant populations and services for which ACP is relevant, have presented challenges for national definitions or a "model" approach to ACP implementation, a topic which is addressed below.

Definitions and Model of Advance Care Planning

There is no definitive model for ACP in Australia, instead, a range of programs, training resources, documents and local initiatives are implemented, often with tailoring for particular sub-groups or local jurisdictional requirements. Initial efforts to implement ACP (particularly those informed by the Respecting Patient Choices program) have tended to use "specialist facilitator" models, often working with hospital inpatients, or people receiving outpatient care in community settings.[9,10] While this approach has been shown to be effective in increasing ACP engagement and uptake,[11,12] and can enable individual practitioners to accumulate substantial skills and experience in ACP, it is also resource intensive. It also may not be as well suited in rural and remote health settings, where populations are more thinly distributed and healthcare is predominantly delivered by generalist health professionals. The recurring challenge being managed across all settings is how best to use limited healthcare resources to reach the right people, at the right time and place, with the right information and ACP conversations.

The Respecting Patient Choices program, along with more recent developments by Advance Care Planning Australia (https://www.advancecareplanning.org.au) have gone some way to identifying agreed standards for best practice in ACP and promoting consistent approaches to implementation across jurisdictions and settings. Position statements from health practitioner professional colleges in support of ACP,[1] and national quality standards for health and aged care providers have also encouraged broader adoption of ACP.[7,8,13] Online training modules provided by Advance Care Planning Australia (https://www.advancecareplanning.org.au/training-and-education/online-courses) aim to provide foundational knowledge for a wide group of health and care professionals, as well as the broader community. A revised *National Framework for advance care planning documents* was produced in 2021, which aimed to support "…uptake of a shared language and common approach to advance care planning and… mutual recognition of Advance

Care Directives across state and territory borders."[6] In addition to addressing issues of terminology for relevant legal documents and advance care directives (ACDs), this framework emphasises the importance of ACP conversations, which are initiated early and revisited regularly across an individual's life course. It also provides guidance on best practice principles for initiating conversations, as well as storing, accessing and enacting ACP documents. While to date this framework has not enabled consistent legislation across jurisdictions, it has provided a common language and shared understanding to inform further research and implementation work.

Implementation of Advance Care Planning in Australia

As one way of quantifying progress in ACP implementation, recent studies led by Advance Care Planning Australia have developed a nationally applicable method for determining the prevalence of ACDs, and other ACP documentation, among older adults in client and/or health records held by hospitals, residential aged care or general practice sites.[14] A nation-wide audit study of 100 sites and 4187 older adult health records determined the weighted prevalence of ACDs to be 14%, while ACP documentation (a broader category also including documents created by health professionals or other people) was estimated to be present in 29% of records.[15] People born in Australia were more likely to have completed their own ACD, while among those born outside Australia, there were higher rates of ACP documents being completed on the person's behalf.[16] While ACP documents are just one indicator of implementation and uptake, these data suggest that efforts to date have had a modest impact on ACP documentation at the point of care, and also that uptake is higher among those from a white, Anglo-Australian background.[16] Given the cultural diversity of the older adult population in Australia, this suggests the need to expand and tailor ACP information and resources for diverse communities.

Following initial efforts focused on implementing "specialist facilitator" ACP models, attention has turned to engaging and building capacity among broader stakeholder groups, including health professionals in diverse settings. A range of projects have been funded to support ACP practice in different settings, a selection of which are included here. The

End of Life Directions in Aged Care (ELDAC) program (https://www.eldac.com.au) and The Advance Project (https://www.theadvanceproject.com.au) are both targeted to staff working in aged care and primary care sectors. The Cognitive Decline Partnership Centre developed resources to guide the practice of supported decision-making for a range of decisions (including ACP) among people with dementia (https://cdpc.sydney.edu.au/research/planning-decision-making-and-risk/supported-decision-making/). The Groundswell Project (https://www.thegroundswellproject.com) aims to empower community members of all ages and health states with knowledge and "death literacy", through grassroots and community-focused initiatives, which align with principles of the public health approach to palliative care.[17]

At a systems level, there are some initiatives to enable storing, accessing and sharing ACP documents.[6] The Australian Digital Health Agency provides the "My Health Record", a digital platform that enables individuals, their authorised representatives and some GPs, to upload ACP documents[b] into a centralised system that can be accessed by registered service providers in the hospital, aged care and primary care settings.[18] The state of Queensland (population of 5.3 million people, or 20% of the Australian population) established a Statewide Office of Advance Care Planning. This office reviews and stores a range of ACP documents, aiming to ensure real-time accessibility of quality documentation across primary, emergency, acute and residential care services. As at 31 March 2023, there were 108,694 relevant ACP documents uploaded to this system.[19] Within both of these systems individuals are able to make revisions to their ACP document, while they have full legal capacity for decision-making.

Impact of COVID-19

The onset of the COVID-19 pandemic in early 2020 has been felt globally, although Australia was arguably fortunate in terms of being able to close international and state borders to slow the initial spread of the virus and

---

[b]Documentation can include statutory (legally-binding) advance care directives (ACDs) outlining preferences for care, statutory ACDs that nominate a substitute decision-maker (SDM) for health or personal matters in the event the person loses decision-making capacity, mental health ACDs and non-statutory ACP documents.

new variants. Despite this, Australia still experienced significant impacts, particularly among vulnerable communities including Aboriginal and Torres Strait Islander communities and those in residential aged care settings. The COVID-19 pandemic impacted the urgency, uptake and use of ACP in a range of ways. The Australian Government's Health Sector Emergency Response Plan outlined strategies for preparing and supporting health systems through the initial stages of the pandemic, including encouraging the completion of ACDs in residential aged-care settings.[20] Telehealth and video-conferencing platforms were increasingly adopted for ACP conversations, and in some jurisdictions, digital witnessing (i.e., by video conference) of legally-binding documents was enabled, through legislative amendments.[21,22] In some jurisdictions in which medical professional witnessing of ACDs was a requirement, this requirement was relaxed, to enable nurse practitioners to undertake this role.[22] In Queensland, the Statewide Office of Advance Care Planning documented an increase in phone consultations about ACP, and an increase in ACP documents received from residential aged care homes.[23] Discussions and contingency planning regarding the criteria for rationing limited healthcare resources (e.g., ventilators and intensive care unit spaces) ensued.[24] In many settings staff were limited to working with a single service provider or hospital ward, and some residential aged care settings became temporary accommodation settings for staff caring for COVID-positive residents. Viral transmission to and between healthcare professionals placed increased pressure on the remaining staff and required the diversion of those staff normally engaged in ACP facilitation, to support acute care teams.

As the pandemic transitions to a new phase, with large proportions of the Australian community now vaccinated, attention has shifted to lessons learned. The widespread shift to digital formats for ACP training, discussions and even document witnessing or distribution has had diverse effects. A range of non-regulated commercial providers now offer digital ACP documents requiring upfront and annual maintenance payments. There has also been greater impetus to increase the number of paper ACP documents uploaded to the My Health Record platform, with trial projects underway to support increased compatibility between the national platform and medical practice software in primary care, residential aged care and community health settings. In most cases, there are no systems in place for identifying document type or enabling quality control of document completion or legal validity, despite data showing a significant proportion of ACDs in health records are not legally valid.[15] Rather than promoting national consistency in ACP, these disparate trials and innovations may in fact result in further fragmentation. Further work will be required to understand the consequences of these various changes on the implementation and uptake of ACP, as well as the protection of patient rights through the ACP process.

Future Research Agenda on Advance Care Planning

A number of ongoing initiatives contribute to progressing the broader work in this area. Advance Care Planning Australia, a peak non-government organisation focused on raising awareness and improving practice in ACP, is funded by the federal government, through recurrent fixed-term grants. Other organisations such as Palliative Care Australia (and state and territory branches) also contribute to local advocacy and training. State and territory government agencies (e.g., Public Guardians or Public Advocates) make available information and resources about ACP and SDM appointments. In 2020, the National Health and Medical Research Council made a Targeted Call for Research in End of Life Care, and four projects (each five years duration) were funded.[25] There is increasing emphasis on ensuring that community members with lived experience (people with life-limiting illnesses and people who provide unpaid care) are actively involved in the design and conduct of research and service delivery projects.[26] There is also a growing focus on addressing the needs of marginalised communities in ACP research, including people from Aboriginal and Torres Strait Islander communities, people from culturally and linguistically diverse communities, rural and remote communities, people at risk of or experiencing homelessness, people in incarceration or in institutional settings, people living with dementia or a disability, adolescents and younger adults and people from LGBTQI+ communities.[27]

Conclusion

This piece has aimed to provide an update on the recent progress in ACP in Australia, and the main issues to address in future work. While a range of programs and resources are available to support practice in ACP, the diverse, ageing and geographically disparate population in Australia presents challenges in adopting a coherent approach or "model" for ACP implementation. The COVID-19 pandemic disrupted standard practice and resulted in a range of innovations, some of which have persisted following the relaxation of public health restrictions. Future directions for research and practice will need to focus on oversight of ACP document quality, and tailoring ACP programs to meet the needs of the diverse Australian community. Continued efforts to promote cross-jurisdictional compatibility of ACP documents and alignment with best-practice principles in ACP, will be important during the next phase of developing ACP in Australia.

References

1. Royal Australian College of General Practitioners. (2012). Position Statement: Advance Care Planning Should Be Incorporated into Routine General Practice. Available from: https://www.racgp.org.au/advocacy/position-statements/view-all-position-statements/clinical-and-practice-management/advance-care-planning.
2. Block B.L., Smith A.K., and Sudore R.L. (2020). During COVID-19, outpatient advance care planning is imperative: We need all hands on deck. *J. Am. Geriatr. Soc.* **68**(7): 1395–1397.
3. Wilson T., Temple J.B. (2022). New Population Projections for Australia and the States and Territories, with a Particular Focus on Population Ageing. University of Melbourne, Melbourne.
4. Australian Bureau of Statistics. (2019). 3412.0 — Migration, Australia, 2017–18. Australian Bureau of Statistics, Canberra. Available from: https://www.abs.gov.au/AUSSTATS/abs@.nsf/DetailsPage/3412.02017-18?OpenDocument.
5. Carter R.Z., Detering K.M., Silvester W., and Sutton E. (2016). Advance care planning in Australia: What does the law say? *Aust. Health Rev.* **40**(4): 405–414.
6. Department of Health. (2021). National Framework for Advance Care Planning Documents. Canberra.
7. Aged Care Quality and Safety Commission. (2018). Quality Standards: Aged Care Quality and Safety Commission. Available from: https://www.agedcarequality.gov.au/providers/standards.
8. Australian Commission on Safety and Quality in Health Care. (2021). National Safety and Quality Health Service (NSQHS) Standards: Australian Commission on Safety and Quality in Health Care. Available from: https://www.safetyandquality.gov.au/standards/nsqhs-standards.
9. Rogers J., Goldsmith C., Sinclair C., and Auret K.A. (2019). The advance care planning nurse facilitator: Describing the role and identifying factors associated with successful implementation. *Aust. J. Prim. Health* **25**(6): 564–569.

10. Detering K.M., Hancock A.D., Reade M.C., and Silvester W. (2010). The impact of advance care planning on end of life care in elderly patients: Randomised controlled trial. *Br. Med. J.* **340**: c1345.

11. Johnson S.B., Butow P.N., Bell M.L., Detering K., Clayton J.M., Silvester W., *et al.* (2018). A randomised controlled trial of an advance care planning intervention for patients with incurable cancer. *Br. J. Cancer* **119**(10): 1182–1190.

12. Sinclair C., Auret K., Evans S.F., Williamson F., Dormer S., Wilkinson A., *et al.* (2017). Advance care planning uptake among patients with severe lung disease: A randomised patient preference trial of a nurse-led, facilitated advance care planning intervention. *BMJ Open* **7**: e013415.

13. Australian Commission on Safety and Quality in Health Care. (2015). National Consensus Statement: Essential Elements for Safe and High-Quality End-of-Life Care in Acute Hospitals. ACSQHC, Sydney.

14. Detering K.M., Buck K., Sellars M., Kelly H., Sinclair C., White B., *et al.* (2019). Prospective multicentre cross-sectional audit among older Australians accessing health and residential aged care services: Protocol for a national advance care directive prevalence study. *BMJ Open* **9**(10): e031691.

15. Buck K., Nolte L., Sellars M., Sinclair C., White B.P., Kelly H., *et al.* (2021). Advance care directive prevalence among older Australians and associations with person-level predictors and quality indicators. *Health Expect.* **24**(4): 1312–1325.

16. Sinclair C., Sellars M., Buck K., Detering K.M., White B.P., and Nolte L. (2021). Association between region of birth and advance care planning documentation among older Australian migrant communities: A multi-center audit study. *J. Gerontol. Ser. B.* **76**(1): 109–120.

17. Kellehear A. (2016). Commentary: Public health approaches to palliative care — The progress so far. *Prog. Palliat. Care* **24**(1): 36–38.

18. Australian Digital Health Agency. (2020). My Health Record: Australian Government. Available from: https://www.myhealthrecord.gov.au/.

19. Queensland Government. (2022). Office of Advance Care Planning Monthly Statistics. In: Office of Advance Care Planning. Queensland Government, Brisbane.

20. Australian Government Department of Health. (2020). Australian Health Sector Emergency Response Plan for Novel Coronavirus (COVID-19). In: Department of Health. Department of Health, Canberra, p. 56.

21. Guardianship Act 1987 No 257 (2023).

22. Powers of Attorney Act 1998 (2023).

23. Queensland Office of Advance Care Planning. (2020). Information provided by Healthcare Purchasing Strategy Unit. Queensland Health.

24. MacIntyre C.R., and Heslop D.J. (2020). Public health, health systems and palliation planning for COVID-19 on an exponential timeline. *Med. J. Aust.* Available from: https://onlinelibrary.wiley.com/doi/abs/10.5694/mja2.50592.

25. National Health & Medical Research Council. Targeted Calls for Research 2023 [16/3/2023]. Available from: https://www.nhmrc.gov.au/funding/targeted-calls-research#download.
26. National Health & Medical Research Council. (2016). Statement on Consumer and Community Involvement in Health and Medical Research.
27. Australian Government Department of Health. (2018). National Palliative Care Strategy 2018. Canberra: Australian Government Department of Health.

Chapter 26

Tō tatou reo — Our Voice: Advance Care Planning in Aotearoa New Zealand*

Jane Goodwin

*Advance Care Planning, Te Tāhū Hauora Health Quality &
Safety Commission, Wellington, New Zealand*

Background on Aotearoa New Zealand

Aotearoa New Zealand (New Zealand) is a collection of islands in the southwestern Pacific Ocean. The country is long and thin, with 15,134 km of coastline and a land mass comparable to that of the United Kingdom and Japan.[1]

The New Zealand population is 5.1 million, and approximately half of the residents live in four main urban areas.[2] The 2018 census reported that nearly 800,000 people (16.5%) living in New Zealand were of Māori descent, and 70% of the population identified as being of European heritage. Other major ethnic groups include Asian (15%) and Pacific peoples (8%).[3]

The Treaty of Waitangi (Te Tiriti o Waitangi) is New Zealand's founding document. Signed in 1840 by Māori chiefs (rangatira) and representatives of the British crown, the Treaty guides the relationship between the

---

*Re-published with permission from special issue of ZEFQ journal; "Advance Care Planning around the World: Evidence and Experiences, Programmes and Perspectives".

Crown in New Zealand (embodied by our government) and Māori. The Treaty promised to protect Māori and Māori culture and to enable Māori to continue to live in New Zealand as Māori despite the increasing arrival of Europeans.

Colonisation, non-adherence to Te Tiriti o Waitangi, institutional racism and a lack of cultural safety has resulted in Māori being significantly disadvantaged compared with the European majority. People who identify as Māori are twice as likely as non-Māori to die from cardiovascular disease and are more likely to be diagnosed with and die from cancer. Māori tamariki (children) have a mortality rate 1.5 times the rate of non-Māori children.[4]

Background of the Health Care System

New Zealand's health care system is predominately funded by general taxation, with an annual budget of approximately $NZ 20 billion (€12,825,400,000)[5] per year.

A health and disability system review in 2019–20 highlighted New Zealand's unacceptable Māori health inequities. This resulted in significant policy change and transformational health reforms, which began in July 2022.[4]

In an effort to centralise health care commissioning and delivery, the previous 20 district health boards were decommissioned and four new entities were established: Te Whatu Ora — Health New Zealand, Te Aka Whai Ora — the Māori Health Authority, Te Pou Hauora Tūmatanui — the Public Health Agency, and Whaikaha — the Ministry of Disabled Peoples. The entities are underpinned by Te Tiriti o Waitangi principles and work in partnership to support a whole-of-country approach to planning and service delivery.[6]

Advance care planning plays a significant role in two of the key outcome priorities of the health system reforms. First, as a tool to elevate person- and whānau[a]-centred care, empowering all people to manage their own health and wellbeing so they have meaningful control over the services they receive and acknowledging that people, their carers and whānau are experts in their care. And second, as a tool to address inequity

---

[a]Whānau: extended family, family group, a familiar term of address to a number of people — the primary economic unit of traditional Māori society. In the modern context, the term is sometimes used to include friends who may not have any kinship ties to other members (Te Aka Māori dictionary).

by tackling the gaps in access and health outcomes between different populations and areas of New Zealand, with a particular focus on outcomes for Māori, Pacific peoples and disabled people.

The reforms provide the opportunity to leverage existing advance care planning ethos and tools to increase consistency and equity in advance care planning systems and delivery across the country. However, the changes and transitions inherent in the reforms have affected organisational decision-making, and many interim entities are unwilling to commit to progressing existing or proposed projects. There is a lot of "waiting" for what might come next.

Policy or Legislative Efforts/Milestones

Te Tiriti o Waitangi and the Code of Health and Disability Services Consumers' Rights (the Code) have led to a unique environment for the evolution of advance care planning in New Zealand.

The four articles of Te Tiriti o Waitangi are kāwanatanga (self-governance), mana motuhake (self-determination), tino rangatiratanga (autonomy) and wairuatanga (spirituality). They promote person and whānau centricity in relationships between Crown agencies and Māori and place responsibility on the health workforce to provide services that are culturally safe and equitable.[7]

Advance care planning provides a tangible way to actualise Te Tiriti o Waitangi in clinical practice. Care and treatment are informed equally by the person and their whānau and health care providers in a relationship modelled on shared decision-making (kāwanatanga). Whānau-centric decision-making recognises Māori authority and autonomy, enabling the right for Māori to be Māori, to exercise their authority over their own lives and to live on Māori terms and according to Māori philosophies, values and practices (tino rangatiratanga). In advance care planning, Māori world views, values and belief systems (what is important to you) are prioritised in care and treatment planning in ways that enable Māori to live, thrive and flourish as Māori.

The Code provides the legal framework for clinical decision-making. Consumers have the right to receive services that respect their dignity and independence, are consistent with their needs, minimise potential harm and optimise their quality of life. If consumers are unable to speak for themselves, they have the right to have clinicians make treatment and care decisions that are consistent with their values, goals and preferences.[8]

In the context of advance care planning, clinicians are required to take a person's values, aspirations and preferences into consideration and are legally bound to follow a valid advance directive.

Definition(s) and Model(s) of ACP Used

Advance care planning in New Zealand is defined as a process of discussion and shared planning for future health care, which involves an individual and their family and whānau and health care professionals.

It gives people the opportunity to develop and express their preferences for future care based on:

- their values, beliefs, concerns, hopes and goals
- a better understanding of their current and likely future health
- the treatment and care options available.

Our vision is to empower all New Zealanders to participate in planning their future care. Our programme develops education, tools and resources to support people and clinicians to optimise the opportunities for a person's voice to be heard and to inform care throughout the person's life.

Our multi-year strategy for 2022–28 was informed and shaped by the recommendations of our Māori partners and is based on the premise that what works for Māori will work for New Zealand.[9] Our strategic priorities and core values (as follows) inform the work we do.

Our Strategic Priorities | Ā mātau kaupapa rautaki matua

Improving experiences for consumers and whānau.

- Embedding and enacting Te Tiriti o Waitangi, supporting mana motuhake.
- Achieving health equity.
- Strengthening systems for high-quality services.

Core Values | Mātāpono

Spirituality | Wairuatanga — the recognition and expression of wairuatanga is valued and encouraged within all processes and domains of advance care planning.

Genealogy and identity | Whakapapa me te tuakiritanga — the unique and full expression of identity is encouraged and valued. The unique mana, whakapapa and ancestry of everyone are respected and accepted through the process of advance care planning. Whānau is the centre of a Māori worldview.

Holistic multi-generational guardianship to keep whānau safe | Kaitiakitanga — an advance care plan is a whānau taonga.[b] Advance care planning combines spiritual, cultural and practical processes to guide and strengthen whānau across generations.

Unity through consensus, collective decision-making | Kotahitanga — advance care planning encourages whānau- and person-centred decision-making processes and supports mana motuhake.

The strategy contains six workstreams that guide our programme delivery. Each includes an objective, strategic overview and actions for both the national advance care planning team and local providers.[9]

Governance and leadership | Mana whakahaere: Supporting cultural safety.

Promotion | Ngā whakatairanga: Normalise person- and whānau-centric care planning.

Tools and resources | Ngā rauemi: Advance care planning is available to all.

Education and training | Whakangungu: A prepared workforce and community.

Monitoring and evaluation | Aroturuki me to aromatawai: Care is based on what matters to consumers.

Implementation | Whakakaupapa: Maximising value.

Groups Addressed

In New Zealand, advance care planning is seen as a process that is applicable across a person's lifetime. It focuses on what is most important to the person and their whānau and is about preparing all people to make decisions now and in the future. Although the advance care plan may contain an advance directive, the plan predominantly focuses on what matters to the person and their goals and values rather than on specific treatment decisions.

---

[b] A taonga is a treasure, anything prized — applied to anything considered to be of value, including socially or culturally valuable objects, resources, phenomenon, ideas and techniques (Te Aka Māori dictionary).

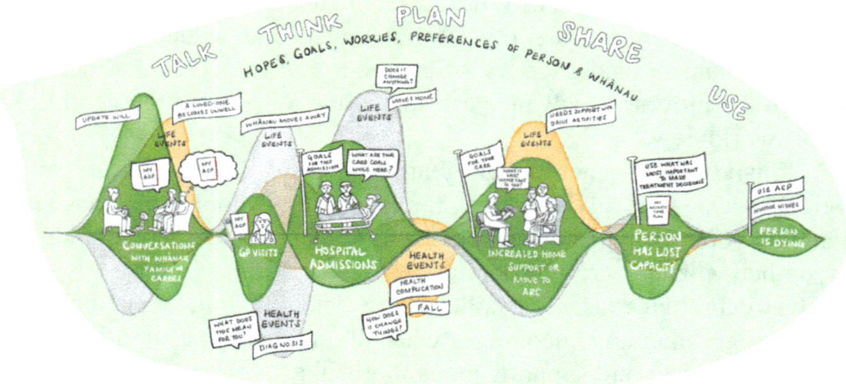

Figure 1.   The advance care planning process in New Zealand. ACP = advance care plan; ARC = aged residential care; GP = general practitioner.

The relevance and prevalence of talking and thinking about, planning around and sharing and using what matters most ebbs and flows through life as health and personal circumstances change (Figure 1).

We use different tools and resources to support different points in a person's advance care planning journey across their lifetime. These include the Advance Care Plan and Guide,[10] Whenua Ki Te Whenua,[11] the Serious Illness Conversation Guide (SICG)[12] and Shared Goals of Care,[13] which is targeted advance care planning for an episode of care in an acute or aged residential care setting.

In New Zealand, an advance care plan is a consumer document. Clinicians and clinical systems are involved and can support its development and sharing, but it belongs to the person and their whānau.

Education/Training of Health Care Professionals and Non-health Care Professionals in ACP

Advance care planning training in New Zealand has evolved over time. It was originally a nationally led workforce training programme delivered by a small group of national trainers, whereas the approach now integrates

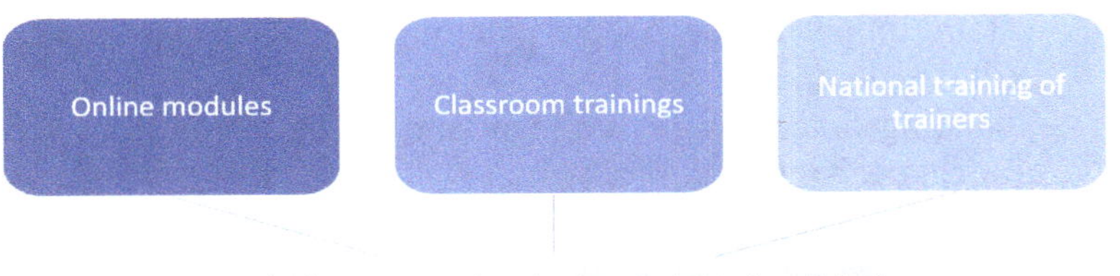

Figure 2.   Education and training — a prepared workforce and community.

online education and a train-the-trainer model, and staff from local Te Whatu Ora teams deliver workshops to their local clinicians.

The focus of education has also shifted from advanced communication training for small groups of senior healthcare professionals to increase the clinical communication competency of the wider workforce. This has been facilitated through online training modules, one-day advance care planning workshops and the SICG programme (see Figure 2).

Online Training

The advance care planning and clinical communication programme offers a suite of online training resources that has been developed over the past 10 years. Some were designed as preparatory learning for in-person workshops, and others were created as additional information and/or training resources in response to requests from the sector. Modules include the following.

1. Basic training ("what is advance care planning?"): a short film that explains what advance care planning is, discusses the benefits from the perspectives of both patients and health care staff and advises where to find further information.
2. Level 1 eLearning training ("how can I start a conversation with a patient or my loved one?"): provided through the following four eLearning modules.
    - Considering advance care planning — completing your own advance care plan, which ensures health care staff have experienced completing a plan before supporting patients with theirs.

- Talking about advance care planning — basic communication skill development.
- Changing outcomes — the legal and ethical framework around clinical decision-making.
- Clarifying advance care planning processes — creating systems and processes to facilitate the recording and retrieving of advance care planning conversations and plans.

3. Implicit bias: Three video-based modules introduce bias for people working in the health care sector who engage directly with consumers or who influence the way health organisations are managed. The modules encourage health professionals to examine their biases and how they affect both the health care they provide and their interactions with consumers and therefore their health outcomes.
4. An introduction to the SICG: This module includes an outline of the problem, the difference good communication and person-centric care can make, an introduction to the SICG and two case studies using the SICG.
5. An overview of the New Zealand legal framework for medical decision-making: A video resource including narrative, closed captions and graphics to explain the New Zealand medical decision-making structure.
6. One-hour SICG training video and supporting webinars: These resources were developed during the COVID-19 pandemic and provide an overview of the SICG, examples of conversations using the SICG, case studies and a guide to documentation.
7. Shared goals of care using the SICG: This module outlines the importance of person-centric discussions and includes an introduction to the SICG, three examples of conversations between an actor and clinicians using the guide and examples of documentation using the shared goals of care template.
8. SICG and shared goals of care for aged residential care: The final module in the current suite demonstrates the use of the SICG and shared goals of care in the aged residential care environment.

Classroom Training

1. One-day advance care planning workshop: This workshop builds on the Level 1 e-learning modules and is targeted at health care professionals and members of the health management team interested in

learning more about advance care planning policies and processes. The workshop is delivered by local trainers and supports participants to:

- take part in basic or uncomplicated advance care planning conversations
- explore the New Zealand legal framework for advance care planning
- explore ethical challenges in advance care planning and how this might impact practice
- capture a patient's voice through conversations and documentation.

2. Serious Illness Conversation Programme: In late 2018, Te Tāhū Hauora Health Quality & Safety Commission (Te Tāhū Hauora) partnered with Ariadne Labs to bring the Serious Illness Conversation programme to New Zealand as a way of increasing the clinical communication competency of the wider health workforce. To ensure the language used in the SICG was appropriate for use in New Zealand, the national programme team led workshops with healthcare professionals, cultural advisors and consumers to adapt the guide to the New Zealand context. The programme provides a system, training and tools to help healthcare professionals improve the quality of their conversations with patients and whānau about what matters to them and incorporate that into treatment planning. The 3-hour workshop is delivered by local district trainers, allowing for an easily scalable training model, targeted delivery and the flexibility to be integrated into existing training structures.

Community Activator Training

Te Tāhū Hauora is currently developing community activator training with Māori champions. We have piloted several different approaches and collected feedback from our Māori and rural community champions through the Kaupapa Hapori project.

We see this project as an opportunity to optimise the huge amount of skill, knowledge and passion for advance care planning that exists in our communities while supporting them to explore advance care planning in a way that works for them.

Information Materials Used, Documentation and Digitalization of ACP Processes in the Health Care Sector and Beyond

Our programme has created resources, tools and education to support people and clinicians to optimise the opportunities for a person's voice to be heard and to inform care throughout the person's life.

These include a website for consumers and clinicians; national hard copy and electronic templates for the advance care plan, SICG and shared goals of care; and promotional resources for the community and clinicians.

New Zealand does not have a unified electronic patient record. Most Te Whatu Ora districts have their own electronic solution that does not integrate with other acute facilities or primary care organisations. A priority of the health reforms is to optimise and make electronic resources compatible, which will provide significant opportunities for sharing advance care planning tools and templates.

Examples of Institutional and Community Implementation

The national advance care planning programme's role in implementation is to provide guidance, direction and connection for the local Te Whatu Ora advance care planning implementation managers actualising the work in their organisations and facilities (Figure 3).

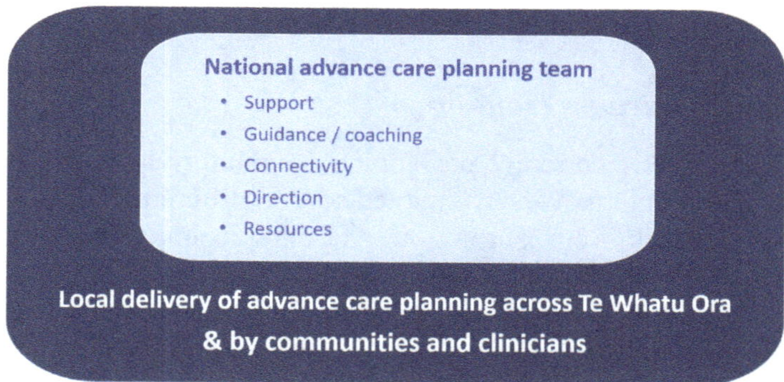

Figure 3.   Implementation — maximising value.

Some Te Whatu Ora districts have dedicated funded staff to support the work, whereas others have passionate people who do their best to champion and promote advance care planning on top of their existing roles.

The national programme team lead 6-weekly virtual hui (meetings) to connect advance care planning and shared goals of care implementation teams across the country. These sessions encourage districts to connect with each other, talk about the different initiatives they are working on and share their successes and challenges. Hui are always well attended and give the national team valuable insight into the daily realities for practitioners and opportunities to support them. These hui are also a great channel to gather feedback and share messaging with those working with consumers.

Feedback and requests from these hui enable the programme to respond to sector and community needs. For example, Te Tāhū Hauora partnered with Manatū Hauora to develop the publication, *Responding when a person raises assisted dying: A conversation guide for health professionals*[14] and an associated handbook for practitioners.[15] It is based on the SICG concept and uses consumer-developed language to help a healthcare professional navigate the conversation while meeting both the person's needs and the legal requirements of the End of Life Choice Act 2019.

Similarly, during the height of the COVID-19 pandemic, Te Tāhū Hauora developed a suite of resources in partnership with Manatū Hauora to support the community response to COVID-19 management.

Research in ACP in New Zealand?

The New Zealand advance care planning programme is funded until 2024 by the now-disestablished district health boards. The budget is small, and there is no provision for dedicated advance care planning research. We leverage research conducted overseas and use our limited resources to support the actualisation of advance care planning across our system and communities.

Patient and Public Involvement (Patient Movement) in Research and Development of ACP

Advance care planning in Aotearoa has always looked to our communities to support and inform our work, and co-design is an important component of our programme resources.

Addressing Diversity and Vulnerabilities (Cultural, Social) Regarding ACP Access and Use

The advance care planning programme actively partners with Māori leaders, experts and whānau Māori to develop solutions and uses information that includes Māori world views, priorities, experiences and solutions to address inequity and advance Māori health.

As described, improving access to services and reducing inequities is a strong driver for the advance care planning programme. Our priority populations are Māori, rural communities and the disability community.

Main Challenges and Barriers

Funding

The advance care planning programme in New Zealand has become proficient at getting maximum value and output from minimal resources and financial investment.

Funding challenges also affect our local teams. Many of these teams are established as part of a short-term project, with funders expecting advance care planning to have been embedded as business as usual at the end of the funding cycle. In reality, advance care planning requires long-term investment to ensure the voice of the person and their family and whānau remains at the centre of their care.

Health Reforms

The ongoing health reforms add another layer of complexity to our service delivery. We are challenged to ensure advance care planning remains visible and that we optimise opportunities to make sure advance care planning and what matters to the person and their family and whānau is woven and considered throughout the infrastructure of the new system.

Health Inequities

We continue to navigate the complexities of our colonial heritage and a predominately Eurocentric and paternalistic health system. Our work is challenging for many of our health professionals. Asking them to consistently align the care they deliver with what matters most to the person is not always well received.

Whose Responsibility Is This?

Although the system and health care professionals are increasingly supportive of the concept of advance care planning, the reality of it being actualised is often not realised. We frequently see the task of introducing advance care planning being passed from service to service with no one committing to supporting the process. This is further exacerbated by a siloed system with frequently poor communication.

Our hope is that an increasing focus on the community supporting these conversations across a person's life journey will act as a counterbalance and reinforce that advance care planning is everyone's business and that we all have a role to play in supporting a person and their family and whānau to share what matters most.

Collaborations with Other Countries/Programmes Regarding ACP

Advance care planning New Zealand regularly collaborates with the team implementing advance care planning in British Colombia, Canada. Both the New Zealand and British Colombian programmes are navigating similar issues and challenges. The opportunity to meet regularly to share experiences and resources has been invaluable. The New Zealand programme also maintains a strong relationship with the training and implementation team at Ariadne Labs, Boston, MA, USA.

Conclusion

Over the last 12 years, the advance care planning programme has created a foundation to support people to think about what matters most to them; to provide them with the support, knowledge, tools and resources to articulate and record this important information; and to engage with a health system that prioritises their values and preferences for care and supports them to live the life they value.

References

1. Encyclopaedia of Nations. (2003). New Zealand country overview. https://www.nationsencyclopedia.com/economies/Asia-and-the-Pacific/New-Zealand.html. Accessed 27 January 2023.
2. Statistics New Zealand. (2023). Estimated population of NZ. https://www.stats.govt.nz/indicators/population-of-nz?gclid=CjwKCAiAo5qABhBdEiwAOtGmbtoGcmPVLsLRBo0r--lWkuz6YyxAVuwRoBxJfC2LZuZSl_J9711H1hoCnz4QAvD_BwE. 10 March 2023. Accessed 16 March 2023.
3. Statistics New Zealand. (2018). 2018 Census ethnic groups dataset. https://www.stats.govt.nz/information-releases/2018-census-ethnic-groups-dataset. Accessed 20 January 2023.
4. Health Navigator New Zealand. (2022). Māori health overview. https://www.healthnavigator.org.nz/clinicians/m/m%C4%81ori-health-overview/. Accessed 20 March 2023.
5. Manatū Hauora — Ministry of Health. (2022). Budget 2022: Vote health. https://www.health.govt.nz/about-ministry/what-we-do/budget-2022-vote-health. Accessed 21 March 2023.
6. Te Kāwanatanga o Aotearoa | New Zealand Government. (2022). Future of Health. https://www.futureofhealth.govt.nz/about-the-reforms/. Accessed 20 March 2023.
7. Archives New Zealand. (2022). Te Tiriti o Waitangi | The Treaty of Waitangi. https://www.archives.govt.nz/discover-our-stories/the-treaty-of-waitangi. Accessed 21 March 2023.
8. Health & Disability Commissioner. (2022). Code of Health and Disability Services Consumers' Rights. https://www.hdc.org.nz/media/6335/code-of-rights_online_5-sept-2022.pdf. Accessed 25 March 2023.
9. Healthy Quality & Safety Commission. (2022). Strategy and road map of actions for advance care planning and clinical communication programme 2022–28. https://www.hqsc.govt.nz/assets/Our-work/Advance-care-planning/ACP-info-for-consumers/Publications-resources/ACP-strategy-and-roadmap_2022-28_final.pdf. April 2022. Accessed 23 March 2023.
10. Health Quality & Safety Commission, My advance care plan and guide. https://www.hqsc.govt.nz/resources/resource-library/my-advance-care-plan-and-guide/. Accessed 30 March 2023.
11. Health Quality & Safety Commission, Whenua ki te whenua: An advance care planning guide for whānau. https://www.hqsc.govt.nz/resources/resource-library/whenua-ki-te-whenua-an-advance-care-planning-guide-for-whanau/. Accessed 30 March 2023.
12. Health Quality & Safety Commission. (2020). Serious illness conversation guide Aotearoa. https://www.hqsc.govt.nz/our-programmes/advance-care-

planning/projects/serious-illness-conversations/aotearoa-serious-illness-conversation-guide. Accessed 20 January 2021.
13. Health Quality & Safety Commission, Shared goals of care. https://www.hqsc.govt.nz/assets/Our-work/Improved-service-delivery/Patient-deterioration/Publications-resources/2021-02-Shared-goals-of-care-777-Form-INHOUSE.pdf. Accessed 30 March 2023.
14. Manatū Hauora | Ministry of Health. (2021). Responding when someone raises assisted dying: A conversation guide for health professionals. www.health.govt.nz/system/files/documents/pages/responding-when-a-person-raises-assisted-dying-a-conversation-guide-for-registered-health-professionals-sep21-v2_0.pdf, Accessed 21 March 2023.
15. Manatū Hauora | Ministry of Health. (2021). Responding When Someone Raises Assisted Dying: A Handbook for Registered Health Professionals, Ministry of Health, Wellington. www.health.govt.nz/system/files/documents/pages/responding-when-a-person-raises-assisted-dying-a-handbook-for-registered-health-professionals-sep21_1.docx. Accessed 30 March 2023.

Chapter 27

Insights from Implementing Advance Care Planning in Five Countries: A Historical Perspective

Bernard "Bud" Hammes

Respecting Choices®, La Crosse, Wisconsin, USA

Introduction

"You can try, but it will never work!" That was the blunt feedback I received when I first proposed creating an advance care planning (ACP) program for chronic dialysis patients in the late 1980s in La Crosse, Wisconsin. This judgement turned out to be wrong.[1] When our program spread to other, more diverse locations, we always faced the same skepticism. The skeptics in every place were also wrong.

The skeptics believed that it was not possible to engage a significant percentage of patients in the process of ACP. This skepticism, I must admit, was not crazy or stupid. At this time, most approaches to ACP had failed or had limited success. This skepticism was grounded in both clinical observations as well as some early reports.[2] Many clinicians had attempted to discuss "end-of-life" issues with patients and often got negative responses, sometimes outright anger, or strong emotional push back. The completion of advance directive documents, after the legal recognition of living wills, was low and the effectiveness of the ones that existed was unclear to disappointing.

So why did the Respecting Choices® (RC) program, created in La Crosse, Wisconsin, work[3,4]? In this chapter, I will analyze why this approach to ACP proved the skeptics wrong, why it worked even in diverse populations, but why the uptake and sustaining of the program remains disappointing.

Needing a New Approach

In the mid-1980s, I was employed by the Gundersen Health System in La Crosse, Wisconsin as a clinical ethicist. One of my roles was to provide ethics consultations. By hospital policy, anyone involved in a complex medical decision, where values seemed to be in conflict or were uncertain, could request a bedside ethics consult. The conflict or uncertainty might involve different individuals or even be experienced by a single person. Through listening, analyzing, and feedback, my role was to help bring a resolution to the conflict or uncertainty so the best decision could be made.

Early in this work, over a two-month period, I was called to three ethics consults that all had the same ethical dilemma. In all three cases, the patients were over 70 years of age, required chronic dialysis, and had suffered a devastating stroke from which there was no expected, neurological recovery. If medical support was continued, these patients would survive but were not expected to recover meaningful interactions with others or their world. They would need 24-hour nursing care, ongoing dialysis, and a feeding tube. The medical/ethical question was clear, "Should we continue dialysis?" The conflict in all three cases was within the families. These families were uncertain about what they should do. Should they stop dialysis knowing that death would be certain and relatively quick, or should they continue medical support knowing their loved one would never recover his or her former place in the world? As I worked through the decision with each family, I heard the same cry, "If we only knew!" What each family desired was a clearer understanding of what their loved one would have wanted. These families were faced with a decision about the life or death of their family members with profound uncertainty about what was best.

As I reflected on these three cases, it became clear to me that these families were not only facing the immediate moral distress of the decision but would live with this moral distress. I had some family members return to talk with me about these past medical decisions. Their question was simple, "Did I murder my family member?" We cannot prevent these decisions from occurring, but I thought we could prepare families to make them, and we could better honor patients' values and preferences. But how? How could we create ACP practices that worked? Because I agreed with the skeptics...the then-existing approach to ACP had failed...I knew we had to reconsider all the assumptions that were being used to design ACP.

Developing a Successful Approach to ACP

At this time in the late 80s, the whole approach and justification for ACP was based on the principle of autonomy...a competent person's legal and moral right to make his or her own medical decisions and especially the right to refuse medical treatment. This foundation for ACP made sense from a historic, legal, and philosophical perspective. Autonomy is clearly a justified way to explain and ground ACP. But in my clinical observations, this was not how patients and families experience decision-making or ACP. Autonomy was seldom their concern or rational. Rather, the question that patients and families struggled with was "What is in my (or my loved one's) best interest?" or simply, "What is good care?"

This different way of thinking about the core of health care ethics had been fleshed out in a book published in 1988, *For the Patient's Good: The Restoration of Beneficence in Health Care.*[5] In this book, Edmund Pellegrino and David Thomasma "...maintain that to be guided by beneficence a physician must perform a right and good health action which is consonant with the individual's values. In order to act in the patient's best interests, or the patient's good, the physician and patient must discern what that good is."

The core message of this book aligned with my observations of what health providers, patients, and families were really struggling with in medical decisions, especially ones where ethical conflicts arose. Could we apply this notion of beneficence to ACP? So rather than asking the autonomy question, "What medical treatment would <u>you want</u> if you had this medical problem?" we would be asking, "What makes life good for you?" and "What is in your best interest when you are very ill?" Autonomy simply says you have a right to decide; beneficence, in the context of health care decisions, says let us think about what is best for you...what type of treatment/care best suits your goals and values? It creates a process that depends on relationships, beliefs, and values; and depends upon a type of practical reasoning with which people are familiar.

The Beneficent Based Approach to ACP

So, as I approached ACP from the principle of beneficence, I framed the process of planning as one where patients would define what was good care, and what was in their best interests. The fundamental question is, "What is best if you had a sudden, serious, and sometimes permanent change in health status where benefits and burdens looked dramatically different?"

Looking back at this re-orientation of ACP, I realize that what we were creating was a process that enabled and supported what is now called person-centre care[6] established through shared decision-making.[7] A process of planning and decision-making for certain future situations that took the articulated values and preferences of the patient, with input from health providers, to define what was in his or her best interest. Conceptualizing ACP this way meant that ACP was firmly part of modern, clinical practice. ACP was not some external, legal, non-clinical activity that a person might consider; but rather it was a crucial part of taking good care of patients. This approach put ACP clearly in the realm of health care rather than a legal transaction,[8] i.e., an obligation that health professionals had to their patients. And this obligation wasn't simply to have a process of planning, but it also required systems and practices to make sure that these plans were available and appropriately utilized. The ultimate outcome of this approach was to know and honor patients' values and preferences even if they became incapable of direct participation in their health care decisions.

So, if we focused on ACP, not as an act of autonomy or legal right to refuse treatment (i.e., simply focused on the source of moral/legal authority to control the decision), but rather as a process of practical reason of how to evaluate future decision (i.e., a focus on best interests when certain medical outcomes existed), we provided a pathway to plan. And if this ACP was done, as a process of shared decision-making, then it more naturally includes others who would help explore these best interests and who would often help carry out these pre-determined best interests. This involvement of family members and providers could help improve the outcomes because we would not only more thoughtfully consider how the person viewed their best interest, but also it would prepare those closest to this person to make decisions based on these expressions. And this more inclusive approach was more affirming of how so many people lived in the world, i.e., in a family unit and community.

Embedding ACP into Clinical Practices

Since this beneficence approach embedded ACP into clinical practice, it became evident that when we did ACP as a conversation with a patient and family, not only did we have a better chance to explore and resolve differences of understanding or values and come to a consensus, but we also could explore other key values like: "sometimes, ongoing treatment might cause more suffering than it is worth"; "it can be a loving act to forego treatment", and "there are limits to what medical treatment can achieve". These are not obvious ideas for everyone, especially in societies that are flooded with stories about "medical miracles." It also became clear that this process of ACP could function as a rehearsal for making future, complicated decisions. Having "practiced" morally complicated decisions when undertaking ACP, a family would be better prepared to face real decisions so they could be more comfortable with the emotions that might be experienced and recognize the "off" ramps and know when it was time to stop certain treatments.

Other Lessons of Seeing ACP as Part of Clinical Practice

As we tried out this beneficence model of ACP, we also clinically learned that it was counterproductive to simply jump to the central decisions about when to stop treatments. We learned that we needed to first identify any fears or concerns that the individual planning might have about the process or its outcome. In the beginning, for almost everyone, ACP was new and unfamiliar. If fears and concerns were not identified, brought to light and addressed, planning often failed to create a useful plan. For example, one frequent barrier was the avoidance of vulnerability. ACP can be very personal. Even within families, sharing one's most basic views of life, meaning, and relationships was not always comfortable. Individuals can fear criticism and rejection. If such a fear is strongly felt, then conversations can remain superficial and the process, at best, is simply checking boxes or may end in bruised feelings and conflict. So, to be effective, it was necessary to first explore and address any fears or concerns about the process of ACP. Having a trained facilitator guide a family through this process often made it both safe and successful.

We also learned that it was more effective to start planning by exploring a person's views of living well rather than jumping right to "end of life" preferences. And when we did consider more specific medical decisions, the question was more focused on when the goals of care should change from prolonging life to focusing on palliation. For example, with the initial program with dialysis patients, after we dealt with any fears regarding ACP and then discussed what it meant to live well, we limited our planning to two questions. (1) if you permanently lost the ability to know who you were and who you were with, should dialysis be continued? And (2) if your heart and breathing suddenly stopped, would you want attempts to restore these vital functions (answering this question required some discussion of CPR outcomes)? We simply didn't have the need to deal with other specific diagnoses like persistent vegetative state or vague prognoses like "terminally ill and death is imminent regardless of treatment." Even the discussion of forgoing feeding tubes was not particularly helpful for chronic dialysis patients.

As we clinically rolled out ACP, we quickly learned that we could not predict who was ready to participate or even was interested in ACP. In fact, when first approached, a significant percentage of people were not ready to have an ACP conversation. Unfortunately, this initial, sometimes strongly expressed refusal, has been used to conclude that people won't do ACP. The simple truth is that in no culture in the world where ACP is first introduced do all individuals quickly embrace it. This type of planning and decision-making is new to humans. To a great degree, a big part of the work was to introduce this process into cultural understanding and competence. We needed to change the cultural behavior by demonstrating the value of ACP for the individual and their family.[9]

Clinical ACP as a Continuum of Behavior Change

We also realized that we did not need to be able to predict who was or was not ready to have ACP conversations. If ACP is built into clinical practice and you design a system around the idea that you might need to approach an individual more than once, the system can be successful. So, in this case, motivational interviewing[10] was the best model. The goal is to move individuals from pre-contemplation to contemplation to preparation and then to action. This can take days, weeks, months or even longer. It became clear that providing some public awareness that ACP was part of good care and to start to shift social expectations was very helpful to achieve success. Understanding that patients may need to be approached several times before they were ready to act, meant that it was important to consider when to initiate planning with specific populations so that even the most resistant would typically complete ACP prior to incapacity. Not surprisingly there will be a small percentage of people who will never plan.

The Focus on When the Goals of Care should Change Helps Prepare for a Broader Ranges of Decisions

It became clear that existing materials and documents were often written at too high of a reading level, focused on decisions that were unimportant or clinically unhelpful, and advance directive documents were often written with a legal vocabulary that was not easy to understand and were off-putting. So, we needed to create other educational materials that were written so they were easy to understand. And we needed to create documents that reflected how patients describe their best interests. For example, many early documents asked patients to express preferences if they were diagnosed to be in a persistent vegetative state (PVS). Explaining PVS is in fact complicated if not impossible. Moreover, getting people to express their preferences about treatment in PVS was not that helpful. PVS affects a relatively small population of individuals. In terms of how individuals talked about their best interests, they were concerned about a much broader range of cognitive losses. So, what individuals were concerned about is the loss of their ability to have true relationships with family, friends, and the world around them. So, the question was, if you permanently lose the ability to relate to yourself, to others, and to the world around you, what would you think the best goal of care would be for you? Answering this question provided a decision for a long list of pathologies/diagnoses but did not require the need to define and inform people planning about each of these different medical conditions.

ACP is not as Helpful for Every Disease Trajectory

It also became apparent that planning for future decisions in certain categories of diseases did not change end-of-life care a great deal. Cancer is probably the clearest example. There are at least two reasons for this reality. Cancer patients most often remain capable to make their own decisions very close to the end of life, so looking at an advance directive or approaching a healthcare agent is seldom necessary. Typically, cancer patients participate in their own decision to enter some type of hospice or palliative care approach. Once this change of goals is established, the role of the health care agent and the advance directive documents becomes rather insignificant. (Of note: when cancer patients decide to focus on palliative care, completing a Physician's Order for Life-Sustaining Treatment can have great value.) Secondly, cancer progresses in a way that most often allows both patients and families to see the uselessness of efforts to prolong life. It becomes overwhelmingly obvious that treatments like CPR, intubation, ICU care and even feeding tubes have no real benefit. This is not to say that completing a power of attorney for health care in a cancer population is worthless, but rather that its impact on outcomes in a population is not as significant. What does become crucial for cancer patients who decided to focus on palliation is to make sure the needed palliative services are available where they reside if they chose not to return to the hospital. And if hospitalization becomes necessary, that the goals of treatment are communicated effectively.

Adopting RC for Culturally Diverse Populations in the USA, Canada, Australia, Singapore, and Germany

Even in Wisconsin, RC had to be tweaked to address the planning needs of different cultures. Some examples. In one cultural group in the La Crosse region, the discussion of future, serious illnesses was complicated because such discussions were believed to create or lead to that reality. So, the RC conversation was changed to discuss these possibilities, not as first-person events, but as third-person events. This change allowed folks in this cultural group to identify their values and preferences…what good care would be…without directly talking about themselves being in this condition. In other cases, individuals had specific, cultural views about who would make medical decisions, for example, "My oldest son." Such a culturally determined choice of a health care agent can constitute good planning and it could lead to a discussion of what good care looks like. It was also assumed that ACP would be rejected by people of color. Yet, when tested in a more diverse, hospitalized population in Milwaukee, Wisconsin the reception by people of color was like patients who were white.[11]

So, this beneficence approach worked in Wisconsin, but could it work in other places with even more diverse populations? La Crosse has largely a white population of people who live in a midsize town surrounded by a rural landscape. It wasn't surprising that everywhere we spread the program we always heard, "Well you can do this in La Crosse, but it won't work here…our population is different." The underlying argument seemed to assume that RC was successful in La Crosse because of some unique characteristics of the population rather than the qualities of the intervention.

I can remember one of the early adopters of the Respecting Choices approach, Fraser Health in Vancouver, British Columbia, Canada. Following our implementation recommendations, the staff at Fraser Health started with a small test of change. They choose one of their dialysis units to implement the program. After several months of implementation, I sent an email to one of the leads and asked two questions. How diverse is the population you are planning with? And what problems or challenges are you facing when having planning conversations?

The response was surprising to me. In the initial population that they had engaged in planning, there were over 25 different cultural groups represented. For example, from India, they identified at least 10 different cultural subgroups. As to challenges, they had two. Planning or facilitating ACP almost always required a translator and facilitation took twice as long as we had experienced in La Crosse (where we almost never needed a translator). Despite the cultural diversity, language barriers, and length of time, planning otherwise was successful. It might be argued that these were the early adopters and that as they approached a larger population they would run into more challenges. But from these initial patients, who successfully planned, Fraser leaders were able to develop a short video of testimonials[12] from a diverse group of patients/families that spoke to the importance and value of ACP to their family. Everywhere, even in La Crosse, where the RC approach to ACP was implemented, there was a need to create cultural change, to introduce and make common a new practice or behavior.

When the program was successfully implemented in Australia at Austin Health[13] there were concerns about the fact that the Chinese population would typically say that the eldest son would make all health care

decisions. In the RC program, if it was clarified that this choice represented the preferences of the person, this would be considered good planning. In Australia, also, there was a concern because the success in La
Crosse was significantly tied to the role of the churches in the community.
The role of churches in Australia was far more limited. In Australia,
people formed social groups based on ethnicity. This cultural difference
was not a real issue. The success in La Crosse was not because of religion,
but rather because RC worked with trusted, community groups and leaders. Ultimately, those implementing the RC program in Australia demonstrated the positive benefits in a randomized control trial.[14]

In Singapore, when we came to implement, we were told that "This
won't work here, our people don't talk about death and dying." As we
undertook the training, it was amazing to see the Singaporean participants
did as well or better than any participants in La Crosse or any other location. At least this group of healthcare providers was comfortable with the
RC process of planning. We also noticed some unique things in Singapore.
The best staff to facilitate ACP conversations were the medical social
workers. (In other places it often was nurses or even chaplains.) They had
the communication skills and clinical roles that enabled them to provide
this facilitation service. And there were language problems. It is clearly
more desirable for the facilitator to deliver the facilitation in the language
of the patient/person and family. Finally, one of the unique challenges
was scheduling a facilitation process. Facilitators in Singapore shared
with me that most planning was focused on elderly persons, many of
whom had numerous adult children. So, scheduling facilitation that gathered all the adult children and the parent in one place at the same time
was often difficult because of the long hours that many Singaporeans
worked.

Finally, in Germany, the program was tested in a largely white community in a handful of nursing homes that all transferred emergency care
to a single hospital.[15] Here the cultural challenges were about creating
new roles and competence for nursing staff to facilitate ACP conversations, to help families understand how these conversations were focused
on best interests rather than limitations of treatment, and adopting new
clinical models so nursing home residents could be successfully provided
with palliative approaches to care in the nursing home.

The RC approach to planning seems to work or be adaptable to any
culture it has so far encountered. The success of the RC's approach to
planning seems to flow from its focus on best interests, a person-centred

approach that both speaks to our common humanity and is respectful of our cultural differences. All humans want the best care, how they define best care will be influenced by their cultural/religious beliefs and how they typically make decisions. Few of us, regardless of culture, want to burden our family or chosen healthcare agents with making our decisions without some sense of what we think is best care. This approach to ACP has value because it helps protect our self-interest and prevents unnecessary distress for our family.

But an Effective Planning Process Is Not Enough

An effective process of planning and recording the plan is not enough to assure that person-centred care will be delivered or that our obligations to act in the patient's best interest are fulfilled. There needs to be a robust clinical redesign. (The most extensive discussion of this systems approach was written by Linda Briggs in her recently published book, *To Know and Honor: Building a Culture of Person-Centered Decision*-Making.[16]) An effective, clinical design requires that there is a standard way to place the advance directive document in the person's medical record(s) so that it is easily found; that the advance directive stays with the patient as he or she moves from one health care setting to another; that the plan is updated and made more specific over time as health status changes; and that physicians are held accountable to review such plans and utilizes the patient's preferences and values in decisions when warranted. It is also necessary to make sure that when a palliative care approach is in the patient's best interest that the needed palliative services in that setting of care can be provided in most circumstances. So, for example, if someone was a resident of long-term care and no longer wanted hospital care aimed at prolonging life, then the long-term care facility must be able to provide palliation of pain and discomfort in most cases at the facility for the plan to work.

Project CARE — Testing the Full Approach

This complete RC model was tested in Singapore.[17] In this study, Project CARE was conducted at seven nursing homes involving residents who were at risk of dying within 1 year. The eligible residents and their families were provided ACP using an RC model of facilitation and preferences were documented using a Physician Orders for Life-Sustaining

Treatment (POLST) form. Using the POLST form and discussing the best interests around the orders on the POLST form was clearly warranted given the subject's short life expectancy. Residents whose preferences included either comfort measures or limited medical interventions were enrolled in Project CARE. The staff of these nursing homes were provided with palliative care training and additional palliative care support. So, this study incorporated a facilitated, RC conversation focused on defining the best interests of the subject, a standardized documentation system, POLST, and the ability to provide palliative care in the nursing home for those who determine their goal were comfort measures or limited interventions.

Project CARE's primary measure was to determine the impact on hospital utilization and related costs. It found that those who received the RC ACP and the delivery of palliative service in the nursing home had significantly lower costs compared to historical controls. Clearly, the cost savings are an important finding given the escalating cost of health care but are particularly appealing given that this cost savings was achieved while promoting and protecting the best interests of the patient. A report in La Crosse, Wisconsin that looked at the use of the POLST form also found that long-term care residents who wanted comfort measures or limited treatment typically died in their facility.[18]

The Challenge of Maintaining an Effective ACP System

Unfortunately, maintaining a person-centred ACP system as proscribed by the RC approach has been a challenging task. In my implementation and consulting work around the world, as well as the success achieved in La Crosse, a crucial factor in building a successful system has been strong, dedicated, and consistent leadership who embrace the person-centred, clinical approach and are provided the needed resources. There is evidence that the RC process of planning and documentation supported by effect ACP clinical systems can improve care for many patient populations. The problem is that these newly developed systems that begin to demonstrate success have often languished, not because of the failure of the concepts or approach, but because of change in leaders, the lack of financial support, and/or the persistent strength of a disease model of health care. Let me explain each of these briefly.

Over the years RC has worked with many organizations that had committed, strong leadership to implement person-centred, clinical-based advance care planning systems. These leaders demonstrated clear success in implementing and spreading these systems. Typically, however, the best of these leaders leave, retire, or take on different responsibilities after a few years.

The leaders who follow are (1) often not as committed to or knowledgeable about maintaining the new, person-centred systems; or (2) get overwhelmed by the many challenges of health care.

When there is a change in leadership, these person-centred systems often get forgotten or put on the back burner and begin to fail or simply fade away.

Another challenge is how the RC systems approach squares with how health care is financed. In so many health systems, the decision about resources is made on a department or unit basis.

Financially, departments are evaluated by how much revenue it brings in relative to the cost of running the department. The challenge here is that effective ACP typically requires some input of trained staff (e.g., facilitators) but there is often little or inadequate compensation for this work. Moreover, the department that might need to provide this service is not the department that might enjoy any cost reduction because of it. So, the cost savings that might accrue from good ACP plus any required systems development and palliative care does not currently square with the way accounting systems often work. As one example, the authors of Project CARE, just reviewed, concluded, "Existing palliative care models are only partially funded by the government while not all nursing homes receive government subsidy." So, the model tested in Project CARE is unlikely to have adequate financial support to be widely implemented. Moreover, as budgets get tight, all too often a department manager will cut or not approve ACP activities because it diminishes the department's financial performance.

Finally, person-centred, ACP systems can run counter to a more traditional, disease-orientated care system where the work is seen as primarily diagnosing and treating diseases rather than caring for people with diseases. In a person-centred approach, it is necessary to make sure that the evaluation and treatment of an ill person is consistent with their values and goals of care at that point in time. In a disease model, decisions can be driven by the protocols and standards of care for treating that disease. Realistically, this dichotomy between a disease and person-centre model is not this clear cut. But honestly, a bias toward one or the other changes how systems operate and how patients are cared for.

Conclusion

The RC model created an ACP process built on beneficence where patients explored how to define their future best interests with their health providers and family and considered when the goals of care might change. Despite the understandable skepticism, this RC model of ACP not only was successful in engaging people but seems to be easily adapted to diverse cultures. Since this approach is part of clinical practice, it also has been committed to building clinical systems so that patients are approached at the right time and assured that their preferences would be known and honored. This resulted in a person-centred, clinical systems approach that has shown success in increasing the number of people whose preferences and values are known and honored.[19] The approach helped not only engage individuals over time but also started to shift culture so that ACP was seen as part of good care.

There are some questions and challenges that remain. How do we implement this model of person-centred care so that it is a sustainable model? Firstly, we need to make a cultural shift from a health system that views quality simply from a disease model to a person centre model. Secondly, we need to provide the needed financial resources because it is good care. One possible tool to help create and sustain this model is clearer and stronger standards from accreditation organizations that credential health systems. Such person-centred standards would keep this model front and centred for all health leaders even when leadership changes; they would make it more difficult to short-change this work simply because it makes budgets look worse; and they would create a bias toward person-centred care so health leaders would not view health care solely through the lens of diagnoses and treatment of diseases.

References

1. Hammes B.J., Dahlberg P., and Colvin E. (1991). Advance directive by dialysis patients: A practical approach to tough ethical decisions. *Nephrology News* **5**: 10–16.

2. Fagerlin A., and Schneider C.E. (2004). Enough: The failure of the living will. *Hastings Cent. Rep.* **34**: 30–42.

3. Hammes B.J., and Rooney B.L. (1998). Death and end-of-life planning in one Midwestern community. *Arch. Intern. Med.* **158**: 383–390.

4. Hammes B.J., Rooney B.L., and Gundrum J.D. (2010). A comparative, retrospective, observational study of the prevalence, availability, and specificity of advance care plans in a county that implemented an advance care planning microsystem. *J. Am. Geriatr. Soc.* **58**: 1249–1255.

5. Pellegrino E.D., and Thomasma D.C. (1988). *For the Patient's Good: The Restoration of Beneficence in Health Care.* Oxford University Press, New York.

6. Institute of Medicine. (2001). *Crossing the Quality Chasm: A New Health System for the 21st Century.* National Academy Press, Washington, DC.

7. Elwyn G., Frosch D., and Thomson R., *et al.* (2012). Shared decision making: A model for clinical practice. *J. Gen. Int. Med.* **27**: 1361–1367.

8. Castillo L.S., Williams B.A., Hooper S., Sabatino C.P., *et al.* (2011). Lost in translation: The Unintended consequences of advance directive law on clinical care. *Ann. Int. Med.* **154**: 121–128.

9. https://www.npr.org/sections/money/2016/10/05/496751771/episode-521-the-town-that-loves-death. Link to an audio story of how the culture in La Crosse, WI was changed and planning for end-of-life became common.

10. Prochaska J.O., and Welicer W.F. (1997). The transtheoretical model of health behavior change. *AMJ Health Promot.* **12**: 38–48.

11. Pecanac K.E., Repenshek M.F., Tennenbaum D., and Hammes B.J. (2014). Respecting choices and advance directives in a diverse community. *J. Pal. Med.* **17**: 282–287.

12. https://www.youtube.com/watch?v=-M31-NiH3yU. Link to video from Fraser Health first aired in 2011. Link checked on 03-21-2023.

13. Lee M.J., Heland M., Romios P., *et al.* (2003). Respecting patient choices: Advance care planning to improve patient care at Austin health. *Health Issues* **77**: 23–26.

14. Detering K.M., Hancock A.D., Reade M.C., and Silvester W. (2010). The impact of advance care planning on end of life care in elderly patients: Randomized controlled trial. *BMJ* **340**: 1–9.

15. in der Schmitten J., Lex K., Mellert C., *et al.* (2014). Implementing an advance care planning program in German nursing homes: Results of an inter-regionally controlled intervention trial. *Dtsch. Arztebl. Int.* **111**: 50–57.

16. Briggs L. (2021). *To Know and Honor: Building a Culture of Person-Centered Decision-Making.*

17. Teo W.-S. K., Raj A.G., Tan W.S., *et al.* (2014). Economic impact analysis of an end-of-life programme for nursing home residents. *Pall. Med.* **28**: 430–437.

18. Hammes B.J., Rooney B.L., Gundrum J.D., *et al.* (2012). The POLST program: A retrospective review of the demographics of use and outcomes in one community where advance directives are prevalent. *J. Pal. Med.* **15**: 1–9.
19. Hammes B.J. (ed.). (2012). *Having Your Own Say: Getting the Right Care When It Matters Most.* CHT Press, Washington, DC.

Section 3

Advance Care Planning in Special Populations and Settings

Chapter 28

Advance Care Planning in Primary Care

Jun Hamano[*] and Ai Chikada[†]

*Department of Palliative and Supportive Care, Institute of Medicine,
University of Tsukuba, Tsukuba, Japan
†Department of Human Health Sciences, Graduate School of Medicine,
Kyoto University, Kyoto, Japan

Introduction

In an aging society such as Japan, it is essential to build a system that can provide comprehensive medical and nursing care in the community.[1] A previous systematic review pointed out that the prevalence of incapacity to consent to treatment or admission was 45% for a psychiatric setting and 34% for a medical setting.[2] Therefore, the importance of advance care planning (ACP) in primary care has been recognized worldwide in recent decades.

However, the nationwide survey conducted in Japan in December 2017 showed that only 1.9% of the general population had ACP with healthcare providers, though 40.6% had ACP with family.[3] In addition, this study showed that the experience of caring for a loved one was significantly positively associated with completion of ACP for oneself (Odds Ratio: 1.88, 95% confidential interval: 1.35–2.64), though there was no significant association with having a family doctor (OR: 1.38, 95% CI: 0.99–1.92). Furthermore, this nationwide survey also showed that the preferred place of end-of-life care differs by the assumed clinical scenario: cancer, end-stage heart disease, and dementia.[4]

A recent systematic review pointed out several barriers to end-of-life care and ACP in primary care: (1) patient factors, (2) personal general practitioner (GP) factors, (3) general practice factors, (4) relational factors, (5) coordination of care, (6) availability of services, and (7) specific circumstances. Regarding personal GP factors, GPs frequently report difficulty with spiritual aspects of care and delivery of culturally appropriate psychosocial care. Some challenges include a perceived lack of time and skill to address these aspects of care.[5] Bernard *et al.* explored the barriers faced by older patients in family practice by talking to their family members and family physicians about ACP. There were eight distinct themes as barriers: (1) Patients thought that they were too young for ACP. (2) The topic is too emotional. (3) The physician should be responsible for bringing up ACP. (4) A fear of negatively impacting the patient–physician relationship. (5) Not enough time in appointments. (6) Concern about family dynamics. (7) ACP is not a priority. (8) Lack of knowledge about ACP.[6]

Current Shift of ACP to Primary Care

A recent systematic review, which focused on ACP in Asia, demonstrated that involving family members with or without the patient was considered crucial in ACP. A previous multicentre cross-sectional observational study in Japan explored the characteristics of the prevalence of patients at risk of deteriorating and dying in primary care. In this cross sectional study of 17 clinics in Japan, 17.3% of the patients in primary care settings seemed at risk of deteriorating and dying.[7] However, another multicentre cross-sectional observational study in Japan indicated that 20.7% of primary care patients had discussed at least one ACP topic with their family physician, though 6.0% had discussed it with their family members and physician.[8] In Singapore, 42% of the general practitioners believed that ACP should be initiated while the patient was still healthy.[9]

Scott *et al.* suggested five plans to facilitate the ACP in primary care: (1) identify patients who may be in their last 12 months of life and add them to the practice's palliative care register, (2) assess their current health and social needs, (3) sensitively raise ACP with patients and their family or carers, (4) provide proactive and personalized care and review this regularly with the patient and family or carers, (5) if patients do not want a specific treatment should incapacity arise, seek specialist help to initiate a legal "advance decision".[10]

Japan's Ministry of Health, Labour and Welfare (MHLW) revised its guidelines on the decision-making process regarding end-of-life care in 2018 when the concept of ACP was formally introduced into the guidelines (MHLW in Japan, 2018). A government-commissioned educational program for healthcare providers called "Education For Implementing End-of-Life Discussion (E-FIELD)" has been launched to promote ACP based on these guidelines. Additionally, ACP is nicknamed "jinsei kaigi" or life meeting to increase public awareness. A logo mark of ACP has been developed, and MHLW is actively engaged in publicity efforts. Various communication skills training programs developed in the US, such as the "Serious Illness Care Program" and "VitalTalk," have also been introduced to Japan. The implementation of ACP has now been listed as one of the certification criteria of designated cancer hospitals in Japan.

Nevertheless, there is no standardized ACP program in Japan, and there is no insurance reimbursement for ACP interventions. Furthermore, advance directives (ADs) and proxies or surrogate decisions are not legally binding and have not been legally established. Therefore, the existence of ADs does not necessarily guarantee that the patient's wishes will be respected and therefore is not given as much weight in Japan as it is in other countries such as the United States, many European countries, Singapore, South Korea, and Taiwan, which have laws regulating ACP and ADs. Therefore, it is necessary to increase public awareness of ACP, including its purpose, content, legal policy, and accessibility, by lobbying the government and local municipalities and establishing legislation.[11]

The critical points for further development of ACP in primary care are as follows: (1) establish the methods to identify the suitable patients and the right time to initiate ACP in the illness trajectory, (2) improve the communication skills of health care providers in primary care, especially in dealing with uncertainties, and (3) facilitate public awareness of the need to initiate ACP in primary care and the knowledge of ACP.

A possible method to identify suitable patients to initiate ACP is using the identification tool, such as Surprise Question (SQ) and Supportive and Palliative Care Indicators Tool (SPICT™). A previous prospective cohort study used 2-year version of the SQ, "Would you be surprised if this patient died in the next two years?", as a screening tool to identify patients at high risk of dying, and they concluded that the 2-year version of the SQ had better performance as a screening tool for a serious illness communication intervention in a heterogeneous primary care population.[12] The SPICT™ is a clinical tool supporting healthcare professionals in identifying people with deteriorating health conditions who may benefit from a palliative approach.[13] Several Asia Pacific countries conducted the translation, cross-cultural adaptation, and content validation of the SPICT™ tool.[14,15] A recent prospective cohort study in general practices indicated that the SPICT™ identifies patients needing palliative care better than the SQ.[16] Therefore, it would be better to establish the best way to identify suitable patients and the right time to initiate ACP in each country and region based on the context.

Conclusion

ACP in primary care is necessary to provide comprehensive medical and nursing care in the community. Each country and region should assess the current situation of ACP, address barriers, and leverage on unique strengths within their own country and region. Moreover, ACP in primary care should be optimized based on the local healthcare system and culture.

References

1. Iwagami M., and Tamiya T. (2019). The long-term care insurance system in Japan: Past, present, and future. *JMA J* **2**(1): 67–69. March 19, 2019 [cited 2023 April 2]. Available from: https://pubmed.ncbi.nlm.nih.gov/33681515/.
2. Lepping P., Stanly T., and Turner J. (2015). Systematic review on the prevalence of lack of capacity in medical and psychiatric settings. *Clin. Med. J. R. Coll. Phys. Lond.* **15**: 337–343 [cited 2023 April 2]. Available from: https://pubmed.ncbi.nlm.nih.gov/26407382/.
3. Hanari K., Sugiyama T., Inoue M., Mayers T., and Tamiya N. (2021). Caregiving experience and other factors associated with having end-of-life discussions: A cross-sectional study of a general Japanese population. *J. Pain Symptom Manage.* **61**(3): 522–530.e5. March 1, 2021 [cited 2023 April 1]. Available from: https://pubmed.ncbi.nlm.nih.gov/32827656/.
4. Hanari K., Moody S.Y., Sugiyama T., and Tamiya N. (2023). Preferred place of end-of-life care based on clinical scenario: A cross-sectional study of a general Japanese population. *Healthcare* (Basel, Switzerland) **11**(3). February 1, 2023 [cited 2023 March 21]. Available from: https://pubmed.ncbi.nlm.nih.gov/36766981/.
5. Rhee J.J., Rhee J.J., Grant M., Senior H., Monterosso L., Monterosso L., *et al.* (2020). Facilitators and barriers to general practitioner and general

practice nurse participation in end-of-life care: systematic review. *BMJ Support. Palliat. Care* [cited 2023 April 1]. Available from: https://pubmed.ncbi.nlm.nih.gov/32561549/.

6. Bernard C., Tan A., Slaven M., Elston D., Heyland D.K., and Howard M. (2020). Exploring patient-reported barriers to advance care planning in family practice. *BMC Fam. Pract.* **21**(1). May 25, 2020 [cited 2023 April 1]. Available from: https://pubmed.ncbi.nlm.nih.gov/32450812/.

7. Hamano J., Oishi A., and Kizawa Y. (2019). Prevalence and characteristics of patients being at risk of deteriorating and dying in primary care. *J. Pain Symptom. Manage.* **57**(2): 266–272.e1. November 14, 2019 [cited 2018 November 18]. Available from: http://www.ncbi.nlm.nih.gov/pubmed/30447382.

8. Hamano J., Oishi A., Morita T., and Kizawa Y. (2020). Frequency of discussing and documenting advance care planning in primary care: Secondary analysis of a multicenter cross-sectional observational study. *BMC Palliat. Care* **19**(1). March 17, 2020 [cited 2023 April 1]. Available from: https://pubmed.ncbi.nlm.nih.gov/32183800/.

9. Tee K.H., Seet L.T., Tan W.C., and Choo H.W. (1997). Advance directive: A study on the knowledge and attitudes among general practitioners in Singapore. *Singapore Med. J.* **38**(4): 145–148 [cited 2023 April 2]. Available from: https://pubmed.ncbi.nlm.nih.gov/9269392/.

10. Murray S.A., Sheikh A., and Thomas K. (2006). Advance care planning in primary care. *BMJ* **333**(7574): 868–869. October 28, 2006 [cited 2023 April 1]. Available from: https://pubmed.ncbi.nlm.nih.gov/17068016/.

11. Chikada A., Takenouchi S., Nin K., and Mori M. (2021). Definition and recommended cultural considerations for advance care planning in Japan: A systematic review. *Asia-Pacific J. Oncol. Nurs.* **8**(6): 628–633. November 1, 2021 [cited 2023 April 1]. Available from: https://pubmed.ncbi.nlm.nih.gov/34790847/.

12. Lakin J.R., Robinson M.G., Obermeyer Z., Powers B.W., Block S.D., Cunningham R., *et al.* (2019). Prioritizing primary care patients for a communication intervention using the "surprise question": A prospective cohort study. *J. Gen. Intern. Med.* **34**(8): 1467–1474. August 15, 2019 [cited 2023 April 2]. Available from: https://pubmed.ncbi.nlm.nih.gov/31190257/.

13. Highet G., Crawford D., Murray S.A., and Boyd K. (2014). Development and evaluation of the supportive and palliative care indicators tool (SPICT): A mixed-methods study. *BMJ Support. Palliat. Care.* **4**(3): 285–290. July 25, 2014 [cited 2013 November 13]. Available from: http://www.ncbi.nlm.nih.gov/pubmed/24644193.

14. Oishi A., Hamano J., Boyd K., and Murray S. (2022). Translation and cross-cultural adaptation of the supportive and palliative care indicators tool into Japanese: A preliminary report. *Palliat. Med. Rep.* (Mary Ann Liebert, Inc.)

3: 1–5 [cited 2022 August 24]. Available from: https://www.liebertpub.com/doi/10.1089/pmr.2021.0083.

15. Effendy C., Silva J.F.D.S., and Padmawati R.S. (2022). Identifying palliative care needs of patients with non-communicable diseases in Indonesia using the SPICT tool: A descriptive cross-sectional study. *BMC Palliat. Care.* **21**(1). December 1, 2022 [cited 2023 April 2]. Available from: https://pubmed.ncbi.nlm.nih.gov/35073869/.

16. Van Wijmen M.P.S., Schweitzer B.P.M., Pasman H.R., and Onwuteaka-Philipsen B.D. (2021). Identifying patients who could benefit from palliative care by making use of the general practice information system: The surprise question versus the SPICT. *Fam. Pract.* **37**(5): 641–647 [cited 2023 April 2]. Available from: https://pubmed.ncbi.nlm.nih.gov/32424418/.

Chapter 29

Advance Care Planning in Australia through the COVID-19 Pandemic

Craig Sinclair[*,†], Liz Reymond[‡,§], and Xanthe Sansome[¶]

*University of New South Wales, Sydney, Australia
†Neuroscience Research Australia (NeuRA), Sydney, Australia
‡Statewide Office of Advance Care Planning, Brisbane South Palliative
Care Collaborative, Metro South Health, Brisbane, Australia
§Griffith University School of Medicine and Dentistry,
Gold Coast Campus, Southport, Australia
¶Advance Care Planning Australia, Victoria, Australia

Advance care planning (ACP) gained traction in Australia when the Respecting Patient Choices program[1] was introduced to one Australian state, Victoria, approximately 20 years ago. Subsequently, all six states and two territories have progressed ACP activities according to local requirements, services available, legislation, and population. Various activities promoting ACP have primarily focussed on older adults and/or those impacted by chronic or life-limiting diseases, given their increased likelihood of clinical deterioration, reduction in decision-making capacity, and requirements for increased functional support and healthcare, including end-of-life care.

Differences in legislation and corresponding documentation across the eight jurisdictions, death-denying societal attitudes, poor quality-control of documentation, a lack of measurable performance indicators/outcomes, and issues with point-of-care accessibility of documentation have contributed to low uptake of ACP and low prevalence of ACP documentation.[a]

Nationally, hospital and aged care quality standards[2,3] include requirements for service providers[b] to facilitate access to ACP. Australia has neither a national measure of ACP conversations nor a definitive database of completed ACP documentation, though the Australian Digital Health Agency provides a platform for individuals, or their authorised representatives, to upload ACP documents to their "My Health Record". The number of ACP documents uploaded is unavailable but they are uploaded as either an "advance care plan" or a "Goals of Care" form.[4]

Advance Care Planning Australia was also established as a peak body to provide a national approach to ACP policy, advocacy, education, research, support, and resources. Widespread national consultation enabled the development of the National framework for advance care planning documents, initially in 2011[5] and most recently in 2021.[6]

National prevalence studies from 2017[7] and 2019,[8] auditing 2,285 and 4,187 medical records respectively, have demonstrated <30% of records included ACP documents and most documents were completed by a health professional (35.8%) or someone else (18.1%)[8] and were non-statutory ACDs (20.9%), statutory ACDs appointing an SDM (10.9%), or statutory ACDs outlining preferences for care (2.7%).[7] Prevalence of statutory ACDs was reported at 14% in people aged

---

[a]Documentation can include statutory (legally binding) advance care directives (ACDs) outlining preferences for care, statutory ACDs that nominate a substitute decision maker (SDM) for health or personal matters in the event the person loses decision-making capacity, non-statutory ACP documents and, some might argue, medical orders completed by a health professional outlining escalation and resuscitation plans in response to adverse clinical deterioration.

[b]Aged care services provide the following: (i) home- or centre-based supports, to meet person-centred needs for cleaning, social support, clinical support, and palliative care in the person's home or the organisation's centre or (ii) long-term care, where a person moves into a room in a residential aged care facility (RACF). A resident of an RACF shares the facility with 10–400 other residents and has access to 24-hour care, inclusive of meals, personal care, activities of interest, clinical care, and end-of-life care.

≥65 years, with the highest prevalence in residential aged care facilities (RACFs) (37.7%), followed by hospitals (11.1%) and general practitioner (GP) practices (5.5%). Only 27% of statutory ACDs included legal requirements for validity (full name, signature, date, and witness' signature).[8] The Australian state of New South Wales performed a local review of 1,006 medical records of adults with chronic diseases in hospital and community settings which showed lower overall prevalence for person-completed documents (2.8%), clinician-completed documents (15%), SDM appointments (4%), and legally binding ACDs (1%).[9] Queensland established a Statewide Office of ACP (hereafter, The Queensland Office) to review and upload both statutory and non-statutory ACP documents to ensure quality documentation is accessible in real time across primary, emergency, acute, and residential care services. As of 31 January, 2023, there were greater than 100,000 documents uploaded in Queensland.[10]

Various clinical barriers contribute to the low prevalence of ACP including the following: (i) lack of knowledge and/or confidence to provide ACP discussions, (ii) life-prolonging focus of health services, and (iii) reluctance on the part of the person or the clinician to commence or progress the discussion.[11] Enablers to conducting ACP include the following: increased public awareness of the importance of ACP, confidence in having ACP discussions, and having skilled and dedicated professionals responsible for ACP.[11]

The impact of COVID-19 in Australia was arguably more manageable than in other countries due to its island status and ability to close international borders to slow initial transmission and control new variant introduction. Table 1 provides a summary of case numbers and deaths and includes a summary of key events in Australia.[12–16]

The emergence of COVID-19 virus placed many, but particularly vulnerable populations, including indigenous, residential, or supported accommodation, older and health-compromised populations, at higher risk of increased morbidity and mortality.

The Impact of COVID-19 on ACP

The COVID-19 pandemic impacted the urgency, uptake, and use of ACP in innovative, positive, and concerning ways. The Australian Government released a Health Sector Emergency Response Plan[17] which included

Table 1.   Summary of COVID-19 progression in Australia: Cases, deaths, and events

Year	Quarter	Cases[12]	Deaths[13]	Australian events due to COVID-19[12-16]
2020	January–March	4,561	20	First case reported (January) First death (March) International and interstate borders close (March) Most elective surgeries postponed (April)
	April–June	8,011	104	Outpatient services commence telehealth (April) Limits on social gathering attendee numbers (April) Hospitals and aged care homes limit visitors then lockdown (May)
	July–September	27,078	886	–
	October–December	28,407	909	
2021	January–March	29,296	909	Vaccinations commence — first dose (February); second dose (March)
	April–June	30,611	910	
	July–September	102,723	1,290	
	October–December	395,506	2,241	International borders re-open to citizens (October) and visa holders (December) Booster vaccine dose commences (November)
2022	January–March	4.263M	5,962	International borders re-open to tourists (February) All interstate borders re-open (March)
	April–June	8.085M	9,897	Fourth vaccine (booster) dose commences (May)
	July–September	10.221M	15,120	
	October–December	11.132M	17,039	

Note: M = millions.

preparing and supporting the health systems through initial stages by encouraging completion of ACDs in RACFs.

Within the first 6 months of the pandemic, five possible opportunities for ACP were identified: reducing the need for rationing, planning for unexpected surges, respecting human rights, enabling proactive care coordination, and leveraging societal change.[18]

To limit exposure to, and severity and transmission of, the virus, telehealth and then video-conferencing platforms were increasingly used for ACP conversations. This progressively enabled relatives separated by distance to be virtually present, a luxury that had previously been limited to a telephone conference call at best.

Related processes of documentation soon followed suit. In some jurisdictions, legislation was introduced to enable digital witnessing of legally binding forms.[19,20] The person witnessing no longer had to be physically present with the principal, instead video calls allowed the principal to sign the document, while the witness performed their usual regulatory clarification requirements, and email it to the witness, who counter-signed and returned the document. This further supported digital transfer of ACP documents between services. The argument to allow nurse practitioners (NPs) to sign ACDs was revisited and enacted in some jurisdictions,[20] given COVID-19 reduced availability of doctors and NPs have long been the only clinician available in many rural/regional centres, prisons, and hospices.

ACP conversations increased by >20% in the first 6-months of the pandemic (January–June 2020), compared to the 12 months prior (green section Figure 1).[21] ACP documents received from Queensland RACFs increased approximately 1.5- to 4-times in the second half of 2019/1920 (January–March and April–June 2020), respectively, coinciding with the start of the pandemic in Australia (Figure 2).[22] Targeted phone calls highlighted awareness within RACFs of their low prevalence of residents' ACP documents and virtual education and support was provided to ensure residents' wishes were known and accessible across sectors. This request for ongoing education through virtual and face-to-face mediums has continued across Queensland.

As the pandemic worsened and without any ACP document, time-poor clinicians shifted their focus to locally authorised, medically completed resuscitation plans or goals-of-care documents, or even coordinated conversational "now-care-planning" discussions, to ensure imminent life-sustaining treatment decisions were known. Further, while it was hoped it

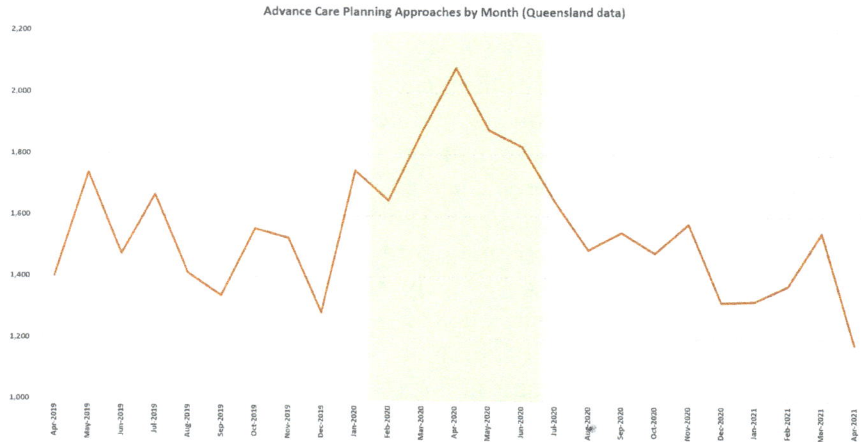

Figure 1.   ACP conversation numbers by month.[21]

Note: Green section shows impact of start of COVID-19 pandemic with increased focus on ACP.

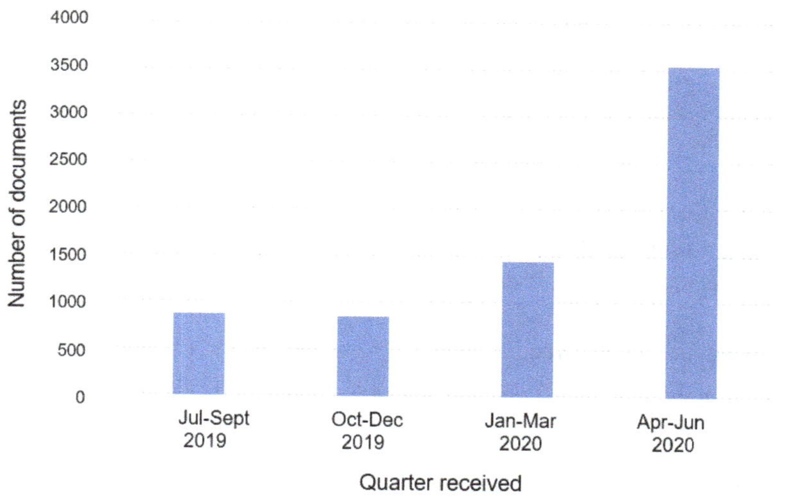

Figure 2.   ACP documents received (by quarter) from RACFs 2019/2020 (Queensland).[22]

would never be required, discussions ensued about criteria for rationing of limited resources, inclusive of hospital and ICU beds and ventilators.[23–26] At a health system level, efforts were made to ensure previously completed ACP documents located at home/RACF were accessible in hospital records

Table 2. Proportion of deaths by location of death: Pre-pandemic (2019 — all deaths) compared to COVID-19 deaths in 2020.[28]

Age group ↓	Place of death →	2019 (all deaths)					2020 (deaths of people with COVID-19)				
		Total number of deaths	Hospital (%)	RACF (%)	Home (%)	Other/ unspec- ified (%)	Deaths due to COVID-19	Hospital (%)	RACF (%)	Home (%)	Other/ unspec- ified (%)
45–64 years		22,406	56.5	3.8	29.3	10.4	36	97	0	np	nr
65–84 years		70,238	59.4	21.2	15.4	4	321	71.3	25.9	2.8	nr
85 years and above		68,149	41.5	50.1	6.9	1.5	509	56.3	43.5	np	nr

Notes: np: not available for publication; nr: not reported.

to ensure people's end-of-life and other healthcare preferences were known, especially regarding hospitalisation, ICU admission, and intubation.

Community-based and residential aged care services also became more aware of the risks of frail elderly people being transferred to and from hospital, and their pre- or peri-pandemic preferences to avoid hospital admissions and to die in their home or RACF. Health service efforts, to enable acute care and dying "in place", were expanded and included acute or palliative in-reach support either in person or via telehealth and geriatric emergency department interventions.[27]

Despite these and other measures, the proportion of hospital deaths of people who died with COVID-19 was higher than pre-pandemic hospital death rates for all ages, yet the proportion of people aged 65–84 years who died in a RACF with COVID-19 was higher than the pre-pandemic proportions of all deaths (Table 2).[28]

To reduce transmission, staff were limited to working with only one service provider, facility, or wing, with some residential services providing temporary accommodation for staff caring for COVID-positive residents. Many specialist staff, including ACP facilitators, were redirected to hospitals or RACFs to support acute COVID management plans or cover staff in furloughed isolation from COVID-19. Specialist ACP staff from hospitals across Victoria were mobilised to focus on RACF residents and complete "Goals of management and deterioration plans", including liaising with appointed medical SDM, family, and GPs.[29] This necessary reallocation of specialty staff into frontline clinical positions reduced normal ACP promotion and facilitation activities.

Unfortunately, due to government restrictions, public health decrees, staff shortages, and transmission risks, people's end-of-life preferences were not always enactable during the pandemic. This was especially apparent if the person/relative was COVID-positive or where preferences included community outings, requests for multiple family members to be present simultaneously, or even transfers to their home, town, or country, which is often requested by Aboriginal and Torres Strait Islander peoples. In some jurisdictions, restrictions were eased to allow visitors when end of life was imminent (i.e., final days).

Lessons Learnt

Recently, clinicians have reported an increased appetite for ACP in all sectors.[29] The general public have become aware their future good health is not guaranteed and medicine cannot cure all. In Victoria, the state most affected by COVID-19 and lockdowns, the focus on promoting ACP has shifted from hospital to community-based efforts. Anecdotally, members of the public who had been considering ACP document completion have been motivated to complete them.[29]

COVID-19 has highlighted that important public health messaging, especially early messaging, is not always broad enough, appropriate for, or well understood by all individuals within culturally and linguistically diverse (CALD) populations, Aboriginal and Torres Strait Islander populations, people with a disability, and people who require easy-read versions of health-related materials. This has facilitated reflection on the need for ACP resources that are easily accessible and understandable by all. Some health professionals from CALD communities have reported how their cultural views on dying and death impact their ability to engage in ACP conversations with residents or patients.

During government-imposed restrictions on travel and gathering numbers, face-to-face education, including workshop training of health or age care professionals and community group education, was unable to be provided. While flexible web-based education has expanded, which increases efficiency for the presenter and resources, recipients of education find it more distracting and less interactive and therefore less effective.[30,31]

Changes to digital engagement and witnessing, have produced an increased appetite for digital ACDs. Numerous unregulated businesses are now offering digital ACP documents requiring initial upfront payments and annual maintenance payments. There is also a push to increase the upload of ACP documents to My Health Record. Projects have commenced to trial facilitated uploading of ACP documents from GP practice software and Aboriginal Community-Controlled Health Organisations. Aside from The Queensland Office, there is no service to quality-check documentation and no delineation of document type to aid clinicians in accessing documents.

The digital completion and processing of ACP documents have raised some concerns about access for all (especially less digitally literate individuals), the voluntary nature of ACP and the lack of integrity and safeguards protecting a person's autonomy.

The Post-Pandemic Future of ACP in Australia

It is hoped and anticipated that lessons learnt and improvements made through the COVID-19 pandemic regarding ACP continue to be developed, given the possibility of similar surges or new pandemics and the recognised benefits of ACP to the person and the health system. Improving equity of access to ACP for all people regardless of their culture, language, ability, education, digital skills, or location has been identified and is being addressed within limited resourcing. Education for individuals and health and care professionals is continuing, and it is anticipated to continue in both virtual and face-to-face modes.

In Australia, improvements in standardised legislation and metrics around ACP conversations and documentation, research, and quality and accessibility of documentation across all sectors require a national approach and support and will hopefully improve clinicians' understanding, confidence, and use of documented ACPs and ultimately the quality of care received by all Australians.

Learning Objectives
- The COVID-19 pandemic increased the urgency of, and community interest in, advance care planning.
- The uptake of telehealth and video-conference platforms for advance care planning discussions has shown that this method is feasible and can enable involvement from family members separated by distance.
- Re-allocation of staff roles to support frontline and acute services during the COVID-19 pandemic negatively impacted routine advance care planning promotion and facilitation.
- The ineffectiveness of some public health messaging during the COVID-19 pandemic illustrates the broader importance of accessibility to resources relating to ACP.

- The increased availability of digital advance care directives and impetus to upload documents into digital storage raises questions about data quality control.

References

1. Silvester W., Stickland E., Adams M., O'Callaghan S., and Kirsner S. (2006). Respecting patient choices. Final evaluation of the community implementation of the respecting patient choices program. *Austin Health*. February 2006.
2. Australian Commission on Safety and Quality in Health Care. (2021). The National Safety and Quality Health Service Standards, 2nd edn. https://www.safetyandquality.gov.au/standards/nsqhs-standards.
3. Aged Care Quality and Safety Commission. (2019). Aged care quality standards. https://www.agedcarequality.gov.au/providers/standards.
4. Australian Digital Health Agency (2023). Advance care planning. https://www.digitalhealth.gov.au/healthcare-providers/advance-care-planning. [Accessed online 3 September 2023].
5. Australian Health Ministers Advisory Council. (2011). A national framework for advance care directives 2011. https://respectingchoices.org/wp-content/uploads/2017/07/a-national-framework-for-advance-care-directives_september-2011.pdf.
6. Australian Government Department of Health. (2021). National framework for advance care planning documents. https://www.health.gov.au/resources/publications/national-framework-for-advance-care-planning-documents?language=en#:~:text=Description%3A%20The%20National%20framework%20for%20advance%20care%20planning,in%20the%20preparation%20of%20advance%20care%20planning%20documents.
7. Detering K.M., Buck K., Ruseckaite R., Kelly H., Sellars M., Sinclair C., *et al.* (2019). Prevalence and correlates of advance care directives among older Australians accessing health and residential aged care services: Multicentre audit study. *BMJ Open* **9**: e025255. https://bmjopen.bmj.com/content/9/1/e025255.
8. Buck K., Nolte L., Sellars M., Sinclair C., White B.P., Kelly H., *et al.* (2021). Advance care directive prevalence among older Australians and associations with person-level predictors and quality indicators. *Health Expect.* **24**: 1312–1325. https://doi.org/10.1111/hex.13264.
9. Jeong S., Barrett T., Ohr S.O., Cleasby P., Davey R., and David M. (2021). Prevalence of advance care planning practices among people with chronic diseases in hospital and community settings: A retrospective medical record audit. *BMC Health Serv. Res.* **21**(1): 303. https://doi.org/10.1186/s12913-021-06265-y.
10. Queensland Government. Office of ACP Monthly Statistics: December 2022.

11. Reymond L. (2021). Statewide Office of Advance Care Planning: ACP Survey Report (unpublished).
12. Tracking coronavirus (COVID-19) across Australia. Cases: States and territories. https://www.covid19data.com.au/states-and-territories.
13. Tracking coronavirus (COVID-19) across Australia. Deaths. https://www.covid19data.com.au/deaths.
14. Tracking coronavirus (COVID-19) across Australia. Covid-19 vaccinations in Australia. https://www.covid19data.com.au/vaccines.
15. Parliament of Australia. (2020). COVID-19: A chronology of state and territory government announcements. https://www.aph.gov.au/About_Parliament/Parliamentary_Departments/Parliamentary_Library/pubs/rp/rp2021/Chronologies/COVID-19StateTerritoryGovernmentAnnouncements.
16. Australian Government, Department of the Prime Minister and Cabinet. (2020). PM Transcripts, Transcripts from the Prime Minister of Australia. Media Release Transcript 42741. https://pmtranscripts.pmc.gov.au/release/transcript-42741.
17. Commonwealth of Australia. (2020). Australian Health Sector Emergency Response Plan for Novel Coronavirus (COVID-19). Department of Health, Publications Number 12723. https://www.health.gov.au/resources/publications/australian-health-sector-emergency-response-plan-for-novel-coronavirus-covid-19?language=en.
18. Sinclair C., Nolte L., White B.P., and Detering, K. (2020). Advance care planning in Australia during the COVID-19 outbreak: Now more important than ever. *Intern. Med. J.* **50**: 918–923. https://doi.org/10.1111/imj.14937.
19. State of New South Wales. (2023). Guardianship Act 1987 No 257. https://legislation.nsw.gov.au/view/xml/inforce/2021-03-27/act-1987-257.
20. State of Queensland. (2023). Powers of Attorney Act 1998. https://www.legislation.qld.gov.au/view/pdf/inforce/current/act-1998-022.
21. Queensland Office of Advance Care Planning. (2020). With information provided by Healthcare Purchasing Strategy Unit, Purchasing & Funding Branch, Queensland Health.
22. Queensland Office of Advance Care Planning. (2020). Graph of RACFs 2019/20.
23. Sansome X. (2022). Personal communication with Victorian clinicians.
24. https://theconversation.com/the-coronavirus-pandemic-is-forcing-us-to-ask-some-very-hard-questions-but-are-we-ready-for-the-answers-132581.
25. https://www.abc.net.au/news/2020-03-31/doctors-ask-for-ethics-guidelines-amid-coronavirus/12107476.
26. MacIntyre C.R., and Heslop D.J. (2020). Public health, health systems and palliation planning for COVID-19 on an exponential timeline. *Med. J. Aust.* https://onlinelibrary.wiley.com/doi/abs/10.5694/mja2.50592.

27. Litton E., Bucci T., Chavan S., Ho Y.Y., Holley A., Howard G., *et al.* (2020). Surge capacity of intensive care units in case of acute increase in demand caused by COVID-19 in Australia. *Med. J. Aust.* https://onlinelibrary.wiley.com/doi/abs/10.5694/mja2.50596.
28. Whiting E., Scott I.A., Hines L., Ward T., Burkett E., Cranitch E., *et al.* On behalf of the Frail Older Persons' Collaborative Program. (2022). A whole-of-health system approach to improving care of frail older persons. *Aust. Health Rev.* **46**: 629–634. https://onlinelibrary.wiley.com/doi/abs/10.5694/mja2.50596.
29. Australian Bureau of Statistics. (2021). Classifying place of death in Australian mortality statistics 3303.0.55.005. https://www.abs.gov.au/statistics/research/classifying-place-death-australian-mortality-statistics.
30. Shah R. (2022). Benchpartner: Face-to-face learning: Benefits, advantages and disadvantages. https://benchpartner.com/blog/face-to-face-learning-benefits-advantages-and-disadvantages.
31. StudyCorgi. (2022). Reasons why face-to-face education is better than online learning. https://studycorgi.com/reasons-why-face-to-face-education-is-better-than-online-learning/.

Chapter 30

Advance Care Planning in Oncology

Kwok-Keung Yuen

Specialist in Clinical Oncology, Hong Kong SAR, China

Introduction

The World Health Organization defines advance care planning (ACP) as a process of "planning in advance for decisions that may have to be made prior to incapability or at the end of life". People may choose to do this planning formally, by means of advance directives, or informally, through discussion with family members, friends, and health care and social service providers, or a combination of both methods.[1] In clinical practice, one important aspect is the completion of an advance directive (AD), a legal document allowing people to choose what they would want in the event that they lack capacity to make their own medical decisions.[2]

More recently, ACP is increasingly considered to be a complex process that "enables individuals who have decisional capacity to identify their values, to reflect upon the meanings and consequences of serious illness scenarios, to define goals and preferences for future medical treatment and care, and to discuss these with family and/or other closely related people, and health care providers. Advance care planning addresses individuals' concerns across physical, psychological, social, and spiritual domains. It may encourage individuals to identify a personal representative and to record and regularly review any preferences, so that their preferences can be taken into account, should they, at some point, be unable to make their own decisions."[3] The goal of ACP is to help ensure that people receive medical care that is consistent with their values, goals, and preferences during serious and chronic illness.[4]

Despite the wide promulgation of ACP in cancer patients, many health professionals are still unfamiliar with ACP. In a scoping review, it was found that professionals could not separate day-to-day care planning and ACP. ACP documentation was scattered and difficult to find and use. Professionals were unfamiliar with ACP, and established practices were lacking. ACP conversations mostly occurred in late cancer. This highlights the need to raise professionals' awareness of ACP.[5]

This chapter aims to provide an overview of the concepts and practices of advance care planning in oncology.

Learning point 1: ACP allows an individual to plan in advance decisions (including medical care and personal arrangements) that may have to be made prior to incapability or at the end of life.

Effects of ACP on Cancer Patient Outcomes

The effect of ACP on aggressiveness of end-of-life care has been evaluated in a prospective trial involving 1,200 patients with metastatic lung or colorectal cancer. Patients who engaged in end-of-life discussions with their physician were significantly less likely to receive aggressive measures at the end of life, including chemotherapy and acute care.[6] Early palliative care is associated with less intensive medical care, improved quality outcomes, and cost savings at the end of life for patients with cancer.[7]

In another randomised controlled trial of 795 terminally ill patients with cancer in one medical centre, it was found that ACP improves psychological symptoms and preferred end-of-life care (life-sustaining treatment including cardiopulmonary resuscitation, intensive care unit care, chest compression, intubation with mechanical ventilation support, nasogastric tube feeding, and intravenous nutrition support).[8] Dedicated ACP documentation is associated with fewer admissions in the last 30 days of life for patients with advanced cancer referred to hospice.[9] There is also evidence to suggest that cancer patients with ACP conversations in primary health care spend more time at home and more often die at home.[10]

In a recent randomised controlled trial, ACP intervention was found to facilitate the issuance of DNR orders among a subgroup of patients with accurate prognostic awareness.[11] ACP and end-of-life conversations have been shown to play a critical role in cancer patients' awareness of their disease and prognosis and help them in making end-of-life care decisions as shown in an integrative literature review.[12]

It has been shown in a prospective multicentre observational study that perceptions of involvement in ACP are positively associated with emotional functioning in patients with advanced cancer.[13] ACP potentially supports hope by being (i) a meaningful activity that embraces uncertainties and difficulties, (ii) an action towards an aware and empowered position, and (iii) an act of mutual care anchored in commitments.[14] In a recent prospective cohort study, it was found that caregivers of patients who completed a do-not-resuscitate (DNR) order experienced reductions in grief, suggesting that ACP may promote grief resolution in caregivers.[15]

Learning point 2: Studies suggest that patients who participated in ACP are less likely to receive aggressive end-of-life interventions. In addition, ACP might have a positive impact on the emotional functioning of patients and grief resolution of caregivers.

Elements and Contents of ACP in Oncology

While patients with advanced cancer may benefit from ACP, there is evidence that their willingness and desire to engage in ACP varies. The reasons for this remain poorly understood. In a systematic review which included 40 studies, it was found that the complex social and emotional environments within which end-of-life care planning occurred are not sufficiently embedded within standardised ACP which focuses on the autonomy of patients.[16] Cancer patients often have deeper concerns and needs and they may experience ACP in a more complex way, with relational, emotional, and social dimensions.[17] In a systematic review of ACP intervention for cancer patients, it was found that interventions that resulted in ACP engagement tended to take a multidisciplinary approach and consisted of multiple consultations staged over time.[18]

In a qualitative study exploring the decision-making process and drivers of receiving palliative care in advance care planning discussions, "choose palliative care" was associated with patients' desire to reduce physical suffering from treatments, avoid being a burden to families and society, reduce futile treatments, and donate organs to help others. Opinions from families are considered to be highly influential and their involvement is important in patients' palliative care decision-making, especially in the Asia-Pacific context.[19] In a systemic review, it was found that mechanisms through which ACP improved outcomes comprised (i) increasing patients' knowledge of end-of-life care, (ii) strengthening patients' autonomous motivation, (iii) building patient's competence to undertake end-of-life discussions, and (iv) enhancing shared decision-making in a trustful relationship.[20]

Factors affecting participants' ACP experiences include gender, educational level, cancer diagnosis,[21] perceptions on the importance of harmfulness of cancer-related information, the way of communicating the bad news, motivation for participating in medical decision-making, and the complexity of future planning.[22] In a focus group study, professionals considered ACP important to address the following: (i) the family's role in medical decision-making, (ii) sensitivity to communication norms, (iii) patients' and families' religious beliefs regarding the control and sanctity of life, and (iv) the availability of a support system for advance care planning (healthcare professionals' education and training, public education, resource allocation, and formal regulation).[23]

In a recent modified Delphi study in Germany, attempt has been made to develop a hospital-based ACP pathway for cancer patients, consensus was reached on a final version of the pathway with 148 elements covering 10 domains: prerequisites, organisation and coordination, identification and referral, provision of information, information sources, family involvement, advance care planning discussion, documentation, update, and quality assurance.[24]

Learning point 3: While the aim of ACP is to promote patients' autonomy, patients may experience ACP in multiple dimensions. Hence, a multidisciplinary approach is essential and the ACP team should be well organised and coordinated, with adequate support in clinical operation, staff training, and quality assurance.

Timing for Initiation of ACP in Oncology

Clinical guidelines recommend early initiation of ACP discussions while the patient is still capable of making an informed decision. However, current evidence suggests that cancer patients infrequently engage in ACP discussions[25] and such discussions often occur late in the course of illness.[26] In an online survey of 118 physicians from 41 oncology institutions, 72% of the participants answered that they had engaged in ACP.

Among these, 33% used a structured format and only 8% used triggers for initiation of ACP. This reflects that there were still substantial variabilities in the timing of ACP communication among oncologists.[27]

A recent prospective study of 54 terminally ill patient and family dyads has shown that nearly 80% of the patients and caregivers agreed that advance care planning should be conducted at the non-frail stage of a disease before the patient experiences significant health problems.[28] In another cross-sectional survey of 200 surgical and medical oncology patients in a tertiary care hospital with a comprehensive cancer centre, it was found that patients preferred to have discussions early before their prognosis worsened (94%).[29]

A prospective study has been conducted to explore the feasibility of the early application of an advance directive at the time of first-line palliative chemotherapy in patients with incurable cancer. Among 64 eligible patients, 44 patients (69%) agreed to conduct the discussion, suggesting the feasibility of early ACP discussion among cancer patients.[30]

Learning point 4: While early initiation of ACP is recommended by clinical guidelines, preferred by patients and caregivers, and seems to be feasible, the optimal timing of initiation of ACP is yet to be defined in clinical practice. There should be a system in place to facilitate ACP discussion in the following time points: (1) when incurable cancer is diagnosed, (2) when anti-cancer treatment is no longer effective, and (3) when there is worsening of health condition with short life expectancy.

Personnel Involved in Oncology ACP

Though different members of the team could conduct ACP, it is important to involve physicians in the process. In a literature review of the implementation of ACP in oncology, ACP sessions were conducted by research assistants (9/26 studies), nurses (5/26 studies), advanced practitioners (5/26 studies), social workers (1/26 studies), clinical psychologists (1/26 studies), and palliative care physicians (3/26 studies). In 7 of the 26 studies, ACP was completed or introduced by an oncologist. While ACP discussion could be conducted by different members of the health care team, the oncologist plays an important role in the introduction and completion of ACP.[31]

It was explicitly and implicitly expressed across the literature that physicians feel they are best placed to determine when patients are ready for ACP and what should be discussed. Twelve out of the 40 included studies addressed the power and the degree of control exerted by the physicians over the patient and over other health professionals, particularly nurses. Unfortunately, physician's influence, such as reluctance in the initiation of ACP discussion, is one of the commonly reported barriers to ACP.[32]

Family involvement in ACP for people with advanced cancer has been investigated by a systemic mixed-methods review. It showed that people with advanced cancer wish to involve family members in ACP if it benefits family members but may be concerned about engaging them in a potentially emotionally laden process. A logic model with two components was suggested: (i) to assess and address family members' concerns and motions and (ii) to facilitate communication between individuals and their family members.[33]

Learning point 5: While ACP could be conducted by different professionals, physicians play an important role in ACP, especially in its introduction and completion. Family involvement is important, especially in the Asian culture.

Clinical Guidelines and Expert Recommendations

There is no standardised approach to ACP for patients with advanced cancer. ACP could take place at different timings of the disease journey, conducted by different health care professionals, and in different settings such as inpatient or outpatient setting.[34] As patient background and family needs vary widely, an individualised, patient-centred, and culturally adapted approach is needed for ACP discussion.[35]

The National Comprehensive Cancer Network (NCCN) guidelines recommend the oncology team to initiate discussions of personal values and preferences for end-of-life care while patients have a life expectancy of years to months. Advance care planning should include an open discussion about palliative care options, personal values, and preferences for end-of-life care, including the congruence between the patient's wishes/expectations and those of the family/caregiver/health care team; followed by formal documents including advance directives, living wills, medical powers of attorney, health care proxy, or any other documents regarding life-sustaining treatments, such as cardiopulmonary resuscitation, medical ventilation, and artificial nutrition or hydration.[36]

The European Society for Medical Oncology guidelines recommend the term "allow natural death" (AND) which focuses more on what is being done and not on what is being avoided, e.g., "Do not resuscitate" (DNR). In the management of patients with far advanced cancer, AND is the preferred term since it presents palliation rather than CPR as the normative default.[37]

The Patient–Clinician Communication: American Society of Clinical Oncology Consensus Guideline[38] recommends the use of an organised framework to guide the bidirectional communication about end-of-life care with patients and families. Before discussing specific treatment options with patients, clinicians should clarify the goals of treatment so that patients understand likely outcomes and can relate the goals of treatment to their goals of care. When reviewing treatment options with patients, clinicians should provide information about the potential benefits and burdens of any treatment and check the patient's understanding. Clinicians should discuss treatment options in a way that preserves patients' hope, promotes autonomy, and facilitates understanding. When patients display emotion through verbal or non-verbal behaviour, clinicians should respond empathetically. Published frameworks including SPIKES,[39] PREPARED,[40] and the Serious Illness Conversation Guide[41] could be adopted for the discussion.

Learning point 6: While the goals of ACP are similar across different clinical guidelines, the ACP process is individualised. ACP discussion involves personal issues and clinicians are expected to respond empathetically with knowledge and skills.

Structured Programmes

Research is ongoing to establish the role of structured programmes of ACP in a clinical setting. In a randomised controlled trial of a structured intervention consisting of an informational pamphlet and discussion involving 120 patients with metastatic cancer,[42] it was found that the intervention was associated with earlier placement of DNR orders and less likelihood of death in a hospital. However, a non-blinded Australian randomised study of a formal ACP intervention based on the Respecting Patient Choices model[43] did not show an increase in the likelihood that end-of-life care being consistent with patients' preferences. Similarly, in a more recent 6-country, cluster-randomised clinical trial of ACP in 665 patients with advanced cancer (the ACTION study),[44] it was found that ACP conversations did not have an impact on patients' quality of life, coping, or involvement in decision-making processes, though patients taking part in ACP conversations were more likely to receive palliative care and more likely to have their documented preferences recorded in their medical records.

In a Randomized Trial of Acceptability and Effects of Values-Based Advance Care Planning in Outpatient Oncology: Person-Centered Oncologic Care and Choices (P-COCC) including patients with advanced gastrointestinal cancer,[45] a novel ACP intervention combining a patient values interview with an informational care goals video was shown to be acceptable to 32 out of 33 participants (97%) but an increased distress score was observed in the intervention arm. In a Korean randomised controlled trial,[46] it was shown that the ACP decision aid reduced the preference for active and life-prolonging treatment and increased the preference for hospice. A recent single-blind, randomised, controlled trial[47] comparing an interactive educational ACP decision aid (Making Your Wishes Known: Planning Your Medical Future) to standard ACP showed no difference in documentation of patient wishes or end-of-life care received.

Learning point 7: There is evidence to suggest structured ACP programmes may benefit various aspects of patient care for those who are engaged in advance care planning. However, results are inconsistent and further research is required.

Overcoming Barriers

Three types of barriers were identified in a focus group study[48]: barriers relating to professionals, to the patient and family, and to the health care system. In a systematic narrative review of Asian healthcare professionals' knowledge, attitude and experience in ACP, healthcare professionals considered ACP difficult to initiate, partly because of their lack of knowledge and skills in ACP, personal uneasiness to conduct ACP, fear of conflicts with family members and their legal consequences, and the lack of a standard system for ACP.[49]

For patients and families, there is evidence to suggest mindfulness-based intervention may enhance the capacity of cancer patients and their caregivers in responding the emotional challenges and decrease their psychological barriers to ACP.[50]

For professionals, the introduction of technology and training may overcome some of the barriers in clinical practice. In a study as part of a quality improvement initiative in medical oncology clinics,[51] a computer prognosis model was used to prompt ACP discussion for those patients who were predicted to have a short life expectancy to have discussion with care coaches who received Serious Illness Care Programme training. An increase in ACP documentation was observed in the intervention arm (35%) as compared to the control arm (3%).

Lack of structural collaboration between the generalist and specialist was expressed as one of the barriers.[48] To overcome the barriers, initiatives have been taken to incorporate palliative care in oncology training and service. Examples include the combined clinical oncology and palliative medicine specialty training in Hong Kong[52] and the European Society for Medical Oncology Designated Centres of Integrated Oncology and Palliative Care.[53]

In Hong Kong, the feasibility to introduce advance directive (AD) in advanced cancer patients was addressed in a prospective cohort study conducted at an oncology palliative care unit in 2009 using a locally designed advance directive form.[54] Of the 191 eligible patients, 120 (63%) signed the advance directive. After the publication of the Hospital Authority guidelines on Advance Directive in 2014, another oncology palliative care unit began engaging cancer patients in advance care planning and 53% of eligible patients completed an advance directive.[55] A structured advance care planning programme has been introduced by a palliative medical unit for patients with advanced malignancy or end-stage organ failure, showing high concordance rate for patients' wish items.[56] In 2019, the Hospital Authority published the HA guidelines on Advance Care Planning[57] and legislation on advance directives is underway.[58] It is hoped that these initiatives, accompanied by professional training and public education, would improve palliative care and end-of-life care in Hong Kong.

Learning point 8: Advance care planning is not only a process of change for the patient but also a process of change for the professionals and the health care system.

Conclusion

Advance care planning allows an individual to plan in advance medical and personal decisions that may have to be made prior to incapability or at the end of life. It is a complex, individualised process with relational, emotional, and social dimensions and requires a multidisciplinary approach with a trained team of skilled professionals to navigate the patient through the uncertainties that one may face in the future. With the advancement of oncological treatment, oncologists could play a more active role in the ACP of their patients, not only to facilitate end-of-life decisions but also to provide holistic oncology and palliative care to the patients.

References

1. WHO Centre for Health Development (Kobe, Japan). (2004). A glossary of terms for community health care and services for older persons. Kobe, Japan: WHO Centre for Health Development.
2. Lindsay A. Dow, Robin K. Matsuyama, V. Ramakrishnan, Laura Kuhn, Elizabeth B. Lamont, Laurel Lyckholm, and Thomas J. Smith. (2010). Paradoxes in advance care planning: The complex relationship of oncology patients, their physicians, and advance medical directives. *J. Clin. Oncol.* **28**: 299–304.
3. Rietjens J.A.C., Sudore R.L., Connolly M., *et al.* (2017). Definition and recommendations for advance care planning: An international consensus supported by the European association for palliative care. *Lancet Oncol.* **18**: e543–e551.
4. Sudore, R.L., Lum, H.D., You, J.J., Hanson, L.C., Meier, D.E., Pantilat, S.Z., Matlock, D.D., Rietjens, J.A.C., Korfage, I.J., Ritchie, C.S., Kutner, J.S., Teno, J.M., Thomas, J., McMahan, R. D., and Heyland, D.K. (2017). Defining advance care planning for adults: A consensus definition from a multidisciplinary Delphi panel. *J. Pain Symptom. Manage.* **53**(5): 821–832.e1.
5. Kuusisto A., Santavirta J., Saranto K., Korhonen P., and Haavisto E. (2020). Advance care planning for patients with cancer in palliative care: A scoping review from a professional perspective. *J. Clin. Nurs.* **29**(13–14): 2069–2082.
6. Mack, J.W., Cronin, A., Keating, N.L., Taback, N., Huskamp, H.A., Malin, J.L., Earle, C.C., and Weeks, J.C. (2012). Associations between end-of-life discussion characteristics and care received near death: a prospective cohort study. *J. Clin. Oncol.* **30**(35): 4387–4395.
7. Scibetta C., Kerr K., Mcguire J., and Rabow M.W. (2016). The costs of waiting: Implications of the timing of palliative care consultation among a cohort of decedents at a comprehensive cancer center. *J. Palliat. Med.* **19**(1): 69–75. January 1, 2016.
8. Tang S.T., Chen J.S., Wen F.H., *et al.* (2019). Advance care planning improves psychological symptoms but not quality of life and preferred end-of-life care of patients with cancer. *J. Natl. Compr. Canc. Netw.* **17**(4): 311–320.

9. Prater L.C., Wickizer T., Bower J.K., and Bose-Brill S. (2019). The impact of advance care planning on end-of-life care: Do the type and timing make a difference for patients with advanced cancer referred to hospice? *Am. J. Hosp. Palliat. Care* **36**(12): 1089–1095.

10. Driller B., Talseth-Palmer B., Hole T., Strømskag K.E., and Brenne A.T. (2022). Cancer patients spend more time at home and more often die at home with advance care planning conversations in primary health care: A retrospective observational cohort study. *BMC Palliat. Care* **21**(1): 61. May 2, 2022.

11. Wen F.H., Chen C.H., Chou W.C., Chen J.S., Chang W.C., Hsieh C.H., and Tang S.T. (2020). Evaluating if an advance care planning intervention promotes do-not-resuscitate orders by facilitating accurate prognostic awareness. *J. Natl. Compr. Canc. Netw.* **18**(12): 1658–1666. December 2, 2020.

12. Goswami P. (2023). Impact of advance care planning and end-of-life conversations on patients with cancer: An integrative review of literature. *J. Nurs. Scholarsh.* **55**(1): 272–290.

13. Kroon L.L., van Roij J., Korfage I.J., *et al.* (2021). Perceptions of involvement in advance care planning and emotional functioning in patients with advanced cancer. *J. Cancer Surviv.* **15**(3): 380–385.

14. Kodba-Čeh H., Lunder U., Bulli F., *et al.* (2022). How can advance care planning support hope in patients with advanced cancer and their families: A qualitative study as part of the international ACTION trial. *Eur. J. Cancer Care (Engl.)* **31**(6): e13719.

15. Falzarano, F., Prigerson, H.G., and Maciejewski, P.K. (2021). The role of advance care planning in cancer patient and caregiver grief resolution: Helpful or harmful? *Cancers*, **13**: 1977.

16. Johnson, S., Butow, P., Kerridge, I., and Tattersall, M. (2016). Advance care planning for cancer patients: A systematic review of perceptions and experiences of patients, families, and healthcare providers. *Psycho-oncology*, **25**(4): 362–386.

17. Johnson, S.B., Butow, P.N., Kerridge, I., and Tattersall, M.H. (2017). What do patients with cancer and their families value most at the end of life? A critical analysis of advance care planning. *Int. J. Palliat. Nurs.* **23**(12): 596–604.

18. Levoy, K., Salani, D.A., and Buck, H. (2019). A systematic review and gap analysis of advance care planning intervention components and outcomes among cancer patients using the transtheoretical model of health behavior change. *J. Pain Symptom Manage.* **57**(1): 118–139.

19. Lin C.P., Evans C.J., Koffman J., Sheu S.J., Hsu S.H., and Harding R. (2019). What influences patients' decisions regarding palliative care in advance care planning discussions? Perspectives from a qualitative study conducted with advanced cancer patients, families and healthcare professionals. *Palliat. Med.* **33**(10): 1299–1309.

20. Lin C.P., Evans C.J., Koffman J., Armes J., Murtagh F.E.M., and Harding R. (2019). The conceptual models and mechanisms of action that underpin advance care planning for cancer patients: A systematic review of randomised controlled trials. *Palliat. Med.* **33**(1): 5–23. January, 2019.

21. Chen Y.C., Huang H.P., Tung T.H., Lee M.Y., Beaton R.D., Lin Y.C., and Jane S.W. (2022). The decisional balance, attitudes, and practice behaviors, its predicting factors, and related experiences of advance care planning in Taiwanese patients with advanced cancer. *BMC Palliat. Care* **21**(1): 189. November 2, 2022.

22. Martina D., Kustanti C.Y., Dewantari R., Sutandyo N., Putranto R., Shatri H., Effendy C., van der Heide A., van der Rijt C.C.D., and Rietjens J.A.C. (2022). Advance care planning for patients with cancer and family caregivers in Indonesia: A qualitative study. *BMC Palliat. Care.* **21**(1): 204. November 22, 2022.

23. Martina D., Kustanti C.Y., Dewantari R., Sutandyo N., Putranto R., Shatri H., Effendy C., van der Heide A., Rietjens J.A.C., and van der Rijt C. (2022). Opportunities and challenges for advance care planning in strongly religious family-centric societies: A focus group study of Indonesian cancer-care professionals. *BMC Palliat. Care* **21**(1): 110. June 22, 2022.

24. Pedrosa Carrasco A.J., Berlin P., Betker L., Riera-Knorrenschild J., von Blanckenburg P., and Seifart C. (2022). Developing a care pathway for hospital-based advance care planning for cancer patients: A modified Delphi study. *Eur. J. Cancer Care (Engl.)* **31**(6): e13756. November, 2022.

25. Narang, A.K., Wright, A.A., and Nicholas, L.H. (2015). Trends in advance care planning in patients with cancer: Results from a national longitudinal survey. *JAMA Oncol.* **1**(5): 601–608.

26. Mack, J.W., Cronin, A., Taback, N., Huskamp, H.A., Keating, N.L., Malin, J.L., Earle, C.C., and Weeks, J.C. (2012). End-of-life care discussions among patients with advanced cancer: a cohort study. *Ann. Intern. Med.* **156**(3): 204–210.

27. Sagara Y., Mori M., Yamamoto S., *et al.* (2021). Current status of advance care planning and end-of-life communication for patients with advanced and metastatic breast cancer. *Oncologist* **26**(4): e686–e693.

28. Lin C.P., Peng J.K., Chen P.J., Huang H.L., Hsu S.H., and Cheng S.Y. (2020). Preferences on the timing of initiating advance care planning and withdrawing life-sustaining treatment between terminally-ill cancer patients and their main family caregivers: A prospective study. *Int. J. Environ. Res. Public Health.* **17**(21): 7954. October 29, 2020.

29. Kubi B., Istl A.C., Lee K.T., Conca-Cheng A., and Johnston F.M. (2020). Advance care planning in cancer: Patient preferences for personnel and timing. *JCO Oncol. Pract.* **16**(9): e875–e883.

30. ParK E.J., Lim Y.J., Kim J.J., Oh S.B., Oh S.Y., and Park K. (2019). Feasibility of early application of an advance directive at the time of first-line

palliative chemotherapy in patients with incurable cancer: A prospective study. *Am. J. Hosp. Palliat. Care* **36**(10): 893–899.

31. Bestvina C.M., and Polite B.N. (2017). Implementation of advance care planning in oncology: A review of the literature. *J. Oncol. Pract.* **13**(10): 657–6624.

32. Johnson, S., Butow, P., Kerridge, I., and Tattersall, M. (2016). Advance care planning for cancer patients: A systematic review of perceptions and experiences of patients, families, and healthcare providers. *Psycho-oncology* **25**(4): 362–386.

33. Kishino M., Ellis-Smith C., Afolabi O., and Koffman J. (2022). Family involvement in advance care planning for people living with advanced cancer: A systematic mixed-methods review. *Palliat. Med.* **36**(3): 462–477.

34. Rietjens J.A.C., Sudore R.L., Connolly M., *et al.* (2017). Definition and recommendations for advance care planning: An international consensus supported by the European association for palliative care. *Lancet Oncol.* **18**: e543–e551.

35. Lin C.P., Cheng S.Y., Mori M., Suh S.Y., Chan H.Y., Martina D., Pang W.S., Huang H.L., Peng J.K., Yao C.A., Tsai J.S., Hu W.Y., Wang Y.W., Shih C.Y., Hsu S.H., Wu C.Y., Chen P.J., Ho H.L., Pang G.S., Menon S., Ng-Han Lip R., Yuen K.K., Kwok A.O., Kim S.H., Kim J.Y., Takenouchi S., Kizawa Y., Morita T., Iwata F., Tashiro S., and Chiu T.Y. (2019). 2019 Taipei declaration on advance care planning: A cultural adaptation of end-of-life care discussion. *J. Palliat. Med.* **22**(10): 1175–1177.

36. National Comprehensive Cancer Network. (2023). NCCN Clinical Practice Guidelines in Oncology — Palliative Care Version 1.2023.

37. Schrijvers, D., Cherny, N. I., and ESMO Guidelines Working Group. (2014). ESMO clinical practice guidelines on palliative care: Advanced care planning. *Ann. Oncol. Off. J. Eur. Soc. Med. Oncol.* **25**(Suppl 3): iii138–iii142.

38. Gilligan, T., Coyle, N., Frankel, R.M., Berry, D.L., Bohlke, K., Epstein, R.M., Finlay, E., Jackson, V.A., Lathan, C.S., Loprinzi, C.L., Nguyen, L.H., Seigel, C., and Baile, W.F. (2017). Patient-clinician communication: American society of clinical oncology consensus guideline. *J. Clin. Oncol. Off. J. Am. Soc. Clin. Oncol.* **35**(31): 3618–3632.

39. Baile, W.F., Buckman, R., Lenzi, R., Glober, G., Beale, E.A., and Kudelka, A.P. (2000). SPIKES-A six-step protocol for delivering bad news: Application to the patient with cancer. *Oncologist*, **5**(4): 302–311.

40. Clayton, J.M., Hancock, K.M., Butow, P.N., Tattersall, M.H., Currow, D.C., Australian and New Zealand Expert Advisory Group, Adler, J., Aranda, S., Auret, K., Boyle, F., Britton, A., Chye, R., Clark, K., Davidson, P., Davis, J.M., Girgis, A., Graham, S., Hardy, J., Introna, K., Kearsley, J., Thoracic Society of Australia and New Zealand. (2007). Clinical practice guidelines for communicating prognosis and end-of-life issues with adults in the

advanced stages of a life-limiting illness, and their caregivers. *Med. J. Aust.* **186**(S12): S77–S105.

41. Bernacki, R.E., Block, S.D., and American College of Physicians High Value Care Task Force. (2014). Communication about serious illness care goals: A review and synthesis of best practices. *JAMA Intern. Med.* **174**(12): 1994–2003.

42. Rhea A. Stein, Louise Sharpe, Melanie L. Bell, Fran M. Boyle, Stewart M. Dunn, and Stephen J. Clarke. (2013). Randomized controlled trial of a structured intervention to facilitate end-of-life decision making in patients with advanced cancer. *J. Clin. Oncol.* **31**: 3403–3410.

43. Johnson, S.B., Butow, P.N., Bell, M.L., Detering, K., Clayton, J.M., Silvester, W., Kiely, B.E., Clarke, S., Vaccaro, L., Stockler, M.R., Beale, P., Fitzgerald, N., and Tattersall, M.H.N. (2018). A randomised controlled trial of an advance care planning intervention for patients with incurable cancer. *Br. J. Cancer* **119**(10): 1182–1190.

44. Korfage I.J., Carreras G., Arnfeldt Christensen C.M., Billekens P., Bramley L., Briggs L., *et al.* (2020). Advance care planning in patients with advanced cancer: A 6-country, cluster-randomised clinical trial. *PLoS Med.* **17**(11): e1003422.

45. Epstein, A.S., O'Reilly, E.M., Shuk, E., Romano, D., Li, Y., Breitbart, W., and Volandes, A.E. (2018). A randomized trial of acceptability and effects of values-based advance care planning in outpatient oncology: Person- centered oncologic care and choices (P-COCC). *J. Pain Symptom Manage.* **56**(2): 169–177.e1. August, 2018.

46. Yun, Y.H., Kang, E., Park, S., Koh, S.J., Oh, H.S., Keam, B., Do, Y.R., Chang, W.J., Jeong, H.S., Nam, E.M., Jung, K.H., Kim, H.R., Choo, J., Lee, J., and Sim, J.A. (2019). Efficacy of a decision aid consisting of a video and booklet on advance care planning for advanced cancer patients: Randomized controlled trial. *J. Pain Symptom Manage.* **58**(6): 940–948.

47. Schubart J.R., Levi B.H., Bain M.M., Farace E., and Green M.J. (2019). Advance care planning among patients with advanced cancer. *J. Oncol. Pract.* **15**(1): e65–e73.

48. De Vleminck, A., Pardon, K., Beernaert, K., Deschepper, R., Houttekier, D., Van Audenhove, C., Deliens, L., and Vander Stichele, R. (2014). Barriers to advance care planning in cancer, heart failure and dementia patients: A focus group study on general practitioners' views and experiences. *PloS One*, **9**(1): e84905.

49. Martina, D., Lin, C.P., Kristanti, M.S., Bramer, W.M., Mori, M., Korfage, I.J., van der Heide, A., van der Rijt, C.C.D., and Rietjens, J.A.C. (2021). Advance care planning in Asia: A systematic narrative review of healthcare professionals' knowledge, attitude, and experience. *J. Am. Med. Dir. Assoc.* **22**(2): 349.e1–349.e28.

50. Cottingham A.H., Beck-Coon K., Bernat J.K., *et al.* (2019). Addressing personal barriers to advance care planning: Qualitative investigation of a mindfulness-based intervention for adults with cancer and their family caregivers. *Palliat. Support. Care* **17**(3): 276–285.

51. Gensheimer M.F., Gupta D., Patel M.I., *et al.* (2023). Use of machine learning and lay care coaches to increase advance care planning conversations for patients with metastatic cancer. *JCO Oncol. Pract.* **19**(2): e176–e184.

52. Yeung, R., Wong, K.R., Yuen, K.K., Wong, K.Y., Yau, Y., Lo, S.H., and Liu, R. (2015). Clinical oncology and palliative medicine as a combined specialty–a unique model in Hong Kong. *Ann. Palliat. Med.* **4**(3): 132–134.

53. Kreye, G., Lundeby, T., Latino, N., Galotti, M., and Kaasa, S. (2022). ESMO designated centres of integrated oncology and palliative care (ESMO DCs): Education, research and programme development survey. *ESMO Open,* **7**(6): 100622.

54. Wong, S.Y., Lo, S.H., Chan, C.H., Chui, H.S., Sze, W.K., and Tung, Y. (2012). Is it feasible to discuss an advance directive with a Chinese patient with advanced malignancy? A prospective cohort study. *Hong Kong Med. J.* **18**(3): 178–185.

55. Kwok, Y.L., Leung, Wai Ming, Agarwal, Arnav, B., and Wong, K.H. (2018). Advance directives in Chinese patients with cancer: A retrospective study in a single palliative care unit. *J. Pain Manage.* **11**(1): 31–40.

56. Chan, K.Y., Chiu, H.Y., Yap, D.Y.H., Li, C.W., Yip, T., Tsang, K.W., Tam, W.O., Au, H.Y., Wong, C.Y., Chan, M.L., and Sham, M.K. (2021). Impact of structured advance care planning program on patients' wish items and healthcare utilization. *Ann. Palliat. Med.* **10**(2): 1421–1430.

57. Hospital Authority of Hong Kong. (2023). HA guidelines on advance care planning. Available from: https://www.ha.org.hk/haho/ho/psrm/EACPGuidelines.pdf. Accessed on 17 April 2023.

58. Tse C.Y. (2021). Advantages of legislation for advance directives in Hong Kong and areas of concern for clinicians. *Hong Kong Med. J.* **27**(4): 309–311.

Chapter 31

Contemporary Cardiology and Advance Care Planning

Tammy J. Pegg[*,†], Rebecca Eddington[†], and Daniel Garofalo[‡]

[*]*Te Tāhū Hauora Health Quality & Safety Commission, Advance Care Planning, Wellington, New Zealand*
[†]*Te Whatu Ora Nelson Marlborough, Nelson, New Zealand*
[‡]*Te Whatu Ora Waikato, Hamilton, New Zealand*

Introduction

Cardiology is often near the forefront of medical technologies and advancements in evidence-based medicine, which has led to significant improvement in survival from cardiovascular disease. However, the net benefit of improving cardiovascular survival is to create complexity in older age, and — although many interventions are less invasive than 20 years ago — ageing is multifactorial, and treating a single condition in older age may lead us to do more without making things better. Understanding advance care planning (ACP) should be a priority for cardiologists; similarly, understanding some aspects of contemporary cardiology practice is paramount for practitioners in ACP.

In particular, advances or care that is really pertinent to the domain of ACP covered here includes resuscitation and cardiopulmonary resuscitation (CPR), cardiac rhythm devices (including internal cardioverter defibrillators and pacemakers), and finally transcutaneous aortic valve replacement (TAVR).

Understanding CPR

Cardiopulmonary resuscitation (defined as chest compressions and rescue breaths) manually empties the heart, offering a degree of cerebral perfusion while the cause of cardiac arrest is reversed.

However, this simple definition has been lost[1] with practitioners grouping broader resuscitation with CPR. Such is the case in the United Kingdom (UK), where the UK Resuscitation Council defines CPR as including chest compressions, high-voltage electric shocks, ventilation, and injection of "drugs".[2] Other groups such as the European, Australian, New Zealand, and Southern African Resuscitation Councils; the Stroke Foundation of Canada; the InterAmerican Heart Foundation; and the American Heart Association retain the original definition of CPR as chest compressions and rescue breaths.[3] Phraseology for withholding these treatments also varies internationally: the USA uses "do not attempt resuscitation" (DNAR), and the UK uses "do not attempt CPR" (DNACPR).

It is therefore unsurprising that the terms "CPR" and "resuscitation" are often used interchangeably by both clinicians and patients. However, CPR is a subset of the broader range of measures that constitute resuscitation. CPR is always a resuscitation measure, but resuscitation is an intent, not a specific treatment. A number of treatments may constitute resuscitation in one context but simply good medical care in another.

Cardiopulmonary resuscitation mostly originated in the operating theatre as a standalone treatment for reversible circulatory collapse after the induction of anaesthesia.[4] Its combination in the 1960s with cardiac defibrillation for the effective treatment of arrhythmic cardiac arrest led to widespread rollout: initially pre-hospital, then to coronary care units where it is recognised as a lifesaver in sudden cardiac arrest.

It continued to spread throughout hospitals and aged residential care facilities, but it is not effective when administered in cardiac arrest resulting from non-cardiac chronic or subacute deterioration. CPR is not a standalone treatment for cardiac arrest and does not provide any meaningful intervention unless there is also a highly reversible cause for the sudden collapse. CPR is largely unhelpful outside those original areas, and clear communication of this message to patients may facilitate better conversations about CPR.[5]

Why Is in-Hospital Cardiac Arrest Different?

Excluding cardiac causes, most cardiac arrest in hospital is simply not reversible, either because of patient factors or the aetiology of the cardiac arrest or simply because cardiac arrest has occurred despite optimal treatment. Importantly, outcomes differ widely between cardiac patients (survival around 40%) and non-cardiac patients (survival only around 10%).[6]

Simply put, CPR is a first aid measure when the heart stops *suddenly*, bridging the time until the patient reaches specialist teams and treatment. But when those teams and treatments are already in play, then cardiac arrest most likely represents failure of medical treatment and the end point of the dying process. In this context, chest compressions and rescue breaths offer no meaningful bridge.

Separating CPR from other forms of resuscitation that may be deployed to prevent fulminant cardiac arrest may help some patients access other evidence-based treatments while restricting futile or unwarranted treatments at the end of life.

Factors That Determine Outcomes of in-Hospital Cardiac Arrest

Several factors impact the outcome of cardiac arrest in hospitals: preexisting health conditions, current illness, aetiology of the cardiac arrest, and whether treatment has already been started. Therefore, despite the immediate availability of health care teams to treat cardiac arrest, survival is poor and overall longer-term survival (cardiac and non-cardiac) is approximately 20%, representing around half of those discharged to a facility instead of home.[6–9] We argue that CPR should be reserved for a few selected patients instead of being a default intervention and offer a clinical decision tree to assist clinicians with such decisions. Importantly, we offer a way for clinicians to consider the value of CPR individualised to the context of the person and their illness to aid decision-making for all parties.

Figure 1 shows a proposed pathway for clinicians considering a plan for clinical deterioration, to provide the medical content for a DNACPR decision as part of discussions around shared goals of care.

How to Talk to Your Patient about CPR?

Conversations with patients about CPR are best undertaken as part of a shared decision-making process, whereby the clinician will first explore the patient's and family's shared goals of care. Understanding the patient's values, priorities, worries, and what they may be prepared to undergo as part of treatment is a fundamental part of shared decision-making. Doing so may also ease the process of communicating clinician concerns around CPR or other advanced treatments.

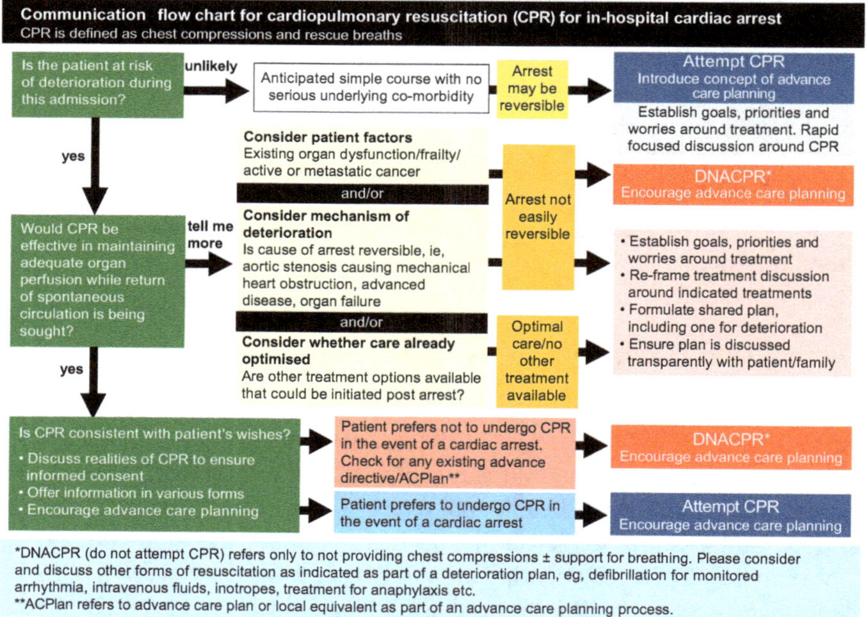

Figure 1.   Communication flow chart to aid DNACPR and shared goals of care discussions.

The balance around decision-making may vary in countries or cultures between weighted for the clinician (benevolent) or more leaning towards the patient/family (autonomous). However, in all respects, communication is central to either discussing the reasons for clinical decision-making in a benevolent culture or facilitating informed decision-making/consent in an autonomous culture. The use of persuasive or manipulative communication techniques using graphic imagery around CPR and associated injuries to dissuade patients away from CPR is well documented in all cultures.[10,11] Simply put, manipulating the patient with descriptions of rib fractures or CPR-associated trauma engages the emotional decision centres and diminishes the capacity for informed decision-making.[10]

We propose a process allowing clinicians to contemplate the value of CPR in any given person, illness, and goals to individualise the information rather than using generic information around CPR and associated harm.

A Three-Step Approach to Help Clinicians Understand the Value and Limitations of CPR for an Individual

The green column in Figure 1 provides a three-step approach for assessing a detailed CPR decision process for a clinician to assist them in undertaking a CPR discussion with a patient or family.

Step 1: Is this patient at risk of deterioration during this admission?

Risk factors for deterioration include age (≥60 years), comorbidities or existing organ dysfunction, and unplanned admissions through the emergency department.[12,13] Other factors include complex or severe presentation with evidence of acute organ dysfunction or raised early warning score.[14,15] Patients deemed at low risk are typically elective admissions for non-complex procedures who are otherwise well; in a time-constrained environment, these patients may not need to be prioritised for a detailed discussion.

Step 2: Would CPR be effective to maintain organ perfusion during attempts to reverse the cause of cardiac arrest?

a.   *Patient factors*: Several factors are known to be associated with worse outcomes after in-hospital cardiac arrest. These include male gender, age >60 years, active malignancy and chronic kidney, liver or pulmonary disease.[12,16–18] Furthermore, clinical frailty is associated with CPR being unsuccessful.[19,20] Swedish registry data suggest that frailty is more important than advanced age: importantly, with good case selection (i.e., non-frail, post-myocardial infarction), older survivors had a good neurological outcome.[21]

b. *Mechanism of deterioration*: The aetiologies of in-hospital cardiac arrest are very different from cardiac arrest in the community. Around 60% of people experiencing cardiac arrest in public spaces present with an initial shockable rhythm,[22] compared with only 25% of in-hospital cardiac arrests.[23] The major determinant of outcomes in hospitals is the potential mechanism of deterioration and whether the process can be reversed in a timely manner. Being monitored for arrhythmia, having a shockable arrhythmia, and being a cardiac patient are all factors associated with favourable outcomes. One-year survival for cardiac patients with an in-hospital cardiac arrest is 39.3% versus 10.7% for non-cardiac patients.[6,7,23]

Beyond the cardiology ward, other causes with good outcomes and survival rates of around 50% generally include adverse drug reactions (especially during anaesthesia), intoxication, and hypothermia.[24] This is inherently logical when we consider the ease of reversing the underlying cause. Conversely, in hard-to-reverse conditions such as sepsis, COVID-19-related hypoxaemia, aortic stenosis, aortic dissection/rupture, neurological causes, and exsanguination, CPR adds very little value once cardiac arrest has occurred. Survival from these conditions is generally much less than 15%.[23–29]

c. *Available treatments*: The final consideration is around whether the treatment has already been optimised at the time of cardiac arrest. If so, the patient has arrested *despite* the best treatment available. Furthermore, if the patient is not suitable for escalation of treatment to the intensive care unit, then — because of the injuries associated with CPR — they are not suitable for CPR either.

Survival of a patient already optimised on intensive care is even lower than in the general ward environment, with survival of 5% and even less for non-shockable cardiac arrest.[16]

The commonest outcome after attempted resuscitation is the return of spontaneous circulation, which occurs in 50–70% of in-hospital cardiac arrests;[9] however, survival is much lower, and 63% of the patients in whom spontaneous circulation returned then made decisions around restricting resuscitation and subsequently died.[8] In many patients already receiving treatment for their underlying disease, the cause of deterioration or cardiac arrest in hospitals cannot be reversed, so they simply have further cardiac arrest later.[7]

Step 3: For the person who may benefit from in-hospital treatment of cardiac arrest, would CPR be something they would want?

In highly selected older patients presenting to hospitals with cardiac disease, CPR is associated with good outcomes, and age alone should not present a barrier to CPR.[21]

Exploring a patient's values, goals, priorities, worries, and what they are prepared to go through for the possibility of more time is better than direct questioning when establishing preferences around CPR or other highly invasive treatments.

It is also important to consider patients who, despite reasonably good health, have a clear sense that CPR is not an intervention they would want. In these situations, it is essential to ensure that the person fully understands the nature and purpose both of CPR and of resuscitation in general so that their informed choice can be accurately recorded and followed. Refusal of CPR does not equate to, for example, refusal of fluid resuscitation for hypotension or of oxygen and antibiotics for respiratory infection.

Empathic Communication with Patients about CPR

Clinicians need to partner with patients to help improve their understanding of CPR or other resuscitation measures. Explaining resuscitation measures and how they relate to the patient's current illness and any current or potential treatments could shift discussions beyond frailty or their existing condition to also account for individualised mechanisms of cardiac arrests or the treatments available. This could shift the emphasis away from graphical illustrations of resuscitation to a more open and honest discussion about what may lie ahead. Table 1 illustrates some examples of conversation starters.

Table 1. Conversation starters around resuscitation based on patient, disease, and available treatments.

Factor	Conversation starter
Patient factors	I am worried that your body is weakened by kidney failure, and it would be difficult for your body to recover if your health worsened. What is your understanding of your health now?
Mechanism of deterioration	Sadly, your dad's health is deteriorating, and his heart is not the problem. If he deteriorates further and his heart stops beating, restarting it won't help him recover. Can we talk about this?
Available treatments	I wish you had responded to the antibiotics better; I worry that you are becoming sicker and could die. I wonder whether we can discuss a plan for if things change.

Summary around CPR and Resuscitation

Clinicians must be able to understand and communicate to patients that CPR:

- consists only of chest compressions and support for breathing,
- manually empties the heart,
- helps maintain brain perfusion while the cause of the arrest is being treated,
- is not effective alone for treating the underlying cause of cardiac arrest.

Most importantly, patients need to hear that, in hospitals, clinicians cannot easily reverse the cause of the arrest with defibrillation or other simple measures. What they may have seen portrayed in television dramas or witnessed at sporting events differs from cardiac arrest inside hospitals. This should be framed within the context of them and their illness and that a cardiac arrest in people sick enough to be in a hospital is usually not related to a fixable problem with the heart. They also need to know that treatments attempting to reduce the risk of cardiac arrest will be given as appropriate: DNACPR is not the same as "do not treat." Absolute clarity about what CPR actually involves is central to changing this culture.

Cardiac Rhythm Devices: Pacemakers and Internal Cardioverter Defibrillators

As patients exert their right to be actively involved in their health care and, as health care teams encourage ACP, shared decision-making and respecting goals of care, requests around the deactivation of cardiac devices have become more prevalent in clinical practice.

As health care providers, our role is to align our care with patient-centred goals. Although deactivation of implantable cardioverter defibrillators (ICDs) is common and may be appropriate to protect a person from painful and futile intervention at the end of life, deactivation of pacemakers is rare because it is rarely appropriate. However, patients, relatives, and other healthcare professionals are increasingly asking about it as part of the dying process.

Ideally, ACP should be discussed when a patient consents to the original implant and at every subsequent generator replacement. However, for several reasons, this is not commonly done.[30]

Device Types

ICDs treat sustained ventricular arrhythmias. Therapy includes anti-tachycardia pacing and cardioversion/defibrillation therapy. An ICD has standard pacemaker functions that are usually programmed to a backup mode (heart rate 30 beats per minute) unless standard pacemaker therapy is also required.

ICDs are implanted in patients who have either had or are at risk of a cardiac arrest or life-threatening arrhythmia (secondary and primary prevention, respectively). These patients often have significant heart disease or heart failure.

Pacemakers can be single- or dual-chamber devices that pace the right heart as part of treatment for bradyarrhythmia.

Cardiac resynchronisation therapy (CRT) is a type of pacing therapy for heart failures and paces both left and right ventricles with the aim of resynchronising cardiac contraction to improve heart function. It is an adjuvant therapy to pharmacotherapy for heart failure and may be combined with defibrillator therapy.

Device Deactivation

ICD therapy may no longer be appropriate as a patient's heart condition progresses (e.g., terminal heart failure) or other disease processes develop (e.g., malignancy and dementia). Retrospective studies have shown that 21% of patients will receive a shock in the 30 days before death.[31]

Deactivation of an ICD does not lead to immediate death, which often needs to be highlighted to the patient and/or their family. Deactivation of an ICD means any ventricular tachycardia or fibrillation will no longer be treated, which may then lead to death; however, this is not universal as these rhythms can be self-reverting.

Deactivating both pacemakers and ICDs is a simple programming change that can be undertaken at the patient's bedside or within the clinic setting, is not painful, and does not involve an invasive procedure. Pacemaker therapy (backup rate) is generally left active. The device can just as easily be reactivated should the patient's clinical condition change substantially. The device is generally not removed.

Pacemaker deactivation can lead to a substantial change in the person's symptoms or well-being, but pacing therapy is still a simple treatment.

Ethical considerations

Ethically, there is no difference between refusing a device and withdrawing its treatment.[32] Most opinions state that turning a pacemaker off is not assisted suicide or passive euthanasia. The central consideration is that, rather than the intervention causing the patient's death, death is caused by the patient's underlying condition.[33,34] Unlike for deactivation of ICDs, deactivation of pacing devices may be subject to legal considerations, particularly around consent and capacity, which are beyond the scope of this piece. It may be advisable to clarify the legal status locally before further exploring deactivation of pacemaker therapy.

Although deactivating a pacemaker device may be no different ethically to withdrawing other therapy, the medical and logistical implications are unique. Deactivating a pacemaker involves an inherent degree of unpredictability and imminence because the scenarios, symptoms, and timeframes that might subsequently unfold vary widely.

Requests for deactivation of pacemaker devices

Generally, pacemaker devices act to alleviate symptoms and improve quality of life, so it is normally unwise and unwarranted to deactivate pacing therapy. Patients may simply be reassured to know that death can ensue naturally with a pacemaker device in place. In most patients, ordinary dying is mediated by progressive acidosis, which will render the device non-functional due to loss of capture.

However, a request for a pacemaker deactivation may still be sent to the pacemaker clinic, an on-call physiologist, a cardiologist, or an electrophysiology specialist. These decisions may take some time to be enacted safely and are ideally untaken with multi-disciplinary support and involvement of the patient's family doctor, palliative care, district or hospice nurses, or mental health practitioners alongside the cardiology/electrophysiology team.

The conversation about deactivating a pacemaker must be fully documented in the clinical records. This conversation and documentation should include the following[35]:

- the patient's views, wishes, and goals of care,
- the patient's awareness of their illness and clinical situation,
- the patient's quality of life, functional status, prognosis, and clinical circumstances,
- the perceived harm from continuous device operation versus its benefits and consideration of how they may align with the goals of care,
- the likely consequences of pacemaker deactivation; however, it is difficult to accurately predict the full consequences of a pacemaker deactivation, and there will be a degree of uncertainty,
- any questions from the patient or family.

If deactivation of the pacemaker is likely to worsen symptoms or discomfort, the patient needs to be made aware of this, and appropriate palliative care or hospice input should be sought.

Medical considerations

From a medical perspective, understanding should include the patient's underlying disease(s) and prognosis and, crucially, the degree of pacemaker dependency. In this regard, there are different potential scenarios and implications.

In a pacemaker-dependent patient (no or very intermittent underlying heart rhythm), deactivation can potentially lead to death or other non-terminal scenarios. In the first situation, extreme bradycardia with loss of output or a bradycardia-induced ventricular arrhythmia can cause rapid or instant death. In a patient with a very slow or intermittent escape rhythm, the clinical situation may include distressing symptoms such as intermittent loss of consciousness, seizures, pre-syncope, fatigue, dyspnoea, falls, and haemodynamic stroke from transient cerebral hypoperfusion. Even with experience, it is often difficult to predict the degree and "adequacy" of an escape rhythm to maintain basic physiological functions.

In a non-dependent patient (underlying heart rhythm exists most of the time), the difference between having the device active or deactivated will generally not be immediately life-threatening. However, deactivation will have an impact on symptoms (as mentioned) and quality of life.

Deactivation of CRT can worsen symptoms of heart failure (orthopnoea, oedema, dyspnoea, acute pulmonary oedema, etc.) without precipitating near dying. As such, CRT should simply be considered as an adjuvant to heart failure pharmacotherapy and should generally not be withdrawn unless in addition to withdrawal of all medical treatments.

Transcutaneous Aortic Valve Replacement

Ageing is the primary cause of aortic stenosis. As we age, calcium deposits form in the aortic valve, leading it to progressively narrow. Once symptoms are present or left ventricular function deteriorates, prognosis is poor.[36] Life expectancy is approximately 2–3 years, with about one-third of this group experiencing sudden death.[36] In addition, once patients become symptomatic, their quality of life may deteriorate quickly, with shortness of breath, angina, and fatigue. Conversely, intervention on the aortic valve carries risk. When considering ACP in patients with aortic stenosis, an understanding of the goals of care is imperative to discussing and planning care that considers overall well-being and quality of life.

In the next 30 years, the number of people aged >65 years is expected to double. Correspondingly, the number being assessed for treatment of severe aortic stenosis is rising, and current data suggest that the prevalence of severe aortic stenosis in those aged ≥75 years is around 3%.[37] The addition of TAVR as an alternative to surgical aortic valve replacement in high-risk older adults has seen substantial exponential growth in aortic valve replacement internationally.[32] Although procedural outcomes are good, with 95% procedural success in high-risk older adults,[38] major complications arise in around 30% of high-risk individuals[32] and may include death, myocardial infarction, cerebrovascular accident, vascular events, bleeding, acute kidney injury, transcatheter valve regurgitation, valve malpositioning, coronary occlusion, and cardiac conduction abnormalities (requiring pacemaker insertion). Furthermore, two in five patients in the original PARTNER I/CoreValve trials of high-risk surgical candidates indicated that they experienced poor health-related quality of life in the following year.[39] Additionally, discharge-to-home rates may be as low as 50%, depending on the level of frailty.[40]

These figures highlight that, although the valve can be fixed, the person is often left with significant health issues that impair independent living or well-being, highlighting the need for more accurate risk-prediction tools and shared decision-making in this complex group. Consequently, frailty has become an essential assessment in this cohort of patients to assist in predicting risk, deciding on optimal treatment pathways, and providing truly informed consent for patients.

To ensure that patients receive care that matches their values as they age and to empower them to have a well-informed role in their health decision-making, it is essential to screen for frailty early on in decision-making to prevent unnecessary and potentially harmful tests and procedures.

Frailty has been described as a syndrome of decreased resistance to stressors due to a decline in physiological reserve. It is widely acknowledged that frailty diminishes the potential for functional recovery after a TAVR or surgical aortic valve replacement.[41,42] Conventional pre-operative risk assessments do not accurately calculate risk in older adults.

Using a simple validated assessment tool, such as the Essential Frailty Tool (EFT), which predicts not only mortality but also other geriatric domains such as functional capacity after aortic valve intervention, will help guide further assessment and conversation.[42] The EFT is a multidomain tool that is simple for any health care professional to administer in less than 5 minutes. It requires recent blood tests, including haemoglobin and albumin, alongside measures of core strength from chair rises and cognition.

Frailty as assessed with this simple tool is a strong predictor of not only mortality but also other meaningful parameters, such as independence and quality of life. Results from the FRAILTY-AVR study indicated that significant frailty is associated with a 65% chance of mortality at 1 year following TAVR.[42]

The point of assessing a patient's overall well-being, including frailty, is to ensure that patients can consider their goals of care with a holistic understanding of their well-being. There is potential for therapeutic misalignment of care, where pathology can take focus in a specialty that is highly focused on intervention.[43] This 5-minute tool shifts the focus away from disease-specific outcomes to guide individualised treatment discussion in the context of recovery, managing expectations, and patient-centred goals.

Conclusion

Cardiology and cardiac intervention have made significant gains in the treatment of heart disease, but effective treatment and improved survival in younger age are creating complexity, comorbidity, and frailty in older age.

The terms CPR and resuscitation are used interchangeably but are distinct entities, and separation of "CPR" from the more general "resuscitation" measures will result in better clinician–patient conversations, clearer medical decisions, and more tailored patient care. In-hospital cardiac arrest is different from out-of-hospital cardiac arrest: in a hospital setting, prevention of cardiac arrest is more important as part of care planning, and cardiac arrest remains difficult to treat once it has occurred.

Withdrawal of cardiac rhythm device therapy often does not precipitate immediate dying and does not prevent natural dying from occurring in most cases. Careful discussion with pacing teams and other specialities as to the implications of withdrawal of cardiac rhythm device therapy is needed to ensure that the implications for the person are fully understood and align with the shared goals of care.

Transcutaneous aortic valve replacement has introduced the option of intervention for aortic stenosis for higher-risk patients. However, complications and loss of independent living are common in these groups, especially in those with co-existent frailty. Risk prediction and goals of care are central to ensuring that treatment aligns with personal goals and that the associated possible outcomes are acceptable.

Acknowledgements

The authors thank Kathryn Mannix for sharing her time and wisdom on CPR and resuscitation in hospitals. We also thank Jane Goodwin, Alex Psirides, and Kate Grundy for developing the three-stage approach for CPR decision-making in hospitals.

References

1. Berry-Kilgour N.A.H., Paulin J.R., Psirides A., *et al.* (2023). A survey of hospital practitioners: Common understanding of CPR definition and outcomes. *Intern. Med. J.* [online ahead of print].
2. British Medical Association, Resuscitation Council (UK), Royal College of Nursing. (2017). Decisions relating to cardiopulmonary resuscitation: Guidance from the British Medical Association, the Resuscitation Council (UK) and the Royal College of Nursing. (3rd edn., 1st rev.). London.
3. Kleinman M.E., Brennan E.E., Goldberger Z.D., *et al.* (2015). Part 5: Adult basic life support and cardiopulmonary resuscitation quality. *Circulation* **132**: S414–S435.
4. Kouwenhoven W.B., Jude J.R., and Knickerbocker G.G. (1960). Closed-chest cardiac massage. *JAMA* **173**: 1064–1067.
5. Adielsson A., Djärv T., Rawshani A., *et al.* (2020). Changes over time in 30-day survival and the incidence of shockable rhythms after in-hospital cardiac arrest-A population-based registry study of nearly 24,000 cases. *Resuscitation* **157**: 135–140.
6. Schluep M., Gravesteijn B.Y., Stolker R.J., *et al.* (2018). One-year survival after in-hospital cardiac arrest: A systematic review and meta-analysis. *Resuscitation* **132**: 90–100.
7. Nolan J.P., Soar J., Smith G.B., *et al.* (2014). Incidence and outcome of in-hospital cardiac arrest in the United Kingdom national cardiac arrest audit. *Resuscitation* **85**: 987–992.
8. Peberdy M.A., Kaye W., Ornato J.P., *et al.* (2003). Cardiopulmonary resuscitation of adults in the hospital: A report of 14 720 cardiac arrests from the national registry of cardiopulmonary resuscitation. *Resuscitation* **58**: 297–308.
9. Andersen L.W., Holmberg M.J., Løfgren B., *et al.* (2019). Adult in-hospital cardiac arrest in Denmark. *Resuscitation* **140**: 31–36.
10. Dzeng E. (2019). Habermasian communication pathologies in do-not-resuscitate discussions at the end of life: Manipulation as an unintended consequence of an ideology of patient autonomy. *Sociol. Health Illn.* 41: 325–342.

11. Eli K., Hawkes C.A., Ochieng C., *et al.* (2021). Why, when and how do secondary-care clinicians have emergency care and treatment planning conversations? Qualitative findings from the respect evaluation study. *Resuscitation* **162**: 343–350.

12. Henriksen D.P., Brabrand M., and Lassen A.T. (2014). Prognosis and risk factors for deterioration in patients admitted to a medical emergency department. *PLoS One* **9**: e94649.

13. Lyons P.G., Klaus J., McEvoy C.A., *et al.* (2019). Factors associated with clinical deterioration among patients hospitalized on the wards at a tertiary cancer hospital. *J. Oncol. Pract.* **15**: e652–e665.

14. Kirkland L.L., Malinchoc M., O'Byrne M., *et al.* (2013). A clinical deterioration prediction tool for internal medicine patients. *Am. J. Med. Qual.* **28**: 135–142.

15. Churpek M.M., Snyder A., Han X., *et al.* (2017). Quick sepsis-related organ failure assessment, systemic inflammatory response syndrome, and early warning scores for detecting clinical deterioration in infected patients outside the intensive care unit. *Am. J. Respir. Crit. Care Med.* **195**: 906–911.

16. Tian J., Kaufman D.A., Zarich S., *et al.* (2010). Outcomes of critically ill patients who received cardiopulmonary resuscitation. *Am. J. Respir. Crit. Care Med.* **182**: 501–506.

17. Reisfield G.M., Wallace S.K., Munsell M.F., *et al.* (2006). Survival in cancer patients undergoing in-hospital cardiopulmonary resuscitation: A meta-analysis. *Resuscitation* **71**: 152–160.

18. Guha A., Buck B., and Biersmith M., *et al.* (2019). Contemporary impacts of a cancer diagnosis on survival following in-hospital cardiac arrest. *Resuscitation* **142**: 30–37.

19. Smith R.J., Reid D.A., and Santamaria J.D. (2019). Frailty is associated with reduced prospect of discharge home after in-hospital cardiac arrest. *Intern. Med. J.* **49**: 978–985.

20. Fernando S.M., McIsaac D.I., Rochwerg B., *et al.* (2020). Frailty and associated outcomes and resource utilization following in-hospital cardiac arrest. *Resuscitation* **146**: 138–144.

21. Hirlekar G., Karlsson T., Aune, S., *et al.* (2017). Survival and neurological outcome in the elderly after in-hospital cardiac arrest. *Resuscitation* **118**: 101–106.

22. Oving I., De Graaf C., Karlsson L., *et al.* (2020). Occurrence of shockable rhythm in out-of-hospital cardiac arrest over time: A report from the COSTA group. *Resuscitation* **151**: 67–74.

23. Andersen L.W., Holmberg M.J., Berg K.M., *et al.* (2019). In-hospital cardiac arrest: A review. *JAMA* **321**: 1200–1210.

24. Wallmuller C., Meron G., Kurkciyan I., *et al.* (2012). Causes of in-hospital cardiac arrest and influence on outcome. *Resuscitation* **83**: 1206–1211.

25. Perman S.M., Stanton E., Soar J., *et al.* (2016). Location of in-hospital cardiac arrest in the United States — variability in event rate and outcomes. *J. Am. Heart Assoc.* **5**: e003638.

26. Radeschi G., Mina A., Berta G., *et al.* (2017). Incidence and outcome of in-hospital cardiac arrest in Italy: A multicentre observational study in the Piedmont region. *Resuscitation* **119**: 48–55.

27. Sulzgruber P., Schnaubelt S., Pesce M., *et al.* (2019). Aortic stenosis is an independent predictor for outcome in patients with in-hospital cardiac arrest. *Resuscitation* **137**: 156–160.

28. Shao F., Xu S., Ma X., *et al.* (2020). In-hospital cardiac arrest outcomes among patients with COVID-19 pneumonia in Wuhan, China. *Resuscitation* **151**: 18–23.

29. Hayek S.S., Brenner S.K., Azam T.U., *et al.* (2020). In-hospital cardiac arrest in critically ill patients with COVID-19: Multicenter cohort study. *BMJ* **371**: m3513.

30. Stoevelaar R., Brinkman-Stoppelenburg A., Driel A.G., *et al.* (2020). Implantable cardioverter defibrillator deactivation and advance care planning: A focus group study. *Heart* **106**: 190–195.

31. Kinch Westerdahl A., Sjöblom J., Mattiasson A.-C., *et al.* (2014). Implantable cardioverter-defibrillator therapy before death: High risk for painful shocks at end of life. *Circulation* **129**: 422–429.

32. Benjamin M.M., and Sorkness C.A. (2017). Practical and ethical considerations in the management of pacemaker and implantable cardiac defibrillator devices in terminally ill patients. *Proc. (Bayl. Univ. Med. Cent.)* **30**: 157–160.

33. Padeletti L., Arnar D.O., Boncinelli L., *et al.* (2010). EHRA expert consensus statement on the management of cardiovascular implantable electronic devices in patients nearing end of life or requesting withdrawal of therapy. *Europace* **12**: 1480–1489.

34. Pitcher D., Soar J., Hogg K., *et al.* (2016). Cardiovascular implanted electronic devices in people towards the end of life, during cardiopulmonary resuscitation and after death: Guidance from the Resuscitation Council (UK), British Cardiovascular Society and National Council for Palliative Care. *Heart* **102**: A1–A17.

35. Lampert R., Hayes D.L., Annas G.J., *et al.* (2010). HRS expert consensus statement on the management of cardiovascular implantable electronic devices (CIEDs) in patients nearing end of life or requesting withdrawal of therapy. *Heart Rhythm* **7**: 1008–1026.

36. Aronow W.S., Ahn C., Kronzon I., *et al.* (1993). Prognosis of congestive heart failure in patients aged ≥62 years with unoperated severe valvular aortic stenosis. *Am. J. Cardiol.* **72**: 846–848.

37. Osnabrugge R.L.J., Mylotte D., Head S.J., *et al.* (2013). Aortic stenosis in the elderly. *J. Am. Coll. Cardiol.* **62**: 1002–1012.

38. Reinöhl J., Kaier K., Reinecke H., *et al.* (2015). Effect of availability of transcatheter aortic-valve replacement on clinical practice. *N. Engl. J. Med.* **373**: 2438–2447.

39. Lindman B.R., Alexander K.P., O'Gara P.T., *et al.* (2014). Futility, benefit, and transcatheter aortic valve replacement. *JACC Cardiovasc. Interv.* **7**: 707–716.

40. Komaki K., Yoshida N., Satomi-Kobayashi S., *et al.* (2021). Preoperative frailty affects postoperative complications, exercise capacity, and home discharge rates after surgical and transcatheter aortic valve replacement. *Heart Vessels* **36**: 1234–1245.

41. Afilalo J., Eisenberg M.J., Morin J.-F., *et al.* (2010). Gait speed as an incremental predictor of mortality and major morbidity in elderly patients undergoing cardiac surgery. *J. Am. Coll. Cardiol.* **56**: 1668–1676.

42. Afilalo J., Lauck S., Kim D.H., *et al.* (2017). Frailty in older adults undergoing aortic valve replacement: The FRAILTY-AVR study. *J. Am. Coll. Cardiol.* **70**: 689–700.

43. Bell S.P., Orr N.M., Dodson J.A., *et al.* (2015). What to expect from the evolving field of geriatric cardiology. *J. Am. Coll. Cardiol.* **66**: 1286–1299.

Chapter 32

Advance Care Planning in Patients with Renal Failure

Yasuhiko Miura

*Division of Adult Nursing, Collage of Nursing,
Iwate University of Health and Medical Sciences, Japan*

Introduction

According to a report by the Japanese Society for Dialysis Treatment, as of December 31, 2021, the number of chronic dialysis patients in Japan was 349700, with 40511 newly introduced patients and 36156 deaths in FY2021, and the number of patients is still increasing, although the rate of increase has slowed down in recent years.[1] In Japan, however, organ transplantation has not progressed, and it is reported that there were 2,057 kidney transplants in 2019, 90% of which were living donor kidney transplants.[2] As for the method of dialysis, 45.9% were reported to be hemodialysis, 50.5% hemofiltration, 0.4% hemoadsorption, 0.2% home hemodialysis, and 3.0% peritoneal dialysis (including combined hemodialysis), indicating that most patients are receiving hemodialysis or hemofiltration at facilities. The average age of chronic dialysis patients at this time was 69.67 years and is getting older every year. The average dialysis history was 7.4 years, but 27.5% of all patients had been on dialysis for more than 10 years, 8.6% for more than 20 years, and the longest reported history of dialysis was 52 years and 8 months. Since less than 1% of patients had been on dialysis for more than 20 years in 1992, the increase in the number of elderly patients on dialysis for a long period of time is a characteristic of dialysis care in Japan.

Advance Directive (AD) for Dialysis Patients

In the diffusion of the concept of AD in Japan, an early start was made in the field of dialysis. In a survey[3] conducted by the author on the attitudes of dialysis specialists in Japan, the US, and Germany toward AD, assuming a dialysis patient with advanced dementia, Japanese dialysis specialists tend to recommend "continue dialysis" in the absence of the patient's AD and the wishes of the patient's family, which was different from the US and Germany. However, there was no difference in the attitude of respecting the patient's AD and family's wishes when they existed. In a subsequent survey of Japanese dialysis patients, more than 80% of patients indicated that they wanted to express their AD, and about 30% of patients actually expressed their AD.[4] However, a later survey revealed statistically that patients' wishes for end-of-life care were understood neither by their families nor by their physicians.[5] In response to these results, in 2003, an advance directive for dialysis patients came into use (Figure 1).[6]

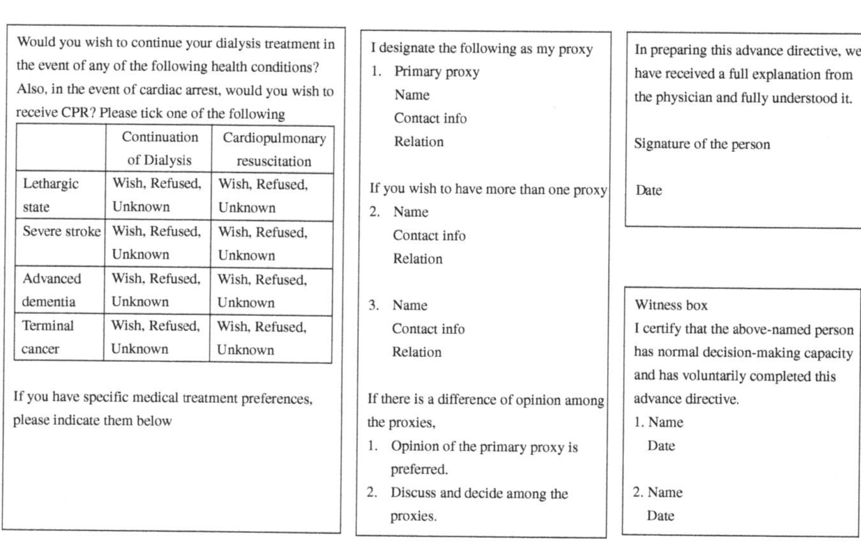

	Continuation of Dialysis	Cardiopulmonary resuscitation
Lethargic state	Wish, Refused, Unknown	Wish, Refused, Unknown
Severe stroke	Wish, Refused, Unknown	Wish, Refused, Unknown
Advanced dementia	Wish, Refused, Unknown	Wish, Refused, Unknown
Terminal cancer	Wish, Refused, Unknown	Wish, Refused, Unknown

Figure 1.   Advance directive form for dialysis patient.[6]

Recent Activities in the Japanese Society for Dialysis Therapy

Although the Japanese Society for Dialysis Therapy referred to advance directives in its 2014 "Recommendations on the Decision-Making Process for the Initiation and Continuation of Hemodialysis",[7] advance directives had been prevalent in many dialysis facilities partly associated with the introduction of advance directives developed by the author. In addition, for the 2020 revision of the recommendations, the concepts of shared decision-making (SDM) and advance care planning (ACP) were introduced. Furthermore, the concept of Conservative Kidney Management (CKM) as an alternative to renal replacement therapy was also presented, and it was stated that appropriate palliative care should be provided in such cases.[8]

SDM in the ACP Process

The concept of informed consent (IC) has long been introduced in Japan as a means to respect the right to self-determination and to break away from the paternalism that has existed since ancient times in the selection of treatment methods. However, over time, it has been pointed out that the doctors "just hand over a written explanation" and the patients "sign the form without understanding it in depth". Against this background, the concept of SDM has begun to spread, and the process recommended in SDM is not to merely list medical options but to also proceed with discussions while checking the reactions of patients and their families, as shown in Figure 2, and to understand their views on life and death, especially their so-called "patient and family narratives". It is a process that an increasing number of Japanese clinical ethics experts refer to as "collaborative decision-making" in reference to the nature of co-creation of treatment plans based on an understanding of the patient's and family's narratives.

ACP in Chronic Kidney Disease (CKD Stage G1-3)

During this period, it is necessary for patients and their families first understand the concept of the disease, to understand the aggravating factors of complications such as diabetes and hypertension, if any, and to

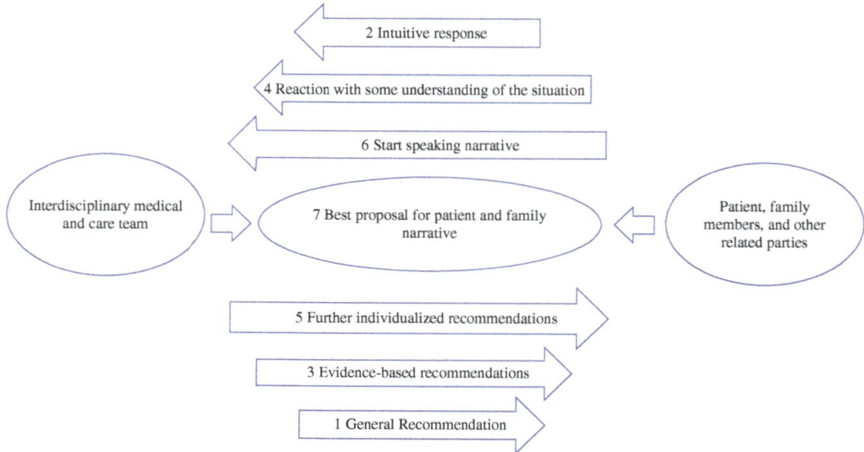

Figure 2.   Schema of desired shared decision making (collaborative making).

understand drug therapy, dietary therapy (potassium restriction, salt restriction, fluid restriction, etc.), and so on. In addition, it is necessary to assess the progress of the disease and plan for the future accordingly (advance life planning, ALP, or ACP in the broad sense of the term). During this period, it is recommended that patients and their families participate in patient education classes (kidney disease classes) held at hospitals specializing in renal disease and receive explanations from not only physicians but also nurses, pharmacists, nutritionists, and other related professionals to deepen their understanding of the disease. In Japan, kidney disease classes have been held at many core hospitals for renal disease since the 1980s.

ACP at the Time When Renal Replacement Therapy Should Be Considered (CKD Stage G 4–5)

As CKD progresses and the patient is approaching Stage G 4–5, he/she needs to understand the impending renal replacement therapies (hemodialysis, peritoneal dialysis, and kidney transplantation) and plan which therapy to choose and what to do with his/her life after the choice is made. The medical staff must ensure that the patient understands and is able to make a decision. The medical staff uses illustrations and videos to help patients understand the renal replacement therapies. Information should also be provided that even after choosing peritoneal dialysis, it is possible to change to hemodialysis due to a decline in peritoneal function and that it is not impossible to temporarily change to peritoneal dialysis after choosing hemodialysis. Some patients have also commented that they were never told about the complications of long-term dialysis, and because this is a long-term treatment, ongoing information and assistance in changing ACP accordingly should be provided during the course of dialysis.

ACP after Starting Dialysis (CKD Stage G5D)

Particularly in Japan, since the dialysis period is long, it is necessary to make a plan for each life stage because, even during stable dialysis, changes in life and work occur as people get older. Changes in academic, work, and family environment may cause changes in dialysis schedule and visiting methods, as well as changes in lifestyle, diet, and medications due to the progression of complications. It is desirable to change the ACP with the patient's consent. In addition, after the introduction of dialysis, "anything can happen at any time," including cardiovascular complications, so it is desirable to start "ACP (≒AD) in case of emergency" in accordance with the patient's state of acceptance. However, advance directives should be handled with caution, as they are likely to change depending on the patient's circumstances and other factors.

How ACP Should Be Tailored to the Japanese Culture

Miyashita *et al.* invited clinicians and researchers in Japan who have a deep knowledge of ACP and investigated "how ACP should fit into Japanese culture" using the modified Delphi method.[9] Based on the results of this study, it was thought that ACP would fit better in Japanese culture if it was considered to begin with advance life planning (ALP), which is the foundation of ACP, as well as the choice of medical treatment in the final stage of life (similar to advance directives), and as mentioned earlier, during the long period of dialysis. Healthcare providers should be willing to discuss the patient's ALP with the patient while the patient is still in good health.

Responding to the Increase in End-of-Life Care for Dialysis Patients

As mentioned in the introduction, the number of elderly dialysis patients is increasing in Japan, and end-of-life care for dialysis patients is also expected to increase in the future. With the presentation of CKM by the Japan Society for Dialysis Therapy, it is expected that the number of patients who choose CKM, complete dialysis, and wish to spend their final hours at home will also increase in the future. In order to provide better end-of-life care, it is desirable not only to have medical knowledge of palliative care but also to understand the narratives of patients and their families. However, in Japan, most dialysis patients receive dialysis at outpatient dialysis-only clinics, and it is difficult for their staff to take charge of end-of-life care at home for dialysis patients. Assuming that dialysis has been completed, the time until the patient's death is as short as around one week, during which time it is difficult for new staff (home doctors and visiting nurses) to build a sufficient trusting relationship with the patient and family. Therefore, the author published a referral form from the dialysis clinic where the patient spent many years for home physicians and other staff providing end-of-life care that includes crucial information, such as the patient's life narrative and ACP (Figure 3). In order to create this information form, the medical staff, together with the patient, must take time to prepare it in advance, and the process itself would be the ACP. In addition to the information form provided by the medical institution, we have also published a "self-introduction sheet" that patients can use to communicate their backgrounds and thoughts (views on life, etc.) to the medical staff (Figure 4). The latter form is intended to be used before the final stage of life (e.g., stage G 1–3). It would be good if patients feel comfortable presenting this sheet themselves when they first see a nephrologist or when they are referred to other facilities so that they can make themselves better understood by the medical staff.

Learning Objectives
- The Japanese Society for Dialysis Therapy (JSDT) advocates the use of Conservative Kidney Management (CKM) as an alternative to renal replacement therapy, which requires the provision of appropriate palliative care, including symptom palliation.

- Decision-making style in health care is changing from paternalism to informed consent, then to shared decision-making, and now to collaborative decision-making.
- A Japanese Delphi study (Miyashita *et al.*, 2022) defined advance care planning as "an individual's thinking about and discussing with their family and other people close to them, with the support as necessary of healthcare providers who have established a trusting relationship with them, preparations for the future, including the way of life and medical treatment and care that they wish to have in the future."

Request Form; Conservative Kidney Management at Home

The patient has been on dialysis at our hospital, but after repeated discussions with the patient and other concerned parties, he has now decided to withdraw dialysis treatment and wishes to receive conservative kidney management at home.

Name ____________   Sex ________   Birth ____________________

Date of Dialysis Introduction __________________   Causative Disease __________________

1. Medical history, complications and previous treatments

(If longer, fill in a separate sheet)

2. Present ADL

3. Current medications

Figure 3.   Request form; conservative kidney management at home.

4. Patient-related information (family, surrogate, acceptance status, etc.)

5. Patient's life history, what is important to him, etc. (Narrative, ACP, advance directives, etc.)

6. Reasons for preferring conservative kidney management at home

7. Assistance that has been developed since the patient announced to withdraw dialysis

8. Information on home care and emergency (when Patient want to resume dialysis)

Ex) Requests have already been made to Visiting Nurse Station A and Home Doctor B.
We have already confirmed that if the patient wishes to resume dialysis or if it is deemed impossible to provide end-of-life care at home, Hospital C, which has inpatient facilities related to our hospital, can accept the patient.

Figure 3.   (*Continued*).

Name   Birth   Sex

Adress   Phone

Family or Surrogate
   Address   Phone

My Life Story
   Young age

   Adult age

   With my family

 Most important things in my life

Plans for the future life (ie. Where, with whom and how to live)

Thoughts on the future medical procedures
(ie. I have an event to look forward to in a few years and would like to be well until then.
I have lived long enough and do not wish to undergo aggressive treatment.)

Figure 4.   Patient self-referral sheet (author's narrative sheet).

Acknowledgement

With special thanks to Dr. Masanori Mori for his work in translating this chapter from Japanese to English.

References

1. Hanabusa N., Abe M., Johki N., *et al.* (2022). 2021 annual dialysis data report, JSDT renal data registry. *Nihon Touseki Igakkai Zasshi.* **55**: 665–723. https://docs.jsdt.or.jp/overview/file/2021/pdf/introduction.pdf.

2. The Japan Society for Transplantation Number of Kidney Transplants and Dialysis Patients in Japan. http://www.asas.or.jp/jst/general/number/.

3. Sehgal A., Weisheit C., Miura Y., *et al.* (1996). Advance directives and withdrawal of dialysis in the United States, Germany and Japan. *JAMA* **276**: 1652–1656.

4. Miura Y., Asai A., Nagata S., *et al.* (2001). Dialysis patients' preferences regarding cardiopulmonary resuscitation and withdrawal of dialysis in Japan. *Am. J. Kidney Dis.* **37**: 1216–1222.

5. Miura Y., Asai A., Matsushima M., *et al.* (2006). Families' and physicians' predictions of dialysis. *Am. J. Kidney Dis.* **47**: 122–130.

6. Miura Y., Asai A., and Hosoya T. (2003). Advance directives for induction of dialysis. In: Japanese Society of Internal Medicine Board Certified Internal Medicine Specialists Group (eds.) *For Better Informed Consent*, pp. 254–258. Japanese Society of Internal Medicine, Tokyo.

7. Working Group for the Development of Guidelines for Hemodialysis Therapy, Japanese Society for Dialysis Therapy. Subgroup to Study Noninduction and Withdrawal of Dialysis. (2014). Recommendations for the decision-making process regarding initiation and continuation of maintenance hemodialysis. *Nihon Toseki Igakkai Zasshi* **47**: 269–285.

8. Committee to develop recommendations on the decision-making process for initiation and continuation of dialysis. (2020) Recommendations on the decision-making process for initiation and continuation of dialysis. *Nihon Toseki Igakkai Zasshi* **53**: 173–217.

9. Miyashita J., Shimizu S., Shiraishi R., *et al.* (2022). Culturally adapted consensus definition and action guideline: Japan's advance care planning. *J. Pain Symptom Manag.* **64**: 602–613.

Chapter 33

Advance Care Planning in Respiratory Medicine

Nittha Oerareemitr

*Pulmonary Department Ekachai Hospital,
Samut Sakhon, Thailand
Koon Palliative Care Specialised Hospital,
Bangkok, Thailand*

Introduction

Chronic respiratory diseases are one of the commonest causes of death, especially chronic obstructive lung disease that has recently grown to be the fourth leading cause of death worldwide.[1] Patients with chronic respiratory diseases face many symptoms that affect the quality of life. Chronic respiratory diseases may have episodes of acute exacerbations that get better with treatment, leading to the misperception that chronic respiratory diseases are "treatable conditions" as a whole. In many cases, patients with exacerbations of chronic respiratory diseases had experienced more than one episode of invasive mechanical ventilator support and had survived the critical conditions. Those patients and their families might perceive that this condition is always treatable with good outcomes. Such therapeutic hubris may not only be expressed by patients and their families but also by healthcare professionals.[2] Patients, families, and healthcare professionals often make medical decisions throughout the disease course without discussing life goals or goals of care in depth. The prognoses of many chronic respiratory diseases are uncertain and difficult to predict, adding to the reluctance of healthcare professionals to discuss advance care planning (ACP) in these conditions.

Although the British Thoracic Society[3] and American College of Chest Physicians[4] acknowledge ACP as a comprehensive part of pulmonary medicine that should be integrated with daily practice by healthcare professionals, ACP is not frequently discussed. In some Asia-Pacific countries, the need for ACP is rarely recognised at the chronic respiratory disease outpatient clinics but becomes relevant when patients are already intubated and when it is difficult to wean off the ventilator. It is always too early, until it is too late.

Like in many countries, it is taboo to talk about death and dying in Thai culture. The initiation of ACP conversation rests on the physician. Even then, the physician may not directly address ACP with patients and it becomes the "elephant in the room".

The Importance of ACP

Chronic respiratory diseases are progressive diseases with variable time courses experienced by different patients with different diseases. Mechanical ventilators are commonly used to prolong patients' life when disease reaches a severe stage.[5] A significant number of these chronically ventilated patients stay in long-term healthcare facilities while some stay at home.[6] In many countries, the majority of chronic ventilator-dependent patients has never discussed about their life goals and their preferences before they become ventilator dependent.[7] After they are connected to mechanical ventilators, discussing ACP becomes even harder as they are physically weaker and experience difficulties in expressing their preferences. Families become the main decision makers and, frequently, the decisions made will be documented as "full treatment and medications, including antibiotics and vasopressors, but deny chest compression", which we call the "do-not-resuscitate" or DNR order. Such medical orders are very commonly misunderstood as ACP among physicians in some countries, but they do not always focus on patients' preferences and goals of care, which are the core tenets of ACP conversations.

Here are some specific reasons why ACP is important for these patients[8–9]:

1. *Clarifies patients' treatment preferences*: Patients with chronic respiratory diseases always require complex medical interventions, such as mechanical ventilation or artificial nutrition and hydration, to sustain their lives when diseases reach a severe stage. ACP allows patients to clarify their preferences regarding these interventions and to choose the level of medical intervention that align with their values and goals of care.

2. *Reduces unwanted medical interventions*: ACP can reduce the likelihood of unwanted medical interventions that may not align with patients' values and goals of care. For example, some patients may prefer to receive palliative care rather than aggressive medical interventions at the end of life, and ACP can help ensure that these preferences are respected.

3. *Decreases patients' and caregivers' stress*: ACP can help decrease stress for caregivers of patients with chronic respiratory diseases. Caregivers who understand their loved one's preferences for medical care can feel more confident in their ability to make medical decisions on behalf of their loved one and may experience less anxiety and distress. ACP will clarify the goals of treatment, rather than just decisions about "using" or "not using" mechanical ventilators. In the event crises happens and patients are mechanically ventilated, the decision-making process with the family will better match the patient's preferences and goals of care.

4. *Improves communication with healthcare providers*: ACP promotes better communication between patients, their families, and healthcare providers. By discussing their treatment preferences, patients can ensure that their healthcare providers understand their values and goals of care and can make informed decisions about their medical care.

5. *Increases patient and family satisfaction*: Patients and their families who engage in ACP often report higher levels of satisfaction with their medical care. ACP helps ensure that patients receive care that aligns with their values and goals of care and can help reduce stress and anxiety for both patients and their families.

The Challenges of ACP

There are many challenges of ACP not only in chronic respiratory diseases but also in other diseases. There has been increasing recognition of the importance of ACP in many countries in the Asia Pacific region in recent years, especially among the ageing population and with the rise in chronic progressive diseases. The Thai government has included ACP in the national palliative care policy, and there are ongoing efforts to promote ACP among healthcare providers and the public. In 2017, the Thai Ministry of Public Health launched a pilot project to integrate ACP into primary care services in selected provinces. The project aimed to increase awareness and understanding of ACP among healthcare professionals and to encourage patients to engage in ACP discussions. The pilot project showed promising results, with increased knowledge and skills among healthcare professionals in ACP and positive attitudes towards ACP among patients.

However, despite the progress made, there are still challenges to implementing ACP in this region. These include the following:

1. *Cultural barriers*: In many countries, there is a cultural belief that discussing death and end-of-life care is taboo and should be avoided. This makes it difficult for healthcare professionals to initiate conversations about ACP with patients and their families.[10] Eighteen percent of pulmonologists are reluctant to start the ACP conversation unless patients initiate conversations about ACP themselves because they are concerned about patients' openness towards this conversation. On the other hand, the literature shows that patients also wait for their doctors to start the conversations.[11,15] In my clinical experience, I have never encountered patients who initiate the conversation themselves. However, when I start the ACP conversation, most of the patients are ready and feel comfortable to talk.

2. *Lack of awareness*: Many people are not aware of the concept of ACP and the benefits it can provide. This means that they may not initiate conversations with healthcare professionals about their end-of-life care preferences. Patients may think that at the end of lifetime, doctors and families will arrange the best treatments for them. Therefore, there are no reasons to overthink about their health at the present moment.

3. *A lack of awareness among healthcare professionals*: Most hospitals do not have ACP facilitators or services in ACP. Doctors know that ACP is important but they do not think that it is their duty to facilitate

ACP. Or they may only start the conversation when patients encounter emergency situations or hospital admissions.

4. *Limited healthcare resources*: The healthcare system in many countries in the Asia-Pacific region, such as Thailand, is under-resourced, particularly in rural areas. This can make it difficult for healthcare professionals to allocate time and resources to implement ACP effectively. From an unofficial survey of 49 Thai pulmonologists, 47% of them cited time constraints.

5. *A lack of skill*: During the 2 years of pulmonary medicine fellowship programme in Thailand, there is no ACP training in the curriculum. Some pulmonologists in university hospitals do not really understand ACP. When senior clinicians do not view ACP as a core skill, this skill set will not be passed on to their trainees.

An Approach to ACP in Chronic Respiratory Diseases

There are many situations that can trigger opportunities for ACP conversation in patients' interactions with the healthcare provider. To allow patients to fully and comfortably express their preferences or their life goals, we need to facilitate ACP when they are ready as well as physically and mentally stable. A trigger for starting the advance care planning process may be when one is not surprised that a patient may deteriorate further and require palliative care consultations.[2,12] Another opportunity is during follow-up after unplanned admission for respiratory events, such as exacerbations of chronic obstructive airway disease (COPD) or pneumonia. This should start during follow-up of stable patients, when they can better deliberate their values and life goals. The third situation is when patients are faced with the possibilities of undergoing new interventions, such as lung volume reduction surgery that have some risks. Discussion about advance care planning will clarify their goals of care. Another trigger is when the overall disease is worsening and patients start to experience increasing health problems. These situations are opportunities to start a difficult conversation and to encourage patients to think about their values and preferences while learning more about their conditions.

Doctors should learn how to start ACP conversations and even facilitate the entire process as patients trust doctors with whom they have a long-term therapeutic relationship, rather than another ACP facilitator.[13]

Opportunities and Strategies

Here are some ways on how to improve[14–15] ACP in Asia-Pacific countries:

1. *Increase awareness*: ACP is still a relatively new concept in some countries, and many people may not be aware of its importance. It is important to increase awareness about ACP through various channels, including healthcare providers, social media, and public awareness campaigns.
2. *Develop culturally appropriate ACP materials*: ACP materials should be culturally appropriate and available in Thai language to reach out to the general public. Culturally appropriate materials will help make ACP more accessible and acceptable to the Thai population.
3. *Train healthcare professionals*: Healthcare providers should be trained in facilitating ACP conversations and documenting ACP discussions with patients. Training programmes could include communication techniques, cultural sensitivity, and the legal framework surrounding ACP.
4. *Encourage ACP discussions*: Encourage families to have discussions about ACP with their loved ones to ensure that their wishes are respected. These conversations should be held in a respectful, supportive environment and should include discussions about values, goals, and preferences for end-of-life care.
5. *Develop a legal framework*: A legal framework needs to be in place to support ACP in each country. The legal framework should include guidelines on ACP documentation, ACP conversation, dispute resolution in ACP, and the role of healthcare providers in the ACP process.

By implementing these strategies, it is possible to improve the adoption of ACP in Asia-Pacific countries and help patients and their families make informed decisions about their end-of-life care.

In summary, ACP is for individuals with respiratory disease, as it can help ensure that their wishes for future medical treatment and care are respected and can help reduce the burden on family members and healthcare providers. It is important to develop the ACP in consultation with the patient's healthcare provider and to involve family members and loved ones in the process. To promote ACP, we need all stakeholders, the government, healthcare providers, and our communities to come together and do their part. The first step is to increase awareness of ACP. It is all hands on deck.

Take Home Messages

1. Chronic respiratory diseases have many symptoms that affect the quality of life. Some diseases may have multiple exacerbations from which patients recover well with appropriate medical interventions. Therefore, patients and their families as well as healthcare providers face much uncertainty and may believe that each episode of deterioration is usually treatable with good outcomes.
2. Early ACP helps family and healthcare providers know about and understand patients' preferences and goals of care. So, they, as much as possible, can make decisions about medical treatment concordant with their loved one's preference.
3. Cultural taboo and lack of awareness are significant barriers to developing ACP in Thailand. Government, organisations, communities, and healthcare providers should all play a part in co-creating viable and sustainable solutions together.

References

1. Global Initiative for Chronic Obstructive Lung Disease. (2021). Pocket Guide to COPD Diagnosis, Management, and Prevention: A Guide for Health Care Professionals.
2. Meehan E. and Foley T. (2020). Advance care planning for individuals with chronic obstructive pulmonary disease: A scoping review of the literature. *J. Pain Symptom Manage.* **59**: 1344–1361.
3. Catherine H., Jenny S., and National Health Service. (2019). Symptom Control, Palliative Care and Referral Guidelines for Patients with Chronic Respiratory Disease, pp. 4–6.
4. Donald S. and Anand I. (2022). Palliative care early in the care continuum among patients with serious respiratory illness. *Am. Thor. Soc.* **206**: e44–e69.
5. Metaxa V. and Anagnostou D. (2021). Palliative care interventions in intensive care unit patients. *Intensive Care Med.* **47**: 1415–1425.
6. Morrison S., and Meier E. (2021). What's wrong with advance care planning? *JAMA* **326**: 1575–1576.
7. Alexander K. and Judy D. (2016). Shared decision making in ICUs: An American college of critical care medicine and American thoracic society policy statement. *Critical Care Med.* **44**: 188–201.
8. Bernacki E. and Block D. (2014). American college of physicians high-value care task force. Communication about serious illness care goals: A

review and synthesis of best practices. *JAMA Intern. Med.* **174**: 1994–2003.

9. Kamal H. and Bull H. (2017). Future of the palliative care workforce: Preview to an impending crisis. *Am. J. Med.* **130**: 113–114.

10. Farquhar M. (2018). Assessing carer needs in chronic obstructive pulmonary disease. *Chron. Respir. Dis.* **15**: 26–35.

11. Quaderi A. and Hurst R. (2018). The unmet global burden of COPD. *Glob. Health Epidemiol. Genom.* **3**: e4–e2.

12. Ferrell R. and Twaddle L. (2018). National consensus project clinical practice guidelines for quality palliative care guidelines, 4th edition. *J. Palliat. Med.* **21**: 1684–1689.

13. Lea J. and Marieke Z. (2018). Advance care planning for patients with chronic respiratory diseases: A systematic review of preferences and practices. *Thorax* **73**: 222–230.

14. Rietjens C. and Sudore L. (2017). Definition and recommendations for advance care planning: an international consensus supported by the European association for palliative care. *Lancet Oncol.* **18**(9): e543–e551.

15. Sinclair C. and Auret A. (2017). Advance care planning uptake among patients with severe lung disease: A randomised patient preference trial of a nurse-led, facilitated advance care planning intervention. *BMJ Open* **7**(2): e013415.

Chapter 34

Advance Care Planning in Geriatric Medicine

Ping-Jen Chen

Department of Family Medicine and Division of Geriatrics and Gerontology, School of Medicine and University Hospital, Kaohsiung Medical University, Kaohsiung, Taiwan

Marie Curie Palliative Care Research Department, Division of Psychiatry, University College London, London, UK

Introduction

The world is facing an unprecedented challenge due to the aging population. The number of people aged 65 years or older worldwide is projected to more than double, rising from 761 million in 2021 to 1.6 billion in 2050. During this period, the population aged 65 or over in Eastern and South-Eastern Asia and in Central and Southern Asia is projected to grow by more than 540 million, accounting for more than 60% of the global increase. The geography of the oldest region in the world is shifting from Europe toward Eastern and South-Eastern Asia by 2050.[1]

Needs for ACP in the Older People

Older people often live with multiple health problems, frailty, and high levels of dependency and experience a gradual decline in cognitive and functional abilities. As these conditions worsen, physical symptoms and existential concerns can go unnoticed and untreated, causing unnecessary distress, increased hospitalizations, and a lower quality of life.[2,3] Older individuals with long-term and fluctuating illnesses have a greater degree of clinical uncertainty and an unpredictable decline in physical health compared to cancer patients, who often have a more predictable decline.[4] Therefore, it is important to provide opportunities for older individuals in long-term care facilities to express their wishes, values, and preferences to ensure that their palliative care needs are met. This has resulted in a growing interest in integrating advance care planning as a critical element of providing excellent continuous patient-centred care.[5]

Advance care planning (ACP) is a process that allows individuals to make informed decisions about their future medical care in the event of serious illness or end of life.[6] The benefits of ACP include identifying and implementing an individual's wishes for medical care, managing personal affairs while one is able, reducing stress and anxiety for family members, improving patient satisfaction and quality of life, and reducing the use of intensive medical interventions at the end of life.[7,8] However, despite these benefits, there are still needs and challenges to consider when it comes to implementing ACP in older people.

Factors Associated with ACP in Older People

Older people's willingness to discuss their future was influenced by their viewpoints of life and death, their health status, experiences, family relationships, and available resources. They may also need to weigh the benefits and burdens of ACP and be supported in decision-making capacity.[9]

Demographic and Health-Related Factors

Large population-based cohort study in Europe showed that one-quarter of community-dwelling older people had discussed ACP. Of those, 90% had discussed it with family/friends, 10% had written ACP documents, and 2% had discussed it with a healthcare professional. Older age (i.e., over 80 years), the female gender, higher educational level, poorer self-rated health, and lower levels of religiosity were independently associated with ACP implementation.[10] In a cross-cultural comparison study in East

Asia, multivariable analysis also revealed that an educational level >12 years was significantly associated with increased ACP awareness.[11]

Among older people who received home-based medical care (HBMC) in our HOme-based Longitudinal Investigation of the multidiSciplinary Team Integrated Care (HOLISTIC study) in Taiwan, multivariable analysis showed that living alone and higher degree of frailty status are associated with better ACP engagement.[12] In a cross-sectional study using American Health and Retirement Study data, older adults with no perceived dementia risk are less likely to participate in ACP, however, many older adults with high levels of perceived risk also had not completed ACP activities.[13]

Health Literacy and Decision-Making Self-Efficacy Factors

Factors such as health literacy and decision-making self-efficacy have significant effects on how older people approach end-of-life discussions and decisions. Communication gaps between physicians and patients regarding end-of-life care arise due to poor health literacy, which often limits patients' understanding of clinical terms, such as diagnoses and prognoses.[14] Furthermore, our finding in the HOLISTIC study demonstrated that older people receiving HBMC with higher self-efficacy in decision-making may engage in ACP better.[12] These factors may contribute to health inequalities. Healthcare professionals and family members may need to enhance older people's health literacy and self-efficacy in the communication process to meaningfully and effectively complete advance care plans.

Cultural, Ethnicity, Religiosity, and Spirituality Factors

Cultural differences played a significant role in their perspectives, and the truthful provision of information, appropriate resources, and family support were important for maintaining dignity at the end of life.[9] Older adults belonging to cultural and ethnic minorities have limited access to palliative or end-of-life care and often do not participate in ACP despite its promotion in several countries. Current strategies to promote ACP neglect engagement with ethnic minorities and religious communities. There is a need for policymakers, medical professionals, social workers, and educators to implement the ethical principle of social justice, to respond to these disparities, and to develop appropriate strategies for promoting ACP.

Challenges for ACP in the Older People in Asia

Awareness of ACP

One challenge in ACP implementation remains the lack of awareness and understanding of ACP among older adults with chronic illnesses. According to an international study in Hong Kong, Japan, and South Korea, around 30% of participants had heard of ACP. A higher proportion of Japanese and people from Hong Kong have heard of ACP/ADs compared to South Korea.[11] Among older people, families, and healthcare professionals in China, low levels of knowledge and awareness about ACP and ADs are also reported.[15] This reinforces the need for public health initiatives that aim to improve awareness and education about ACP among older adults, their families, and healthcare professionals to recognize its benefits.[16]

Death as a Taboo Topic with a Low Value

In some Asian cultures, such as traditional Chinese culture, death and dying are taboo topics that are not openly discussed. This can make it difficult for healthcare providers to bring up the subject of ACP with older people and their families, leading to a lack of understanding and awareness of ACP.[17] Older people may refuse to understand the concept of ACP, and their family members may not be aware of the importance of having these conversations. Moreover, the communication barriers among older people and their families can further complicate the situation. This can result in a lack of understanding of the older person's preferences.

In addition, in many Asian cultures, there is a strong emphasis on maintaining hope and prolonging life, which can conflict with the intent of ACP, such as clarifying the person's values, goals of care, and what quality of life means to the individual. This can lead to a lack of consensus on end-of-life care decisions and create challenges for healthcare providers to initiate the ACP conversation.[18]

Collectivism and Filial Piety

Many Asian cultures place a strong emphasis on family-centred collectivism rather than person-centred individualism. The harmony of the whole family or group of people is often prioritized over personal autonomy in the decision-making process.[19] A cross-cultural survey in Asia showed that the most preferred decision maker and person with whom to discuss end-of-life care issues was a family member, especially in people living in Chinese culture. More than 70% of the participants indicated that they would not prefer to leave an advance directive but may prefer family members to act as decision makers when older people become incapable of deciding for themselves.[20]

In East Asian countries where Confucianism and the notion of "filial piety" are prominent, there is a strong social obligation for children to care for their aging parents. Older people may perceive that their families are responsible for making the best end-of-life care decisions for them, and physicians tend to discuss the patient's poor prognosis and treatment options with a male family member rather than with the patient directly.[21] Family values and physician authority often take precedence over patient autonomy in the cultural norm in Asia.

Delivery of Goal-Concordant Care

Another challenge is the poor correlation between wishes expressed in advance directives in the medical record, and the care individuals receive at the end of life. While the number of older adults completing advance directives has increased over time, the presence of an advance directive had little effect on hospitalization rates.[22] A study found that only 41% of patients with advanced cancer who completed an advance directive had their end-of-life wishes documented in the medical record, and only 21% had their preferences communicated to their healthcare team.[23] These findings highlight the need for improved communication and implementation of advance care planning to ensure that patients receive care that is aligned with their wishes at the end of life.

Lessons Learnt from My Clinical Experience of ACP in Geriatric Medicine

Before the Patient Right to Autonomy Act (PRAA), which defines the official process of ACP consultation, was enacted in 2016, many clinicians in Taiwan, including myself, were having conversations with patients and their family members about their preferences for care and treatment at the end of life or in the event the patients are not able to make decisions. The following are points that I learned about ACP during my clinical practice in geriatric medicine.

Timely Initiation of ACP in Any Occasion across Different Settings

Ideally, ACP often involves multiple brief discussions over time. Timely initiation of the conversation about patient's viewpoints of disease and its trajectory may benefit in identifying personal values and preferences.[24] This is particularly important when considering patients who may move between different care settings including home or long-term care facilities, clinics, and hospitals. For instance, a patient with a complex medical history may require care from various specialists, primary care providers, and hospital teams. In such situations, having a clear understanding of the patient's preferences and goals of care can help ensure that their wishes are respected regardless of the setting in which they receive care.[25] These discussions can enable patients and their families to receive consistent and coordinated care which aligns with their individual needs and values, and the ongoing communication can help ensure that care plans are updated as needed.

Identify the Trajectory of Main Disease and Multimorbidity

If clinicians have a prior understanding of the typical patterns of decline in the underlying health conditions of patients, they can define and comprehend the main trajectory of the patient's health.[26] This knowledge can facilitate discussions with the patient and their family about their expectations regarding possible future scenarios and assist in planning for what is important to them. Evidence suggests that a comprehensive approach to advance care planning that considers complexity and emphasizes meaningful conversations about outcomes that are significant to the individuals and their families is beneficial.[27]

Embrace the Uncertainty and Normalize the Talking about Death

Uncertainty of disease or the trajectory of multimorbidity in older people is often seen as an "enemy" to be constrained by medical science. Anxiety about future disability, a sense of lack of control, and receiving insufficient or excessive medical care can also be fueled by uncertainty.[4] However, an unpredictable but obvious risk of deteriorating and dying should be a valuable chance to initiate ACP with all people who have progressive and advanced conditions.[28]

It is crucial for health professionals to acknowledge that normalizing death is essential to make ACP ordinary and a default conversation with patients and family members.[29] ACP can be normalized by communicating with patients that this topic is routinely broached with every patient and encouraging patients to reflect on their preferences in various hypothetical scenarios. Normalizing ACP reduces the stigma of dialogue among patients and their family members and removes the taboo from the conversation.

Involve Family Members and Facilitate Relation Autonomy

Regarding collective decision-making style in Asian societies which stems from the cultural value of familism, early involvement of family members of older people in the ACP conversation is important.[30] In Taiwan, PRAA stipulates that at least one relative of first or second degree of affinity should participate in the official process of ACP counseling with multidisciplinary professionals. Inviting family members does not mean that they supplant their loved one in decision-making but listen to their senior relatives' preferences, support them if they have low health literacy, and reach a consensus with family harmony.

The concept of "relational autonomy", a balanced and multidimensional concept of personhood, highlights the interdependence between patients, families, medical professionals, and the community.[17] This concept can assist Asian patients, particularly older adults, in shared decision-making with their families and significant others while maintaining the collectivism paradigm in Asia. Although the adoption of relational autonomy may increase the complexity of the decision-making process, good interpretation and effective communication with families and significant others can help minimize this drawback.

An Approach to ACP and Person-Centred Care in Geriatric Medicine

It is essential to develop a practical approach that integrates ACP and goal-concordant care across different diseases, specialties, settings, and dimensions of need to avoid fragmentation of care. A four-stage cyclical process is recommended, which includes timely identification for enhanced support and care planning, multidimensional assessment, care planning conversations that consider the individual's opinions, concerns, expectations, and priorities, and coordination of care through the reliable sharing and updating of care plans. This process is repeated as the individual's situation and needs change.

1. Identification (individual or population screening)

The initial step in the process is to evaluate people who are at risk and initiate proactive and personalized care planning when a severe illness is diagnosed or the person's health starts deteriorating progressively due to multiple health conditions. This identification is referred to as the "first transition," and it occurs much earlier than the "second transition," when the individual is typically identified as dying, and formal palliative care is considered. The decline of patients along each trajectory can vary, and the rate of decline may also differ. As a result, individual patients may die at different stages along each trajectory.[31]

Assessment tools such as Supportive & Palliative Care Indicators Tool (SPICT) that is based on the burden of illness and clinical indicators, rather than prognosis, have been created and confirmed as reliable to recognize individuals with declining health in various settings, irrespective of the illness they have.[32] ACP for older people should be person-driven and individualized, initiated at time points important to older people and their families. This requires a sensitivity to conversation triggers or cues from individuals.[29]

2. Assessment (of patient and carers)

The evaluation process involves assessing the current multidimensional needs of the patient and their primary caregiver while considering their cultural context and family situation. Additionally, the stage or point that the patient has reached in their illness trajectory should be identified. With this "situational diagnosis" and an understanding of the expected trajectory of the illness, we can anticipate future needs and events proactively.[33]

The frailty index that utilizes a comprehensive geriatric assessment (CGA) can assist professionals in determining the level of overall vulnerability, leading to a more comprehensive understanding of the patient's general situation.[34] Multidisciplinary team-based approaches to gather the information and identify various needs of the patient are beneficial for the process and outcomes.[24]

3.   *Planning (with shared decision-making)*

It is then appropriate to have conversations with the patients and their family about their values, concerns, and expectations. It is also essential to share information based on the patient's illness trajectory while taking into account all of their conditions to discuss potential future events and uncertainties.[28] To plan ahead, we need to have a conversation with the person to understand their values, concerns, and expectations. We then discuss available options, taking into account their potential illness trajectory. This conversation can cover predictable events such as hospital admissions and making emergency care plans, as well as what to do if the person loses the capacity to make decisions. We may use a problem-oriented approach to personalize care and support in different settings and make shared decisions about the benefits and risks of tests and treatments. Standardized process with illustrated image templates or visual decision aids may facilitate patients' understanding and improve the quality of communication.[35]

To ensure that ACP is carried out effectively, a collaborative and multidisciplinary approach should be adopted. This would involve building a network of staff members from different levels of healthcare who can work together toward a common goal. It is important that each member's role is clearly defined to promote active engagement in the process.[29] Furthermore, conducting a collaborative negotiation that involves older people, family members, and staff may bridge communication gaps between all parties involved and enhance coherence and shared responsibility in decision-making. As the patient's circumstances, values, and preferences change, we adjust the goals of care by engaging with them and their caregivers in discussions. Caregivers may have additional concerns about their own health and responsibilities, so it is essential to evaluate and manage their needs as well.[36]

4.   *Care coordination (record, share, and update)*

Globally, there are ongoing efforts to create electronic systems for coordinating care that enable information sharing among various healthcare teams and locations.[37] In Taiwan, a person can have his official advance directive after the ACP process, and the AD can be uploaded to the National Health Insurance (NHI) cloud and registered in the NHI smart card. The NHI smart card is used for every health service everywhere at any time so that the AD can be identified in any agency in the healthcare system. This kind of coordination system should enable pertinent clinical data to be electronically updated, exchanged, and accessed by all essential healthcare providers.

In the USA, the Physicians Orders for Life-Sustaining Treatment (POLST) which provides a concise summary of the patient's decision about specific treatments, can be transferred across different settings. Such a summary of the care plan is helpful for clinicians or carers in various settings to consistently provide care concordant with the patient's preferences. This kind of summary, which takes into account patients' illness trajectory influenced by multimorbidity and the choice of intervention treatments for acute events, may improve the quality of medical decision-making when receiving unplanned care.[38]

Given the inherent uncertainty in future care planning, ACP should involve ongoing discussions instead of a single instance. It is important to continuously review and modify the conversations and documentation based on feedback, especially when there are changes in the person's health status or capacity.[29]

Conclusion

ACP should be a default conversation involving multiple brief discussions over time to ensure care plans are updated as needed. Identifying the trajectory of the patient's major disease and multimorbidity is crucial to facilitate discussions and assist in planning. Embracing uncertainty, involving family members, and using a practical approach to ACP and person-centred care are also vital. A four-stage cyclical process for ACP is suggested, including timely identification, multidimensional assessment, care planning conversations, and coordination of care through reliable sharing and updating of care plans. Overall, ACP is essential to ensure individualized care for older adults, and the involvement of family members and multidisciplinary professionals can enhance the decision-making process.

References

1. United Nations. *Leaving No One Behind in an Ageing World.* World Social Report 2023.
2. Evans C.J., Bone A.E., Yi D., *et al.* (2021). Community-based short-term integrated palliative and supportive care reduces symptom distress for older people with chronic noncancer conditions compared with usual care: A randomised controlled single-blind mixed method trial. *Int. J. Nurs. Stud.* **120**: 103978.

3. Stephens C.E., Hunt L.J., Bui N., Halifax E., Ritchie C.S., and Lee S.J. (2018). Palliative care eligibility, symptom burden, and quality-of-life ratings in nursing home residents. *JAMA Intern. Med.* **178**(1): 141–142.

4. Etkind S.N., Lovell N., Bone A.E., *et al.* (2020). The stability of care preferences following acute illness: A mixed methods prospective cohort study of frail older people. *BMC Geriatr.* **20**(1): 370.

5. Sharp T., Moran E., Kuhn I., and Barclay S. (2013). Do the elderly have a voice? Advance care planning discussions with frail and older individuals: A systematic literature review and narrative synthesis. *Br. J. Gen. Pract.* **63**(615): e657–668.

6. Rietjens J.A.C., Sudore R.L., Connolly M., *et al.* (2017). Definition and recommendations for advance care planning: An international consensus supported by the European association for palliative care. *Lancet Oncol.* **18**(9): e543–e551.

7. Martin R.S., Hayes B., Gregorevic K., and Lim W.K. (2016). The effects of advance care planning interventions on nursing home residents: A systematic review. *J. Am. Med. Dir. Assoc.* **17**(4): 284–293.

8. Weathers E., O'Caoimh R., Cornally N., *et al.* (2016). Advance care planning: A systematic review of randomised controlled trials conducted with older adults. *Maturitas* **91**: 101–109.

9. Ke L.S., Huang X., Hu W.Y., O'Connor M., and Lee S. (2017). Experiences and perspectives of older people regarding advance care planning: A meta-synthesis of qualitative studies. *Palliat. Med.* **31**(5): 394–405.

10. Breslin L., Connolly E., Purcell R., Lavan A., Kenny R.A., and Briggs R. (2022). What factors are associated with advance care planning in community-dwelling older people? Data from TILDA. *Eur. Geriatr. Med.* **13**(1): 285–289.

11. Kawakami A., Kwong E.W., Lai C.K., Song M.S., Boo S., and Yamamoto-Mitani N. (2021). Advance care planning and advance directive awareness among East Asian older adults: Japan, Hong Kong and South Korea. *Geriatr. Gerontol. Int.* **21**(1): 71–76.

12. Liao J.Y., Chen P.J., Wu Y.L., *et al.* (2020). Home-based longitudinal investigation of the multidisciplinary team integrated care (HOLISTIC): Protocol of a prospective nationwide cohort study. *BMC Geriatr.* **20**(1): 511.

13. Lee Y.K., Fried T.R., Costello D.M., Hajduk A.M., O'Leary J.R., and Cohen A.B. (2022). Perceived dementia risk and advance care planning among older adults. *J. Am. Geriatr. Soc.* **70**(5): 1481–1486.

14. de Vries K., Banister E., Dening K.H., and Ochieng B. (2019). Advance care planning for older people: The influence of ethnicity, religiosity, spirituality and health literacy. *Nurs. Ethics.* **26**(7–8): 1946–1954.

15. Zhang X., Jeong S.Y., and Chan S. (2021). Advance care planning for older people in mainland China: An integrative literature review. *Int. J. Older People Nurs.* **16**(6): e12409.

16. Kozlov E., Llaneza D.H., and Trevino K. (2022). Older patients' and their caregivers' understanding of advanced care planning. *Curr. Opin. Support. Palliat. Care* **16**(1): 33–37.

17. Cheng S.Y., Lin C.P., Chan H.Y., *et al.* (2020). Advance care planning in Asian culture. *Jpn. J. Clin. Oncol.* **50**(9): 976–989.

18. Chen Y.H., Ho C.H., Huang C.C., *et al.* (2017). Comparison of healthcare utilization and life-sustaining interventions between elderly patients with dementia and those with cancer near the end of life: A nationwide, population-based study in Taiwan. *Geriatr. Gerontol. Int.* **17**(12): 2545–2551.

19. Brossoie N., Hwang E., Song K., Jeong J.W., and Young-Woo K. (2022). Assessing age-friendliness: Individualistic vs. collectivistic cultures. *J. Aging Soc. Policy* **34**(2): 311–334.

20. Ho L.Y.W., Kwong E.W.Y., Song M.S., *et al.* (2022). Decision-making preferences on end-of-life care for older people: Exploration and comparison of Japan, the Hong Kong SAR and South Korea in East Asia. *J. Clin. Nurs.* **31**(23–24): 3498–3509.

21. Lai C.F., Tsai H.B., Hsu S.H., Chiang C.K., Huang J.W., and Huang S.J. (2013). Withdrawal from long-term hemodialysis in patients with end-stage renal disease in Taiwan. *J. Formos. Med. Assoc.* **112**(10): 589–599.

22. Barnato A.E., Chang C.C., Farrell M.H., Lave J.R., Roberts M.S., and Angus D.C. (2010). Is survival better at hospitals with higher "end-of-life" treatment intensity? *Med. Care* **48**(2): 125–132.

23. Johnson S., Butow P., Kerridge I., and Tattersall M. (2016). Advance care planning for cancer patients: A systematic review of perceptions and experiences of patients, families, and healthcare providers. *Psychooncology* **25**(4): 362–386.

24. Lum H.D., Sudore R.L., and Bekelman D.B. (2015). Advance care planning in the elderly. *Med. Clin. North Am.* **99**(2): 391–403.

25. Abu A.l., Hamayel N., Isenberg S.R., Sixon J., *et al.* (2019). Preparing older patients with serious illness for advance care planning discussions in primary care. *J. Pain Symptom Manage.* **58**(2): 244–251.e241.

26. Kendall M., Carduff E., Lloyd A., *et al.* (2015). Different experiences and goals in different advanced diseases: Comparing serial interviews with patients with cancer, organ failure, or frailty and their family and professional carers. *J. Pain Symptom Manage.* **50**(2): 216–224.

27. Hopkins S.A., Lovick R., Polak L., *et al.* (2020). Reassessing advance care planning in the light of Covid-19. *BMJ* **369**: m1927.

28. Kimbell B., Murray S.A., Macpherson S., and Boyd K. (2016). Embracing inherent uncertainty in advanced illness. *BMJ* **354**: i3802.

29. Zhou Y., Wang A., Ellis-Smith C., Braybrook D., and Harding R. (2022). Mechanisms and contextual influences on the implementation of advance care planning for older people in long-term care facilities: A realist review. *Int. J. Nurs. Stud.* **133**: 104277.

30. Lin C.P., Cheng S.Y., and Chen P.J. (2018). Advance care planning for older people with cancer and its implications in Asia: Highlighting the mental capacity and relational autonomy. *Geriatrics (Basel)* **3**: 43.

31. Downar J., Goldman R., Pinto R., Englesakis M., and Adhikari N.K. (2017). The "surprise question" for predicting death in seriously ill patients: A systematic review and meta-analysis. *Cmaj.* **189**(13): e484–e493.

32. Maas E.A., Murray S.A., Engels Y., and Campbell C. (2013). What tools are available to identify patients with palliative care needs in primary care: A systematic literature review and survey of European practice. *BMJ Support. Palliat. Care* **3**(4): 444–451.

33. Amblàs-Novellas J., Espaulella J., Rexach L., *et al.* (2015). Frailty, severity, progression and shared decision-making: A pragmatic framework for the challenge of clinical complexity at the end of life. *Euro. Geriat. Med.* **6**(2): 189–194.

34. Rockwood K., Song X., MacKnight C., *et al.* (2005). A global clinical measure of fitness and frailty in elderly people. *Cmaj* **173**(5): 489–495.

35. Frechman E., Dietrich M.S., Walden R.L., and Maxwell C.A. (2020). Exploring the uptake of advance care planning in older adults: An integrative review. *J. Pain Symptom Manage.* **60**(6): 1208–1222.e1259.

36. Carduff E., Jarvis A., Highet G., *et al.* (2016). Piloting a new approach in primary care to identify, assess and support carers of people with terminal illnesses: A feasibility study. *BMC Fam. Pract.* **17**: 18.

37. Leniz J., Weil A., Higginson I.J., and Sleeman K.E. (2020). Electronic palliative care coordination systems (EPaCCS): A systematic review. *BMJ Support. Palliat. Care* **10**(1): 68–78.

38. Polak L., Hopkins S., Barclay S., and Hoare S. (2020). The difference an end-of-life diagnosis makes: Qualitative interviews with providers of community health care for frail older people. *Br. J. Gen. Pract.* **70**(699): e757–e764.

Chapter 35

Partnering with tāngata whenua, the People of the Land: Advance Care Planning in Aotearoa New Zealand

Maarie Hutana (Ngāi Tahu)

*Māori Engagement Manager, Advance Care Planning National Team,
Te Tāhū Hauora Health Quality & Safety Commission,
Wellington, New Zealand*

Key Messages

- Develop genuine relationships with Indigenous people and their communities.
- Deliberately nurture the growth of your Indigenous workforce.
- Tailor services to meet the needs of Indigenous communities.
- Indigenous leadership is needed at all levels of decision-making.
- Be prepared to share power and do things differently.
- Reflect upon what institutional mechanisms need to change to achieve health equity for Indigenous peoples.
- Success does not occur without a strategy and mobilisation of the strategy.
- Sit in the problem, even if you don't have an answer.
- Be kind to yourself — decolonising a system will take time.
- Be bold. Be brave. Commit to standing up when you see injustice and inequity.

Introduction

No Hea Koe? Where Are You From?

When I'm having a tough day in the office, Daniel's[a] words remind me why I work in healthcare:

> "Hey Maarie, did you see the news on telly last night?"
>
> "No. What's happening?"
>
> "They said that Māori[b] (the Indigenous people of Aotearoa New Zealand) get cancer more than Pākehā (New Zealanders of European descent). Is that true?"
>
> "Yes, that's true"
>
> "They said that Māori get less tests and medicines than Pākehā too. Is that right?"
>
> "What else did they say, Daniel?"
>
> "They said that Māori are more likely to die of cancer than Pākehā. Should I tell them that I'm not Māori?"

I was a nurse at the time, working with Māori patients and their families affected by blood cancer. My role was to walk alongside Daniel to guide and support him through the months of chemotherapy, radiation, bone marrow transplant, and consolidation treatment. I was part of a larger team that helped him navigate the health system and the social complexities that came from having to stop work, manage home life without family support, and travel to multiple hospital treatments. I also allayed his fears that he'd be treated differently, and die, because he was Māori.

Māori are the Indigenous peoples of Aotearoa New Zealand (Aotearoa). We make up 17.4%[1] of the national 5 million population[2] on a small collection of islands in the South Pacific Ocean.

Kupe was the first Māori explorer to arrive in Aotearoa, nearly 800 years ago.[3] He navigated from east Polynesia using the prevailing winds, ocean currents, and stars and landed on what was later named Aotearoa, "the land of the long white cloud".

---

[a]This is a pseudonym.

[b]A glossary of Māori words is provided at the end of this chapter.

The Polynesians who had migrated to Aotearoa were not known as Māori. Rather, they identified themselves as hapū (extended family groups or sub-tribe), which usually held the name of a tupuna (ancestor). When Europeans arrived nearly 400 years later, they gave the tāngata whenua (people of the land) a single name to help them identify and associate the natives as a single people. It's thought that the word Māori is derived from the words tāngata Māori, which means normal or native people.

The Māori Worldview

This chapter highlights the steps taken to elevate te ao Māori and mātauranga Māori (Māori knowledge) across the advance care planning (ACP) programme in Aotearoa. It speaks of the depth and richness that can be gained from integrating a worldview that is different to the mainstream approach.

This is a story about sharing power to influence the well-being of a nation, and it reveals how a treaty signed in 1840 is driving social and political change to decolonise the health sector and contribute to health equity for Māori.[4–6]

How Are You?

Significant health inequities exist between Māori and non-Māori New Zealanders across most health indicators, including life expectancy, health outcomes, and quality of care.[4,6–9]

Colonisation, racism, and marginalisation are well recognised as key drivers of the health inequities that affect Māori and Indigenous people globally.[10–13]

Power dynamics

To understand the health inequities that affect the contemporary realities of Māori in Aotearoa, it is helpful to first reflect upon the historical journey that has brought them to the present day.

Failure to explore the roots of the health inequities, namely colonisation, places Indigenous peoples at risk of being subjected to racist or stereotypical assumptions and bias.[10–13] However, an understanding of the historical and societal context provides insight into the persistent power imbalance and unequal position of Māori within society and rejects deficit framing.[11,13]

For example, when Māori are "blamed" for not attending outpatient clinics, they are often labelled "non-compliant", "distrusting", or "typical". This places the person at fault and releases the health professional and health service of any obligation.[10]

This type of "patient blaming" does not serve anyone. Rather than deficit-framing in this way, it is more useful to recognise the realities that impact Indigenous peoples following generations of racism, marginalisation and dispossession.

Colonisation

Globally, colonisation is acknowledged as a fundamental health determinant for Indigenous peoples[4,6–9] and is directly linked to the burden of disease and poverty.[14] The inception of colonisation occurred many generations ago, but the impact is still felt by Indigenous peoples within our health structures, systems, legislation, policy, and programme strategic plans, which are engineered by the ethnocentric worldviews of the dominant culture.[4,5,7,15]

The differing values, beliefs, and norms between the dominant culture and the Indigenous population are reflected in the persistent and pervasive health inequities that shape Indigenous people's health experiences and outcomes[4,7]:

> That Indigenous peoples and cultures have survived in these hostile environments speaks to the strength and resilience of the people.[7]

Te Tiriti o Waitangi: The Treaty of Waitangi

In 1840, a founding document of Aotearoa — the Treaty of Waitangi (Te Tiriti o Waitangi; Te Tiriti) — was written by representatives of the British Crown and translated into te reo Māori (Māori language). It was signed by Crown representatives and some but not all rangatira (Māori tribal leaders). It was intended to foster unity and a partnership between the Crown and Māori so that settlers and Māori could live together in peace. However, the two texts differed significantly[3] and left the parties with dissimilar expectations of the treaty's terms.[16] It was also rapidly disregarded by the Crown, who declared sovereignty and began the systematic process of colonising the country. Rangatira travelled to England to petition the Queen to no avail, and complaints voiced internationally over decades remained unaddressed.[17] Māori were disenfranchised, disempowered, and demoralised and entered into 180 years of seeking redress for breaches of Te Tiriti by the Crown:

> Kia whakatōmuri te haere whakamua
>
> *I walk backwards into the future with my eyes fixed on my past*

This whakataukī (a Māori saying by an unknown author) recognises that we cannot see into the future, but we can look to the wisdom of the past, from our tūpuna, to inform how we move forward.

Broken promises

By 1860, most Māori land had been lost to the Crown or to settlers,[16,18] and laws that marginalised Māori were passed, including the following:

- the Education Ordinance 1847, which dismantled use of the native language[19]; by 1975, only 5% of Māori children could speak their language,[20]
- the New Zealand Settlements Act 1863, which allowed the Crown to confiscate the land of any iwi (tribe) "engaged in rebellion" against the government; Pākehā settlers were given the confiscated land,[21]
- the Native Schools Act 1867, which established a national system of village schools under the control of the Native Department as part of the government's policy to assimilate Māori into Pākehā society,[22]
- the Tohunga Suppression Act 1907, which outlawed Indigenous health practices.[4]

Māori have suffered economically, physically, spiritually, and culturally from colonisation.

Paradoxically, from the 1880s, Pākehā included Māori performers, traditions, images, and art forms as displays of a national identity abroad and as key attractions for the tourism industry. By the early 1900s, important foreign visitors were greeted with a formal Māori welcome.[23]

The Māori population significantly increased during the post-war era that began in 1945. Māori migrated in droves from rural family communities to the cities in search of work.[22,24] This meant more Māori children entered mainstream schooling and then continued on to university and trade schools.

The 1970s saw a new generation of young Māori who had been raised and educated in the cities. There was a revival of protests by both Māori and Pākehā demanding recognition of Te Tiriti and redress for the dispossession and marginalisation of Māori lands and culture.[17]

Political shifts saw the passing of the Treaty of Waitangi Act 1975, which established a legal process for Māori to raise breaches of Te Tiriti for resolution and reconciliation by the government.[25,26] In 1989, legislation was written with guiding principles on how the government and the public sector would honour Te Tiriti o Waitangi.[27]

Te Tiriti remains fundamental to health and social policy in Aotearoa, and health and disability services are committed to honouring the Crown's responsibilities by the following:

- enabling Māori to exercise authority over their health and well-being,
- achieving equitable health outcomes for Māori,
- enabling Māori to live, thrive, and flourish as Māori.[28]

Currently, the Aotearoa health sector is undergoing a major restructure[29] in which Te Tiriti o Waitangi forms the basis of change.

How does this relate to ACP?

In Aotearoa, a Tiriti-based future is one where Māori people thrive and succeed as Māori. It is a world where Māori feel safe to be Māori and where cultural differences are acknowledged and embraced.

Te Tiriti is a powerful tool that we use in the ACP programme to ask ourselves whether our processes and actions are dismantling, perpetuating, or even creating health inequities. We acknowledge that we are still learning how to authentically apply Te Tiriti to our work. The obstacles we most often encounter are health system processes, or ways of thinking, that are set in a Western paradigm and do not serve Indigenous peoples. Rather, these ethnocentric systems and rigid thinking continue to cause unjust and avoidable health inequities for Indigenous peoples:

> We need to open our minds as there are more ways than one approach.
> If you are able to look at the world from different approaches, then you
> will be better able to help people.[10]

Who Are You?

ACP in Aotearoa

The aim of ACP is to give people the opportunity to think, talk, and write about what matters to them most and consider their wishes for healthcare now, in the future, and at their end of life. Understanding what matters most to a person and their whānau (family, including extended family and friends) is central to our health system being able to deliver whānau- and person-centric care that enhances mana (prestige or honour) and supports well-being.

Many Māori families feel disempowered. They feel that their knowledge is undervalued and that they are not involved in decision-making about their care and treatment. This leads to whānau feeling distanced from both healthcare professionals and their own health. ACP provides an opportunity for their voice to be heard. It supports people to be participants in their healthcare while also ensuring that they feel their input is respected and valued.

ACP supports consumers, their whānau, and clinicians to have conversations to gain a shared understanding of the person's values and goals. An advance care plan enables these wishes and aspirations to be documented so this information can be used to support future care planning and shared decision-making.

There is significant value in having ACP conversations even if they are not documented. However, ideally, people would document their wishes and preferences and share copies of their advance care plan with friends, whānau, and healthcare teams. The national ACP programme supports consumers, clinicians, and health managers with this process. The programme develops resources and education for consumers and clinicians and guides implementation across the health sector.

Past and present

We've come a long way since the inception of ACP in Aotearoa in 2011.

Today, the ACP programme is guided by the mātāpono (core values) of our 2022–2028 strategy[30] and encompasses a range of tools and processes to gather, share, and integrate people's health goals and preferences at different points in their health journey.

In the past, Māori leaders have been sought to provide cultural guidance for the programme. For example, a rangatira Māori carefully chose

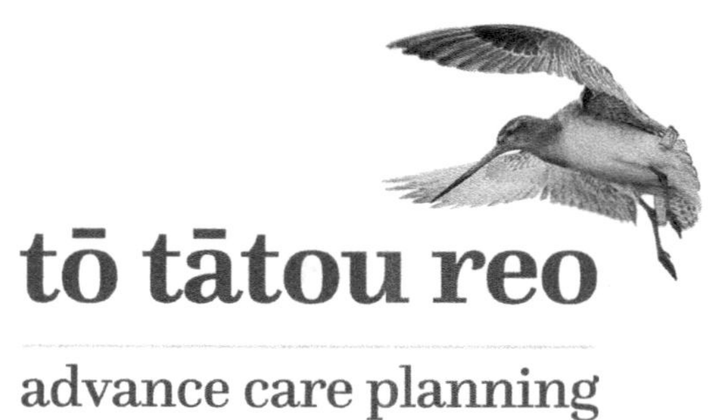

Figure 1.   The words "tō tātou reo" translate from te reo Māori to "our voice" and reflect the collectivist nature of Māori and the importance of whānau and community.

and gifted the words *tō tātou reo (our voice),* which have been part of the programme's visual identity from the beginning (Figure 1). These words succinctly define ACP for Māori as they reflect the collectivist worldview of Māori rather than the individualistic perspective of the Western world.

The ACP programme has a Māori leadership group and Māori representation on the national steering group, and we seek participation from Māori health professionals and consumers for national projects.

In 2020, a Māori project manager was employed in the national team to drive the programme's commitment to embed and enact Te Tiriti in support of Māori health outcomes.

Build Authentic Partnerships

Indigenous leadership is required at all levels of decision-making.

Low Māori representation in an ACP team, governance group, steering group, or advisory group requires people in these groups to be bold and courageous about highlighting issues for Māori. This requires considerable effort and assertiveness and risks Māori perspectives being overlooked and ignored.

Our Aspirations

- Shift cultural norms; if we do what we've always done, we'll get what we've always got.
- Ensure advisory and strategic planning groups truly reflect a Te Tiriti partnership in terms of power and decision-making.

- Reflect on our own bias, assumptions, and stereotyping and apply a cultural approach to our work.
- Build on our Māori workforce at all levels, including governance and strategic planning.
- Validate and affirm Māori solutions and mātauranga Māori.
- Apply a community-led approach to ACP projects and initiatives.
- Accept that Māori have a collectivist worldview, which is different to the Western individualistic worldview, so timelines will be different.

What We've Learned — Be Prepared to Share Power and Do Things Differently

Although Māori perspectives are sought, they are often not listened to, overlooked, misunderstood, or changed to suit the organisation. This can be frustrating and undermining for the Māori people we interact with and can impact ongoing relationships. It is important to actively listen, check to ensure we understand what we have heard is correct, and then collaborate in a relationship of partnership (i.e., shared power) to seek solutions.

It is important to engage with Māori leaders and stakeholders early in the development process of a project or initiative to ensure they are tailored for, and relate with, Māori communities. One of the reasons for this is to acknowledge the diversity within Māori culture and that a "generic" Māori resource may not be relevant for all Māori. As with any cultural group, there is diversity among Māori iwi, hapū, communities, and whānau. Therefore, what may suit a Māori community in one part of the country may not be relevant or appropriate for Māori from a different part of the country.

The ACP national team have learned that a broad approach is required when seeking Māori leaders, health professionals, and communities to participate in the planning and design stages of an initiative. This is to ensure that we develop resources, education, and ACP tools that are accessible to and relevant and appropriate for Māori communities. This has required more people to be involved in the planning and design teams and more consultation sought to gain te ao Māori perspectives, which has a downstream effect on programme target timelines and budget. While this can be challenging to the "usual ways of working", if we continue to do what we've always done, we'll get what we've always got, and we are aiming for meaningful progress.

Our Growth

The employment of and investment in a Māori project manager to lead Māori ACP projects and initiatives were pivotal for the ACP programme. It supported a strategic and concentrated effort to identify and enable factors that would increase the accessibility of ACP for Māori.

The first responsibility of the project manager was to form a group of Māori leaders to work in partnership with the national ACP team. The aim of this group is to ensure that Māori worldviews, values, and beliefs are prioritised across the programme.

In 2021, the Mana Enhancing Design Partners (Mana-E) for ACP group was formed. Mana-E provides advice and guidance on the ACP training materials and tools and the development of resources to ensure that they are tailored for and relatable to Māori communities.

The initial focus of Mana-E was to contribute to the strategy development of the national programme to improve the accessibility, acceptability, and uptake of ACP.

Mana-E used a Māori-centred approach to think about and document their recommendations for the ACP strategic plan. This included pūrākau (storytelling), karakia (prayer), waiata (singing), and whanaungatanga (connection) and ensuring that only Māori voices contributed to the process to prevent the dominant culture from having an influence. This was a new way of working for the ACP team, who sat through the discomfort and experienced first-hand the challenges and rewards of sharing power. This work culminated in a document named *Kaupapa Pīkau: A Māori perspective of advance care planning.*

All the recommendations made for Māori within *Kaupapa Pīkau* were included in the ACP programme's 2022–2028 strategic plan and roadmap of actions,[30] highlighting the authentic commitment from the ACP national team to partner with Mana-E and improve Māori health outcomes.

Te ao Māori, mātauranga Māori perspectives, and equity-focused initiatives are now woven throughout the programme's strategic plan.[30] The national programme's team of project managers are now working to bring the strategic intent alive to embed and enact Te Tiriti across the programme and improve Māori health outcomes.

Fostering Indigenous Self-determination

We aspire to consistently support mana motuhake (self-determination for Māori according to Māori philosophies, values and practices) in the design, delivery, and monitoring of projects and initiatives across the ACP programme.

We acknowledge the following:

- Māori know what is best for Māori.
- Non-Indigenous people cannot be experts on Indigenous peoples' health priorities.
- Indigenous people are not homogenous, rather they have rich and diverse ways of understanding the world.
- The cultural identity of Indigenous peoples has been undermined and marginalised and is a key health determinant for wellness and engagement with healthcare.

We work to:

- use a community-driven approach to create sustainable and enduring change,
- strengthen our capacity and capability to elevate mātauranga Māori across the ACP programme,
- authentically partner with Māori leaders and communities to hear and action their priorities,
- listen carefully and gain clarification when we don't understand,
- collaborate with local communities and people to ensure we understand,
- ensure Māori perspective is gained from the outset of all new projects and initiatives,
- seek advice on what cultural protocols exist to support effective engagement and communication,
- increase efforts to attract, develop, and retain our Māori ACP workforce.

What We've Learned — Deliberately Nurture the Growth of an Indigenous Workforce

Clear strategic direction is required to build on and strengthen an Indigenous ACP workforce, and it is essential that this development be adequately resourced and underpinned by investment in infrastructure and Indigenous leadership.

Māori are under-represented in the Aotearoa ACP workforce in all areas of the programme. This includes people in advisory groups, specialised Māori groups, communities that are accessed for research projects, and healthcare professionals.

Although the health sector reports growth in the capacity and capability of the Māori health workforce, the pool of people is still relatively small, and those working in this specialised area are in high demand.

Our Growth

Case *study: A Māori-centred approach to gain Māori perspectives of ACP*

A Māori-led project was initiated to gain Māori perspectives of ACP and identify solutions to support and improve Māori access and uptake of ACP.

The project leaders collaborated with local ACP health workers to connect with local Māori communities and hear their stories about, needs from, and aspirations for ACP. Advice was sought from local Māori elders to ensure that the proposed tikanga Māori (Māori philosophy and customary practices) were correct for the local community, and Māori-centred methodologies of engagement were used when meeting with the Māori community groups.

Three main themes emerged from the community meetings as as follows:

- *Elevate mātauranga Māori*: Participants were clear that ACP resources, promotion, online tools, and education should reflect a Māori worldview through images, stories, concepts, and practices to make them more accessible for Māori.
- *Develop a community Māori ACP workforce*: All community groups voiced the desire for a community-based Māori ACP workforce. It was identified that these people would need to be set up to succeed, which would require a Māori-centred approach to training and for them to have access to the appropriate resources and ongoing support.
- *Normalise ACP for Māori*: It was thought that social media could be used to promote ACP to a younger demographic, who would in turn introduce ACP to their whānau. The use of technology to make a voice recording of an ACP was a common theme across all groups, as was the development of an ACP phone app.

Many positive outcomes have arisen from this initiative:

- An ACP change manager role was established to coordinate the development of culturally relevant ACP education resources and tools for the Māori community workforce. This initiative is led by Māori leaders from across the health sector and non-government organisations. The training will provide a platform for Māori ACP champions to facilitate ACP conversations with Māori families in their communities.

- A monthly national ACP promotional campaign named *Kia Whakarite — Be Prepared* has been established that features images and stories about ACP from a younger demographic. There is a strong drive for the featured campaign champions to be Māori. The campaign is presented via social media and our website,[31] through stakeholders, and in poster form. Several of the articles from the promotion have been run in national magazines, and the whānau stories have been shared more broadly. The campaign aims to bring whānau stories on how ACP has supported people and their whānau to be heard and feel respected in the healthcare environment. It has now been embedded into the programme's business.

A particular challenge throughout all three of these initiatives — in the community meetings, during the development of tools for a Māori ACP community workforce, and in the national ACP promotional campaign — has been difficulty finding Māori participants. With this in mind, we are working on specific strategies to build on and strengthen our connections with Māori stakeholders and community groups.

The Power of Data to Effect Meaningful Change

The collection of robust, high-quality data that measure and monitor people's ACP activities is essential for creating meaningful change. Accurate health data could provide insight into how ACP services are being used and by whom. This knowledge would help with strategic planning so that finance, workforce, training, resources, and promotional campaigns can be channelled to where they are most needed.

For example, over the years 2018–2021, Māori health professionals made up only 7.8% of the total number of people who completed online ACP training modules in Aotearoa. These data have led the team to reflect on what needs to be done to make ACP more accessible and appropriate for our health workforce and what actionable steps we will take to support equitable participation.

Our Aspirations

Data to support equity-focused action are needed in the following areas:

- *The Indigenous ACP workforce*: How many Indigenous people have ACP-specific roles, where are they located, and what resources do they access for their communities?
- *Consumer preferences*: How do people access advance care plans (i.e., in hospitals or in the community), what health resources are being used (i.e., what is and is not working) and are people primarily accessing digital or paper-based ACP consumer resources?
- *Ethnicity comparisons*: Does the number of advance care plans uploaded to medical records or accessed by medical teams vary?
- *Appropriateness of material*: How do responses to questions within the advance care plan vary and why?
- *Engagement with ACP material*: How does use of resources vary among regions?

Our Challenges

In Aotearoa, the collection of national datasets on ACP activity is limited, and the data captured varies across regions. There is hope that the dynamic reforms[29] currently taking place within the Aotearoa health system will address these system issues:

> He iti hoki te mokoroa, nāna I kākati te kahikatea
> *The grub may be small, but it cuts through white pine.*

This whakataukī speaks to how perseverance and determination will see us succeed and urges us to not be deterred by seemingly complex or large obstacles.

The Study

Case *study: Building and sharing information*

An audit in the Canterbury region of Aotearoa aimed to understand the impact of ACP after the first 3 years of implementation in this region.[32] Findings revealed that, although uptake had steadily increased within the general population, minority ethnic populations, including Māori, were significantly under-represented and that culturally relevant Māori-specific resources were needed. These findings aligned with those from ACP studies in east Taiwan,[33] Australia,[34] and Canada.[35]

The Canterbury audit's findings and recommendations led to the creation of a national ACP resource to support Māori families to think and talk about ACP (see the following case study).

The Growth

Case *study: Community-led development of consumer resources*

A Māori advisory group was formed to lead the planning, design, and delivery of an ACP consumer resource for Māori named *Whenua ki te whenua* (from the womb to the earth). This group was made up of Māori leaders from within the health sector and Māori community. The advisory group held wānanga (series of workshops to meet, discuss, and deliberate) with local Māori communities to discuss and explore whakaaro Māori (thoughts from a Māori worldview perspective) about what was needed to support families to start ACP conversations.

An Indigenous writer and an Indigenous designer were contracted to bring the whakaaro Māori from the wānanga to life. The designer began by writing a whakatauākī (a Māori saying by a known author) to establish a rationale for the project and feel the essence of the kaupapa (purpose) (Figure 2). He then created a tohu (Māori design) as a visual expression of the whakatauākī (Figure 3).

The *Whenua ki te whenua* resource was tested nationwide to gain consumer feedback, which was overwhelmingly positive across ethnicities and age groups:

"It has a sense of freedom."

"Our whānau felt heard."

"This has many examples that will be relevant for people. I think many will connect with this."

"When I look at it, I see Māori. Very empowering and capturing to the eye. Seeing Māori designs and the significant manu (bird) brings out the beauty of our culture, language and identity."

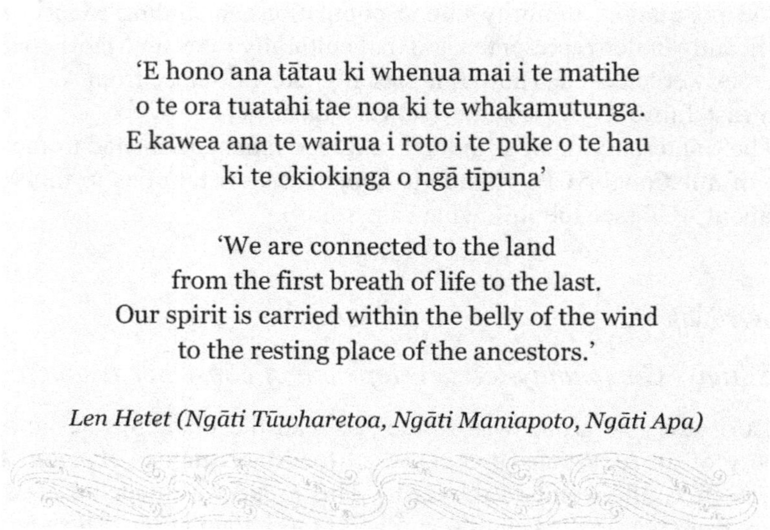

'E hono ana tātau ki whenua mai i te matihe
o te ora tuatahi tae noa ki te whakamutunga.
E kawea ana te wairua i roto i te puke o te hau
ki te okiokinga o ngā tīpuna'

'We are connected to the land
from the first breath of life to the last.
Our spirit is carried within the belly of the wind
to the resting place of the ancestors.'

Len Hetet (Ngāti Tūwharetoa, Ngāti Maniapoto, Ngāti Apa)

Figure 2. This whakatauākī speaks of the journey of life and end of life — from the womb of our mother (whenua), we return to the land (whenua). The Māori worldview holds the land as sacred, as the land is our earth mother, Papatūānuku.

We officially launched *Whenua ki te whenua* using a Māori-centred approach that was infused with tikanga Māori. It was blessed by a Māori elder, and all those who were involved in its development were acknowledged. Karakia were said and waiata sung to uplift the wairua and enhance the mauri (life force) of *Whenua ki te whenua* as she was given flight:

"The doorway has been opened to let the light in. Mind though, the opening is just a crack. This is just the beginning. It's a great start." (Mana-E member)

The resource is available in both English and te reo Māori (see Figure 4). Following the launch, public reaction continued to be very positive, and interactions with our social media and website[31] spiked:

"Thank you so much. I am Filipino but have become a naturalised citizen of NZ. I feel a special affinity to the Māori culture because we have exactly the same values and principles. It is in our blood too what you have written ... making me feel we are brothers/sisters sharing the same hopes."

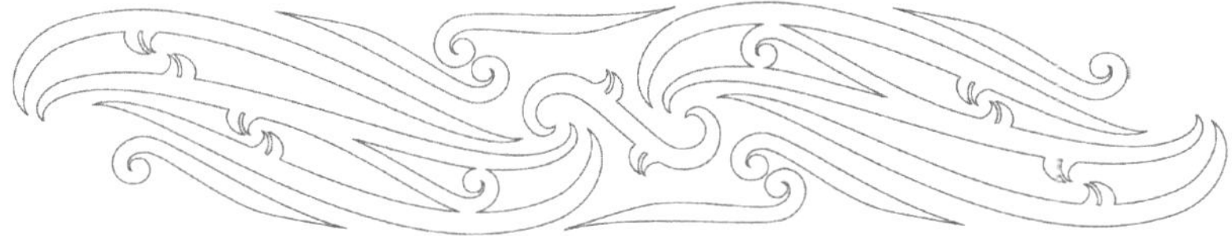

Figure 3.   This tohu was borne from the whakatauākī. They are intricately connected, and as such this tohu represents the journey of life — whenua ki te whenua (from the womb to the land). At the centre of the tohu is the person and their whānau. The koru (coiled) patterns depict the winds that carry us through the journey of life "… our spirit is carried within the belly of the wind …".

Given this success and the favourable reception of both the wairua and the look and feel of *Whenua ki te whenua*, the national ACP programme has:

- revitalised the programme's visual identity and brand narrative with the resources, whakatauākī, and tohu,
- conducted a further study that resulted in a strong community call to integrate the resource into the development of our new consumer advance care plan document,
- used the community approach to develop an ACP resource specifically for Pacific people.

Conclusions

Internationally, it is recognised that the health inequities that affect Indigenous peoples are driven by the legacy and continued impacts of colonisation.

It is important that healthcare professionals understand the historical and societal realities of Indigenous peoples to gain insight into how the power imbalance affects health behaviours and engagement with health services. With this knowledge, we can move forward to eliminate health inequities and work to decolonise the systems within which we work.

The ACP programme in Aotearoa is committed to:

- elevating mātauranga Māori to enable Māori to live, thrive, and flourish as Māori,

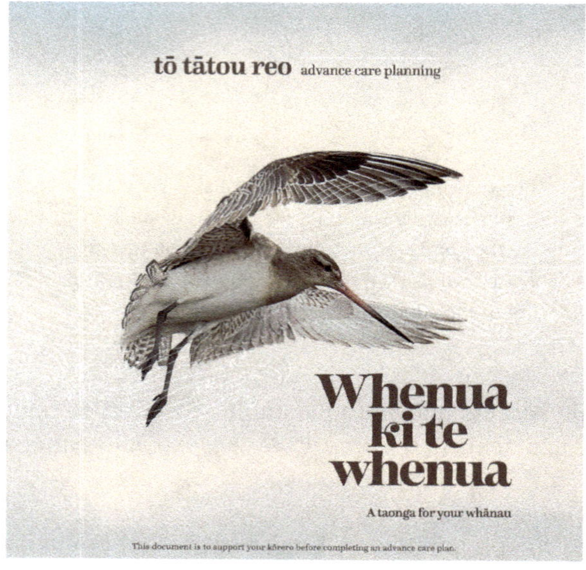

(a)

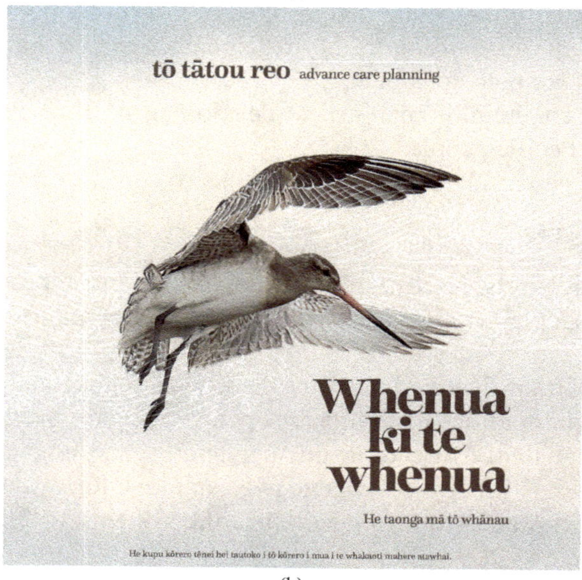

(b)

Figure 4.   (a, b) The bird used in this resource is a kuaka (bar-tailed godwit). Ancestral stories from northern iwi say that kuaka accompany the wairua of the departed back to Hawaiki (ancient homeland, the final resting place of wairua).

- embedding and enacting Te Tiriti o Waitangi, supporting mana motuhake,
- strengthening and nurturing the ACP Māori workforce,
- maintaining authentic partnerships with Māori stakeholders, consumers, and clinicians,
- strengthening our systems for high-quality equitable services.

It is understood that these activities must be adequately resourced and underpinned by investment in infrastructure and Indigenous leadership at all levels of decision-making.

With the process of "Indigenising" the health landscape gaining more momentum, and the Aotearoa health reforms focused on eliminating health inequities by honouring and enacting Te Tiriti, we have some exciting times ahead.

Acknowledgements

Ko te amorangi ki mua,

Ko te hāpai ō ki muri,

Te hei mauri ora!

Leaders to the fore; we all have important roles to play

Behold, there is life!

To my tūpuna who have set the path and provided guidance and reassurance along the way, you are my inspiration.

To all those who have worked to advance Māori and Indigenous peoples' health and well-being in the past, present, and future, I send you my deepest regard and respect.

To my ACP colleagues across the motu (country) both past and present, I'm grateful to be part of a passionate and motivated team. I acknowledge all that we've done and all that lies ahead of us to bring people's voices to the centre of their healthcare so they feel valued and heard.

References

1. Stats NZ: Tatauranga Aotearoa. (2022). Māori population estimates. 30 June 2022. https://www.stats.govt.nz/information-releases/maori-population-estimates-at-30-june-2022/. Retrieved 10 April 2023.

2. Stats NZ: Tatauranga Aotearoa. (2022). Population. https://www.stats.govt.nz/topics/population. Retrieved 10 April 2023.

3. Wilson J. (2020). History — Māori arrival and settlement. Te Ara — The Encyclopedia of New Zealand. http://www.TeAra.govt.nz/en/history/page-1. Retrieved 10 April 2023.

4. Came H., O'Sullivan D., Kidd J., *et al.* (2020). The Waitangi Tribunal's WAI 2575 report: Implications for decolonizing health systems. *Health Hum. Rights* **22**: 209–220.

5. Talamaivao N., Harris R., Cormack D., *et al.* (2020). Racism and health in Aotearoa New Zealand: A systematic review of quantitative studies. *NZ Med. J.* **133**: 55–68.

6. Came H., McCreanor T., Manson L., *et al.* (2019). Upholding Te Tiriti, ending institutional racism and Crown inaction on health equity. *NZ Med. J.* **132**: 61–66.

7. Jones R., Crowshoe L., Reid P., *et al.* (2019). Educating for Indigenous health equity: An international consensus statement. *Acad. Med.* **94**: 512–519.

8. Medical Council of New Zealand, Te Ohu Rata o Aotearoa. (2020). *Baseline Data Capture: Cultural Safety, Partnership, and Health Equity Initiatives.* Medical Council of New Zealand, Wellington.

9. Wilson D., Moloney E., Parr J., *et al.* (2021). Creating an Indigenous Māori-centred model of relational health: A literature review of Māori models of health. *J. Clin. Nurs.* **30**: 3539–3555.

10. Durie M. (2018). Mauri ora practice and mauri ora practitioners. In: Kingi T.K., Durie M., Elder H., *et al.* (eds.) *Maea te Toi Ora: Māori Health Transformations,* pp. 223–246. Huia Publishers, Wellington.

11. Reid P., Paine S., Te Ao B., *et al.* (2022). Estimating the economic costs of Indigenous health inequities in New Zealand: A retrospective cohort analysis. *BMJ Open* **12**: e065430.

12. Hyett S., Gabel C., Marjerrison S., *et al.* (2019). Deficit-based indigenous health research and the stereotyping of Indigenous peoples. *Can. J. Bioethics.* **2**: 102–109.

13. Fogarty W., Bulloch H., McDonnell S., *et al.* (2018). *Deficit Discourse and Indigenous Health: How Narrative Framings of Aboriginal and Torres Strait Islander People Are Reproduced in Policy.* The Lowitja Institute, Melbourne.

14. Smallwood R., Woods C., Power T., *et al.* (2021). Understanding the impact of historical trauma due to colonization on the health and well-being of Indigenous young peoples: A systematic scoping review. *J. Transcult. Nurs.* **32**: 59–68.

15. Harris R.B., Paine S., Atkinson J., *et al.* (2022). We still don't count: The under-counting and under-representation of Māori in health and disability sector data. *NZ Med. J.* **135**: 54–61.

16. Fox C. (2010). Change, past and present. In: Mulholland M., and Tawhai V. (eds.) *Weeping Waters: The Treaty of Waitangi and Constitutional Change*, pp. 41–61. Huia Publishers, Wellington.

17. van Meijl T. (2020). Culture versus class: Towards an understanding of Māori poverty. *Race Class* **62**: 78–96.

18. Orange C. (2023). Te Tiriti o Waitangi — the Treaty of Waitangi — Dishonouring te tiriti — 1860 to 1880. Te Ara: The Encyclopedia of New Zealand. https://teara.govt.nz/en/interactive/36363/maori-land-loss-south-island. Retrieved 5 April 2023.

19. Calman R. (2012). Māori education — mātauranga — Missionaries and the early colonial period. Te Ara: The Encyclopedia of New Zealand. https://teara.govt.nz/en/zoomify/34874/education-ordinance-1847. Retrieved 20 March 2023.

20. Te Tai Treaty Settlement Stories. (2023). 1945–1978 Language under threat. New Zealand Government. https://teara.govt.nz/en/te-tai/te-mana-o-te-reo-maori-chapter5. Retrieved 28 March 2023.

21. New Zealand History. (2021). Land confiscation law passed 3 December 1863. https://nzhistory.govt.nz/the-new-zealand-settlements-act-passed. Retrieved 7 April 2023.

22. Calman R. (2012). Māori education — mātauranga — The native schools system, 1867 to 1969. Te Ara: The Encyclopedia of New Zealand. http://www.TeAra.govt.nz/en/maori-education-matauranga/page-3. Retrieved 7 April 2023.

23. Pool I., and Jackson N. (2018). Population change — Māori population change. Te Ara: The Encyclopedia of New Zealand. http://www.TeAra.govt.nz/en/population-change/page-6. Retrieved 14 April 2023.

24. Derby M. (2011). Māori–Pākehā relations — Māori renaissance. Te Ara: The Encyclopedia of New Zealand. TeAra.govt.nz/en/maori-pakeha-relations/page-6. Retrieved 9 April 2023.

25. Waitangi Tribunal: The Rōpū Whakamana i te Tiriti o Waitangi. (2017). Past, present & future of the Waitangi Tribunal. History of the Waitangi Tribunal. https://waitangitribunal.govt.nz/about/past-present-future-of-waitangi-tribunal. Retrieved 30 March 2023.

26. Derby M. (2012). Waitangi Tribunal — Te Rōpū Whakamana. Te Ara: The Encyclopedia of New Zealand. https://teara.govt.nz/en/waitangi-tribunal-te-ropu-whakamana. Retrieved 20 March 2023.

27. Hayward J. (2023). Principles of the Treaty of Waitangi — ngā mātāpono o te Tiriti o Waitangi. Te Ara: The Encyclopedia of New Zealand. http://www.TeAra.govt.nz/en/principles-of-the-treaty-of-waitangi-nga-matapono-o-te-tiriti-o-waitangi/print. Retrieved 7 April 2023.

28. Ministry of Health. (2020). *Whakamaua: Māori Health Action Plan 2020–2025*. Ministry of Health, Wellington. https://www.health.govt.nz/publication/whakamaua-maori-health-action-plan-2020-2025.

29. Future of Health: Te Anamata o te Oranga. (2022). About the health reforms. https://www.futureofhealth.govt.nz/. Retrieved 4 April 2023.
30. Healthy Quality & Safety Commission. (2022). *Strategy and Road Map of Actions for Advance Care Planning and Clinical Communication Programme 2022–28.* https://www.hqsc.govt.nz/assets/Our-work/Advance-care-planning/ACP-info-for-consumers/Publications-resources/ACP-strategy-and-roadmap_2022-28_final.pdf.
31. Te Tāhū Hauora Health Quality & Safety Commission. Te whakamahere tiaki i mua i te wā taumaha: Advance care planning. www.myacp.org.nz.
32. Goodwin J., Shand B., Wiseman R., *et al.* (2021). Achievements and challenges during the development of an advance care planning program. *Australas. J. Ageing* **40**: 301–308.
33. Li I.-F., Huang S.-M., Lee C.-F., *et al.* (2021). Perceptions of behavioral awareness, intention, and readiness for advance care planning: A mixed-method study among older indigenous patients with late-stage cancers in remote areas of Eastern Taiwan. *Int. J. Environ. Res. Public Health* **18**: 8665.
34. Sinclair C., Williams G., Knight A., *et al.* (2014). A public health approach to promoting advance care planning to Aboriginal people in regional communities. *Aust. J. Rural Health* **22**: 23–28.
35. Hyett S., Marjerrison S., and Gabel C. (2018). Improving health research among indigenous peoples in Canada. *CMAJ* **190**: E616–E621.

Kuputaka: Glossary

Hapū: extended family group, sub-tribe

Hawaiki: ancient homeland and final resting place of wairua

Iwi: tribe

Karakia: prayer

Kaupapa: purpose

Kia whakarite: be prepared

Koru: coil

Mana: prestige, honour

Mana motuhake: self-determination for Māori according to Māori philosophies, values and practices

Manu: bird

Māori: Indigenous people of Aotearoa New Zealand

Mātāpono: core values

Mātauranga Māori: Māori knowledge

Mauri: life force

Motu: country

Pākehā: New Zealander of European descent

Papatūānuku: earth mother from ancestral Māori creation narratives

Pūrākau: storytelling

Rangatira: Māori tribal leaders

Tāngata whenua: people of the land, the Indigenous people of Aotearoa

Te ao Māori: Māori worldview

Te reo Māori: Māori language

Tikanga: Māori philosophy and customary practices

Tohu: Māori design

Tō tātou reo: our voice

Tupuna: ancestor

Tūpuna: ancestors

Waiata: singing

Wairua: life force; spirit or spiritual body

Wānanga: series of workshops to meet, discuss and deliberate

Whakaaro Māori: thoughts from a Māori worldview perspective

Whakatauākī: a Māori saying by a known author

Whakataukī: Māori saying by an unknown author

Whānau: family, including extended family and friends

Whanaungatanga: connection

Whenua: land, womb

Chapter 36

Advance Care Planning in Children and Young People

Nobuyuki Yotani[*] and Poh-Heng Chong[†]

*Department of Palliative Medicine, National Center for Child
Health and Development, Japan
†HCA Hospice, Singapore

Introduction

This chapter focuses on advance care planning (ACP) in children and young people (CYP). In terms of age spectrum, the population in question is diverse. It can range from newborns, neonates, and infants, beyond teenagers, to young adults below 25 years[1]; all still under the care of pediatric providers for life-shortening conditions diagnosed before 18 or 21 years (age of majority, depending on jurisdiction).

ACP in pediatric practice is described as a "process of discussions between families and healthcare providers about preferences for care, treatment and goals in the context of the patient's current and anticipated future health."[2] On the surface, elements highlighted within that quote parallel those in the adult setting. Whether this is indeed true is debated further in the following section comparing ACP across both populations.

Given inherent uniqueness in context (both clinical and socio-cultural) between these two groups, the primacy of ACP as a critical service intervention among CYP living with any serious illness is outlined in the following section. This is followed by the "nuts and bolts" of how ACP is typically conducted in pediatric palliative care (PPC). With common deliverables like care plans yet bearing significant impact on stakeholders in mind, the stages and processes of ACP within the pediatric domain will be comprehensively explicated for those who may be unfamiliar.

Despite a growing body of literature informing its implementation and many resources providing practical guidance, completion, or for some healthcare professionals, even the initiation of ACP discussions remains challenging. Before concluding this chapter, practice "pearls" gleaned from empirical experience in the clinical setting will be shared. All types of healthcare professionals would find them helpful to navigate delicate and emotional conversations expected. To deepen overall understanding, key concepts and effective strategies expounded will be reiterated through two real-life case studies (one centred in pediatric oncology and the other non-cancer) to close this chapter.

Why Is Pediatric ACP Important?

As pediatric medicine advanced over the years, treatment options for previously incurable conditions increased. This resulted in an increasing number of children living with chronic conditions. In the US, children with chronic conditions (CCC) are defined as those with the following: serious medical conditions reasonably expected to live beyond 12 months (unless death intervenes), involving several organ systems or one organ system severe enough to require specialty care, and needing hospitalization in a tertiary care centre. They now account for 10% of hospitalized patients.[9] The same trend is observed in Asia. Future care planning in this group of vulnerable children is now undeniably urgent to safeguard all types of positive outcomes.

Every child and family have individual needs, and each child goes through a unique process of development. For children with serious illnesses, ongoing growth and development are closely linked to the course of the illness as well as the treatment and care received. The approach that professionals adopt when discussing future care plans with children and families is first to explore how the child and parents perceive the current state and then ask what they consider important for the future. These types of discussions strengthen the autonomy of the child and parents and is congruent with contemporary best practice promoting shared decision-making — all core elements of ACP in the CYP setting.

A key feature of ACP in adults is to "repeatedly discuss future treatment and care while the patient is still capable of making decisions, before he or she is no longer capable of making decisions."[10] In the case of children, it is not uncommon for them to lack (or have insufficient) decision-making capacity. It is hence difficult to translate concepts of ACP in adults directly to the pediatric domain. As highlighted previously, it is also important in pediatrics to support the young person to "confirm his/her own values, fully consider the meaning and outcome of serious illness, clarify goals and intentions for future treatment and care, and discuss these with family and medical caregivers" while "discussing concerns through the physical, psychological, social, and spiritual aspects of the individual."[11]

Next, following the family-focused and child-centred philosophy elaborated, ACP in the CYP setting ensures that care and treatment are always tailored to everyone's preference. It also prepares families both cognitively and psychologically for critical situations in future, reducing uncertainty and anxiety if they should arise. The completed ACP document can prevent unwanted acute hospital admissions and invasive medical procedures during a crisis. The sense of control it accords to parents, who are already managing anticipatory grief at the time, has been raised as important to families.[6] On a different note, an advance care plan provides clarity in the acute situation for prompt and appropriate actions. In our experience, for example, at the children's emergency or intensive care, this is most helpful for attending healthcare professionals who may be unfamiliar with the child or family.

Given all of the above, ACP in particular is most relevant for children whose futures are limited or threatened. Prognostic uncertainty notwithstanding, the need for ACP and its priority increases as the child's condition deteriorates.

The following questions are helpful signposts:

- Would you be surprised if this child dies within the next 12 months?
- Would you be surprised if this child dies from the illness or its complications?
- Would you be surprised if this child dies from the condition before reaching adulthood?

If the response to any of the above is "no," the time is now! Thinking about how the family would like to spend time together as the child's condition worsens will help them to think about how they might cherish the present. Despite wide hesitancy or even reluctance that is understandable in this instance, timely but compassionate engagement in these future-oriented discussions ultimately minimizes later regrets in child bereavement.

Difference between Adult and Pediatric ACP

Despite processes and deliverables that are conceptually similar, the administration of ACP in CYP living with life-shortening conditions is operationally disparate. As mentioned before, it differs from adult ACP in clinical and socio-cultural perspectives. This has implications for how (and when) ACP is initiated, engaged between stakeholders, and applied when completed. Five areas of divergence are shared here. They support the argument that a different approach may be indicated when it comes to ACP in the CYP population. We start with selecting the right patient groups to promote ACP.

Contrary to the adult setting where different groups are targeted to extend its benefits (almost like a public health movement), ACP is never discussed in the context of children or young people who are healthy and well. This is easy to understand. While opening an ACP conversation with an older person on what "living well" means may not be strange or perceived hard, doing the same with the family of a healthy young person is neither intuitive nor appropriate. In fact, even when the CYP is seriously ill or even dying, ACP often gets brought up late in the course of illness. Possible reasons underpinning this phenomenon are discussed next.

The *process* (serial discussions on values and preferences, and achieving alignment of goals between stakeholders) takes priority, rather than the *deliverables* (creating a "form" that sets care limits or its wider dissemination afterwards). To our knowledge, this is prevalent across all types of PPC services internationally. Forging mutual understanding over time, instead of ticking off boxes on a form, is evidently more acceptable to parents or even their clinicians; both stakeholders do not readily "seal" the ACP document as "final" most of the time. Before exploring why, yet another feature exclusive to doing ACP with the CYP needs to be appreciated first.

While the spotlight is obviously on the CYP, family stakeholders meeting clinicians at the table are usually their parents or legal guardians.

The adults are assumed to act in the "best interest" of the CYP to make important decisions on their behalf. In other instances where the patient is a young adult that lacks mental capacity or is unable to communicate his or her wishes for whatever reason, again their respective legal surrogates (like appointed deputies, for example) will decide for them, this time based on the principle of "substituted judgment" or what the young person would have preferred or chosen for themselves if they could decide and communicate.[3] Notwithstanding the above however, if any CYP is able to participate, and wishes to do so when asked, no effort should be spared to involve them.[4] "Bringing out" or "listening to" the voice of the CYP is now best practice, if not already the norm in routine pediatric care. The child life specialist (trained allied health worker that helps the CYP who is unwell cope with their medical experience) or leveraging appropriate technical aids are ways to make this feasible.

Next, distinct from adult palliative care, there is wide preponderance of non-oncological conditions versus cancer in PPC. This directly contributes to pervasive uncertainty surrounding illness trajectory in general and patient prognosis in specific.[5] In addition, with "letting go" less easy in a young person who is seriously ill, intensive treatments are often aggressively pursued despite decreasing the likelihood of success.[6] All these factors prevent timely ACP in this setting. Again, this relates to informal as well as professional caregivers. Signifying how little things have moved (and inherent challenges in ACP among CYP), the top three barriers identified by clinicians surveyed more than a decade ago are still relevant today: unrealistic parental expectations, differential prognostic understanding between clinicians and parents, and lack of parental readiness for ACP.[7]

Putting everything together, it is definitely not an overstatement to say ACP in the context of CYP is an intricate and complex endeavor. It was described by one study group as "the delicate dance of figuring it out!"[8] Before ending this section on differences, two additional facets unique to ACP with CYP are raised to substantiate aforementioned claims of intricacy and complexity. Peculiar to PPC, the primary physician or specialist very often continues to be involved in supporting the child (and family) jointly with clinicians on the PPC team, whereas in the adult patient, the oncologist, for example, might have "handed over" the patient's care to the palliative care team in hospital or hospice. Hence, as ACP is in progress, the primary clinician of the CYP may need to be looped in. In fact, the family may expect or actively seek their participation, given robust and longstanding relationships built before PPC even got involved. On a related note, particularly as Pediatric Medicine as a discipline becomes more advanced and subspecialized, the primary clinician's involvement could be pivotal for another reason. For instance, there might be situations where certain medical interventions in a cardiac patient are deemed still appropriate late in the disease course and need specific mention in the ACP. Therefore, the pediatric ACP may require specific inputs from subspecialty clinicians or at least get signed off by a palliative specialist working in collaboration with colleagues from other pediatric disciplines caring for the same patient.

Adding further to the complexity in this context, documented advance care plans have been known to undergo frequent changes, or were deliberately kept "under wraps" by parents during a medical crisis. As mentioned before, prognostic uncertainties as well as difficulty in "letting go" are likely contributory factors. However, in our experience speaking with many bereaved parents, the need to ensure that *everything possible is indeed done* is most likely the singular concern in those situations.[6] This is partly the reason why stakeholders in ACP for the CYP focus predominantly on the "process" rather than the "output". More about both of these in the following sections — on the importance of pediatric ACP and how it is performed among CYP with serious illnesses.

How Is It Conducted in the Pediatric Setting?

Most medical providers probably immediately think of Do Not Attempt Resuscitation (DNAR) if asked what might be a priority to discuss with families when a young patient's condition deteriorates. While DNAR is important to avoid futile treatments or minimize preventable suffering, discussions about the future go beyond DNAR orders and need to start early. If a discussion only begins during a crisis, there is a rush to make decisions. On the other hand, when the disease is stable, stakeholders could reflect and think about the conversation without feeling pressured to decide right away. Timing is therefore critical.

Prior preparation on the part of the medical provider is equally important. One ought to be familiar with or appraised of the child's latest condition, treatment and care options, expected clinical outcomes, and align with all clinicians involved in the child's care. It is important to consider the child's current and future developmental levels, including projected risks and potential consequences in the event that aggressive interventions are chosen. Ahead of the discussion, it is good to plan specific discussion items (agenda), familiarize with them, and possibly rehearse beforehand.

Whether in a medical crisis or during periods of stability, meetings to discuss the future will be a little different from regular meetings to provide medical updates. ACP discussions would be exploratory and listening types of conversations, centred on the perspectives of the child and the parents. It is pivotal here for the child and parents to talk about how they are coping, what they think is important (in treatment and care), and why they think those are important and to share their hopes and concerns. The goals of treatment and care and if requested a specific treatment plan will then be decided together with all relevant healthcare professionals. Sometimes, the discussion may need to be broken into several smaller meetings (for timeouts or cooling off) to allow information assimilation and emotional processing before achieving final consensus as aspirational outcomes. These types of discussions can be "heavy" for both clinicians and families. The following algorithm is a recommended way to proceed, divided into a sequence of five steps:

Step 1: Learn more about the child and family before the ACP discussion
The medical provider needs to learn what the child and family valued so far and if these would change in future. These may include the following areas:

(1) *About the child*
Inquire about parents' perception of the child:
- What kind of child is he/she?
- What does your child like or dislike?

(2) *About the illness*
Explore what the illness means to (or how it impacts) the child and the family:
- What does this mean for your child and your family?
- How do you think your child's illness or condition will change?

(3) *Quality of life (QOL)*
Explore perceptions on QOL for the child and the family:
- What would you describe as a good day for your child and/or your family?

(4) *The parental role*

Explore what is important for parents to be "good parents":

- What do you value as a parent for your child?

These discussions should be held on a regular basis, not just before an impending medical crisis. It is also important to highlight what we value can change with time and events. By capturing the evolution in priorities over the illness trajectory, medical providers can better appreciate the child and family's lived experience and tailor management that is congruent with individual needs and wishes.

Step 2: Explore the family's understanding of the child's illness

It is critical that the family understands the progressive nature of the current illness. If there is a gap, it would be impossible to have fruitful discussions as the family's wishes for the future are being sought. Therefore, first, explore how the family understands the present circumstances and future trajectory of the child's illness.

It might be helpful to have someone other than the primary care physician verify the family's understanding. For example, during the palliative care consult, the following can be asked: "I think I have a fair understanding of your child's condition through his/her chart and information from his/her primary care physician. However, I would like to know what the family has heard and how you understand your child's medical condition. So, if you don't mind, may I ask you to tell me what you have been told about your child's current situation as well as future plans?"

When asked this way, many families are most willing to tell us their story. As they share, we might notice subtle lapses in understanding. Further discussions to correct or clarify may then be indicated.

Step 3: Explore readiness for ACP discussion

Discussing the future can be emotionally difficult for everyone, as the child, parents, and medical providers are universally confronted with the reality of the child's condition worsening. Therefore, it is very important to explore the other party's readiness when initiating the discussion. For example, the following can be used to explore receptivity:

"We too hope that (child)'s condition will progress well. However, have you ever thought about what would happen if his/her condition worsens as it did last time and he/she could no longer maintain his/her current condition (i.e., if the situation does not improve and he/she can no longer maintain his/her current condition)?"

There are really two main objectives at this point of the discussion: The first objective of communicating uncertainty is hinted when the following phrase is articulated in any variation: "Hope for the best, prepare for the worst."[12] Second, ask about the child/family's wishes and what may be important to them. Seek to explore, empathize, and understand. Open the discussion with "what ifs" in preparation for future changes in the patient's condition. This can help make the discussion less "invasive" or awkward. An alternative is to ask, "Have you ever thought about what happens when your child's condition gets worse?" instead of asking, "What will you do if your child's condition worsens?" By asking this way, if the child/family does not want to talk about it, he/she can say, "I have not thought about it," to signal that he/she is not ready. A compassionate approach is key. It is important to facilitate these discussions very gently by confirming every step of the way the readiness of the child/family to proceed, especially when discussing high-stakes scenarios with profound implications.

Step 4: Discuss management plans that are compatible with shared goals of care

If a family is ready to move forward, treatment specifics will be discussed next. The traditional approach in family meetings of such nature is to talk about future treatment plans such as cardiopulmonary resuscitation and intubation in terms of medical benefits and burdens before further decisions are made. However, the family as lay people may not fully appreciate the intention or implications of various interventions the same way as medical professionals. It may be more productive or even meaningful to set the goals of treatment and care together. This could involve deciding if it should be "to live as long as possible" or "to live as long and as well as possible." Shared decision-making can then take place on the most appropriate treatments that match the goals of care. Additionally, there are benefits in asking the family how or why they feel the way they do about mutually agreed treatment plans. Understanding the basis behind various preferences provides rich insights into priorities or concerns from the family's perspective. Uncovering hidden thoughts or feelings can help bridge communication gaps as well as foster opportunities for enhanced support. Even as families expressed readiness to come to the table, topics discussed here are ultimately difficult and emotionally challenging. This makes the next step especially crucial.

Step 5: Foster hope

As they begin sharing their thoughts about the future, it is vital to listen to the hopes of the family. Children and families do not just have a single hope but rather a collection of many little hopes.[13] In exploring the first hope the family articulates — what it is and why it is there — we may be able to uncover other underlying hopes. Ultimately, for many parents of a young child, the hope in miracles does not disappear. Maintaining the hope of miracles is both an adjustment to adversity and loss, as well as a positive way of communicating love for oneself and one's child. During a life-threatening situation or for that matter at the end of life, persistent hope for a miracle expressed by the child and family can be confusing to the medical staff. It is important to validate the family's hopes and, in many instances, also appropriate to hope together with families. Practically, asking "what other hopes do you have?" opens opportunities to talk about further hopes in a dire situation. This can be comforting to everyone, as the hurt of grief and loss is shared tacitly, while the ever-evolving hope remains very much alive.

Discussion, Documentation, and Dissemination

What ensues after "discussion" are processes around "documentation" and "dissemination". Though equally important to the steps in discussion outlined above, there are many variations in practice across settings, both internationally and regionally. Only a brief account covering essential points is provided here, to be flexibly adapted to local systems and processes. Generally, the ACP discussion is documented clearly in the medical records after the meeting. There are different ways the report is structured; broadly, it contains a summary of the discussion and describes care and treatment goals elicited. If particular instructions for treatment or their limitations have been agreed, these are also documented on the form and included in the medical record. Care and treatment orders must be specific and clear to all healthcare professionals involved. Parents may be asked whether external healthcare professionals like family doctors or general physicians will also receive a copy on top of one for themselves. Some countries use digital versions or operate sophisticated systems that allow storage, sharing, and also versioning when changes are made.

Experience and Tips from the Field

Having reached this point of the chapter, it would be clear that completion of ACP with any CYP is always individualized; tailored to the unique needs of the young person concerned; and informed by values, beliefs, and preferences of the family within which he or she is situated socio-culturally; care plans are arrived at by consensus between multiple stakeholders, then crystallized, documented, and shared where relevant. In the previous section, the way it is normally performed in pediatric practice is made explicit and explained. That should support many practitioners in initiating and completing most ACP (including the CYP where possible). Nonetheless, given the intrinsic intricacy and complexity mentioned before, it may be helpful to highlight a few more considerations to maximize overall chances of success, while optimizing the experience for everyone. The following recommendations in five key areas are organized from contemporary evidence and our practice experience:

First, ACP is often a misunderstood term or a challenging activity. It can mean different things to different people, whether informal caregiver or healthcare professional.[14] It may be prudent to define explicitly what we mean, or at least specify the agenda, when an appointment is made to do ACP. Anecdotally, families have been known to promptly decline attendance, as in their minds their sick child is not yet dying. Albeit less common, other families with previous positive experience looked forward to talking about future plans. Among some clinicians, the ACP is still perceived to be synonymous with DNAR or the extent of care order. Those of us in palliative care who work in the acute in-patient setting would not be unfamiliar with urgent calls for us to facilitate ACP discussions with parents whenever a "complex" case is newly admitted into the Intensive Care Unit (ICU) before the weekend. Fortunately, these misconceptions are gradually corrected over time, with greater awareness and relevant training. Ultimately, clarity of purpose all around will lead to goal alignment, paving the way for positive outcomes and meaningful impact. The benefits of ACP have already been outlined previously.

Second, not all families will be receptive to ACP. Carr *et al.* described aptly: "*Parents who accepted they could not change the outcome but could control other aspects were open to pACP (pediatric ACP) whereas those who fought to change the outcome and did not accept the prognosis did not reach a point of accepting pACP initiation.*"[15] There may be untoward consequences if the CYP or the family is hastily or worse, harshly invited to participate in this "delicate dance" when they are not ready. Not only do we risk subverting tenets of patient or family-centred care that governs modern pediatric practice, we could bring undue distress or even trauma to all involved. In the current zeal across the healthcare sector to embrace ACP, pediatric providers at managerial or commissioning levels should hence exercise restraint and refrain from setting ACP completion rates as a key performance indicator for any PPC service. We firmly believe that *empathy*, *humility*, and *patience* on healthcare professionals' part are most critical.

Third, the same authors that reported those two groups of families above also described two types of triggers for initiation of ACP discussions: "proactive" and "reactive."[15] *Proactive* approaches accord the luxury of time to revisit problematic issues and ensure that meetings are held only when parental caregivers are psychologically ready or receptive, for best results. Less effective were discussions described as *reactive*, in a sudden or unexpected crisis where quick assessment of parental goals is required, to establish limits of care at the emergency department, for example. That said, we have observed positive elements even in the "reactive" category. After "the storm had blown over", in many instances, opportunities to open ACP discussions became available where families were never receptive before. We posit that in the process of seeking active treatments, the cost of preserving life, and the burden of physical suffering becomes apparent to parents, provoking the search for alternative care goals. That is exactly the moment when the watchful patience of healthcare professionals gets rewarded.

Fourth, since trust plays a large part in setting the scene for serious conversations during ACP, it may be assumed that only clinicians that are known to CYP or their families for a significant period are able to engage them effectively. This may not always be true. PPC clinicians, for example, are called in at various times to support these conversations. Apart from the right attitude and timing, we believe there are other qualities and skills involved that all pediatric practitioners can learn and possibly strengthen under expert guidance. The literature has highlighted a few of these.[14] The family must feel that the provider shares the same goals as them. The underlying assumption is that both parties will work closely in the best interest of the seriously ill young person. As much as they need to trust the provider, the family must also feel that the provider trusts them too. This relates to qualities of empathy and humility mentioned previously, again within a trusting relationship — with a single goal to do everything possible while minimizing suffering. The provider is also expected to be capable, confident, and comfortable with the tasks anticipated during ACP. Needing to be "comfortable" acknowledges the hefty emotional burden of holding a safe space for both partners working on a critical yet delicate project. These pointers from extant evidence are very much consistent with our empirical experience.

Fifth, and last but certainly not least, we return to the discussion point on parents requesting frequent changes to existing ACP or deliberately withholding the ACP in a medical crisis. It is worth examining this peculiar phenomenon a little deeper, based on past experience supporting CYP and their distraught parents, during the tumultuous journey of dying and grief. Through sharing this, we aim to illuminate the path toward compassionate and personalized care, for all pediatric providers privileged with the responsibility of caring for them. We learnt to accept ambivalence (and turnarounds) among grieving parents who struggle between preservation and letting go.[16] Therein lies reasons for indecisiveness, such as minimizing regrets through "leaving no stones unturned". What has remained firm though is the fact that parental caregivers are definitely not in denial. With this insight, it is imperative to ensure that the first two components of any ACP (*eliciting family beliefs and values* followed by *capturing the goals of care*) are performed well, instead of focusing solely on completing *documentation and dissemination* (often mislabeled by parents as "signing off" their own child). In our opinion, the most helpful thing we can do as healthcare providers at this most difficult time is to affirm them as good parents and cede them the "control" they should rightfully own.

Hopefully, these nuggets of practice wisdom come in useful as the novice clinician ventures into the relatively new practice of pediatric ACP. Before the conclusion, principles and concepts introduced thus far are illustrated using two case studies to consolidate learning.

Two Case Studies

Case 1

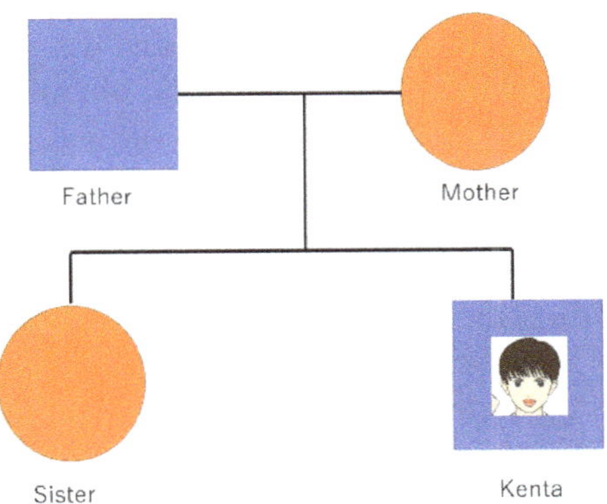

Our palliative care team first met Kenta in the emergency room. He was 16 years old then, had severe neck pain from a cervical sarcoma and could not stand up. Through his primary oncologist, we promptly prescribed an analgesic regimen for rapid pain relief.

After one course of treatment, his symptoms improved and Kenta was able to sit up and talk. It was then that he told us a story about his past. He had been a member of a soccer team but dropped out of mainstream school to join a correspondence school due to a problem with a friend. He also stopped playing football since. Given that it was over nothing really big, it was something that he had regretted to this day. After Kenta related his story, I spoke with him about his illness. "You have heard that this disease can metastasize, do you want to know more about that yourself?" Without hesitation he answered, "Of course I would like to know. I want to know about the metastasis. Even if it is not curable, I want to know that too, because it is about me!" His eyes locked with mine as he uttered earnestly.

Thankfully, Kenta responded well to the oncological treatment. His condition improved, and he was able to go home and spend time with his family for a few months. However, his condition flared once more during a relapse and he needed to be hospitalized again. This time, he did not respond as well to the cancer treatments. Radiation therapy was added, but the disease remained resistant to treatment. The tumor invaded his spinal cord and he soon became paralyzed in the lower half of his body.

The primary oncologist had other secondary treatment options but was not confident that they would work for his type of aggressive sarcoma. The oncology team decided that it might be better to terminate treatment altogether and allow him to spend more time with family at home instead. We informed his parents about our plans and sought their consent to talk to Kenta about his condition and discuss his future. They were concerned that he would lose all hope and initially declined. I shared with his parents what was discussed before — his desire to know everything about himself. The parents eventually relented.

Before the ACP discussion, we confirmed with Kenta the intentions for us to talk about his condition. His oncologist shared the bad news: "I can't cure your disease. There are treatment options to moderate your condition, but they may be temporary. I would like to propose the other option for you to stop further cancer treatments and go home with painkillers if that is what you would like." He listened quietly throughout, kept his eyes in the air and didn't say a word. Only his mother's sobbing echoed in the room. The medical staff left the room in the end, thinking that he would need some "space" in the meantime.

A few days later, in front of his parents, he informed the oncologist of his decision. He wanted to continue further treatment to fight the disease, even if it means in the process, he should die in the hospital. He did finally die while undergoing chemotherapy a few weeks later, albeit without suffering too much pain.

Despite the unfortunate circumstances, it is critical that we ascertain how much the young person with serious illness wants to know about the disease and where appropriate given the autonomy to plan his future. It is impossible when approached late. This case reminds us the importance of performing timely ACP, to ensure that the wishes of the young person have a chance of being realized, without lingering regrets.

Case 2

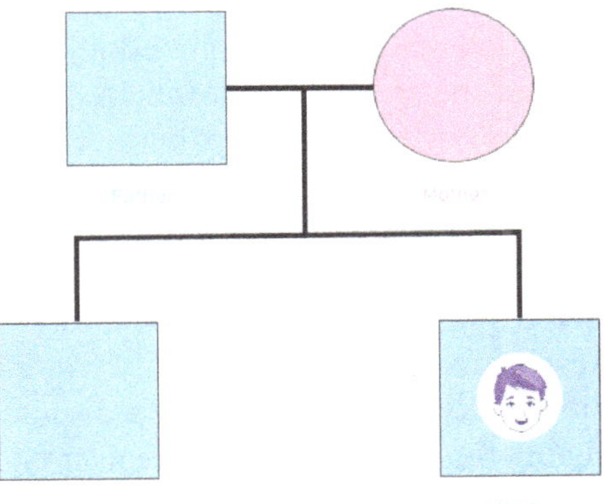

Kyle was a 14-year-old boy with quadriplegic cerebral palsy when the hospice team first met with him and his lovely family at home. He had just been discharged from the hospital after a month's stay for management of aspiration pneumonia.

In the letter of referral for community palliative care, we were informed he had a "stormy" admission. Kyle had developed a parapneumonic pleural effusion that required drainage under radiological guidance, but the procedure was complicated by a pneumothorax causing a collapsed lung requiring chest tube insertion and a period of observation in the intensive care unit. His oxygen saturation did not improve, and he eventually required non-invasive ventilatory support. While he was able to feed orally with mom's help before, his swallowing was assessed to be poor during the admission and a feeding tube was promptly inserted.

After all that had happened, his mother (and family) was obviously much relieved to bring their little boy home. Kyle himself looked tired. Mom even more so. She also brought back three additional things that now became routine in Kyle's life: a BIPAP ventilator, suction machine, and nasogastric tube.

The community palliative care team was asked to continue caregiver training at home and perform one more important piece of work — to create an advance care plan. Though he was stable previously, it was perceived by clinicians in the hospital that Kyle had become very "vulnerable" and might not survive another hospitalization in the future.

Initially, mom had refused to hear anything about ACP. The team reluctantly put that aside and sought to learn more about him during happier times. Though Kyle stopped schooling for some years due to his susceptibility to viral infections, he had had no hospital admission in the last decade! The team soon realized his mom felt miserable and conflicted then. She perceived that the series of unfortunate events was due to her carelessness, causing her boy to choke. Furthermore, while staying in the hospital with Kyle throughout what seemed like a never-ending ordeal, she had sometimes prayed for God to "take him".

In contrast, Kyle's dad and eighteen-year-old brother were very keen to document their wishes for active treatment in a formal medical plan, in case attending professionals gave up prematurely. Their request prevailed, despite mom's hesitation to even sit down for a discussion. An ACP was drawn up specifying aggressive therapy if Kyle ever encountered a medical crisis. That was in fact tested a few times when he got readmitted for recurrent bouts of pneumonia and urinary tract infections.

A urine catheter was soon added to the medical paraphernalia around Kyle as he gradually developed bladder dysfunction. During the same period, Kyle also developed intestinal problems and lost significant weight. He began developing pressure sores on his buttocks, ears, and heels. Though he was non-verbal and never regained his smile in his oft-drowsy state, he moaned in pain every time dressings were changed. This distressed everyone at home greatly.

The team was called in one day and Kyle's mom asked for the ACP to be changed. She did not want him to be readmitted again and hoped that any emerging medical issue could be managed at home. She had apparently convinced dad and their older son, as both nodded in agreement.

As staunch Christians, they came to the consensus that Kyle was near the end of his existence on earth and would soon be reunited with God in heaven.

The week after a new plan was inked. Kyle developed a new fever that he never recovered from despite enteral antibiotics prescribed. He died peacefully at home with his loving family surrounding him.

Conclusion

1. While processes and deliverables may be conceptually similar to ACP in the adult setting, sensitive and effective implementation of ACP among CYP is necessarily nuanced, intricate, and complex and ultimately different in many aspects.
2. The number of children with complex chronic conditions is increasing, and ACP will likely become even more important than before. ACP discussions not only strengthen autonomy of the child and parents, but they also promote the concept of shared decision-making in serious illness.
3. Timely ACP discussions for future care planning ensures that vulnerable children receive prompt and appropriate care during a medical crisis, without parental caregivers having to decide under duress and in haste, the types of care the CYP should receive in an emergency.
4. ACP in CYP is more than a DNAR discussion. It covers more scope and needs to be done early, sometimes over a few meetings. Preparation, sensitivity, and hopefulness are key features. The five-step algorithm offers practical guidance.
5. Not every child or family is receptive to the idea of ACP. It should never be imposed systemically or rushed. Both proactive and reactive approaches have been described. Nonetheless, the process is often more important than the outcome.
6. Everyone can learn the art of successful yet compassionate ACP with CYP and their families. Empathy, humility, and trust are key qualities that the healthcare worker can foster and practice over time in this art.
7. All ACP written in the CYP setting should be considered perpetual drafts. Be prepared to change individual preferences within the ACP or even have families revoke ACP at times of crises. As healthcare professionals supporting families of CYP with serious illness, sensitivity to their needs and respect for their desire for control are key.

8. As difficult medical decisions are being made, all parents (or their legal guardians) are expected to act in the best interest of the young person with serious illness. In the rare instance that the medical professional feels that the well-being of the CYP is threatened or where ethical boundaries are crossed, the respective clinical ethics panel providing oversight may be consulted for advice. Tools for ethical analysis such as the "Zone of Parental Discretion" may be used in such instances.[17]

References

1. Kim C.H., Song I.G., Kim M.S., Lee J.Y., Lim N.G., and Shin H.Y. (2020). Healthcare utilization among children and young people with life-limiting conditions: Exploring palliative care needs using national health insurance claims data. *Sci. Rep.* **10**(1): 1–10.
2. Spicer S., Macdonald M.E., Davies D., Vadeboncoeur C., and Siden H. (2015). Introducing a lexicon of terms for paediatric palliative care. *Paediatr. Child Health* **20**(3): 155–156.
3. Weaver M.S., Boss R.D., Christopher M.J., Gray T.F., Harman S., Madrigal V.N., *et al.* (2022). Top ten tips palliative care clinicians should know about their work's intersection with clinical ethics. *J. Palliat. Med.* **25**(4): 656–661.
4. Yotani N., Kizawa Y., and Shintaku H. (2017). Differences between pediatricians and internists in advance care planning for adolescents with cancer. *J. Pediat.* **182**: 356–362.
5. Yotani N., Kizawa Y., and Shintaku H. (2017). Advance care planning for adolescent patients with life-threatening neurological conditions: A survey of Japanese paediatric neurologists. *BMJ Paediatrics Open* **1**: e1–8.
6. Chong P.H., Walshe C., and Hughes S. (2021). A good death in the child with life shortening illness: A qualitative multiple-case study. *Palliat. Med.* **35**(10): 1878–1888.
7. Durall A., Zurakowski D., and Wolfe J. (2012). Barriers to conducting advance care discussions for children with life-threatening conditions. *Pediatrics* **129**(4): e975–e982.
8. Kobler K., Bell C., Kavanaugh K., Gallo A.M., Corte C., and Vincent C. (2020). Health care professionals' awareness of a child's impending death. *Qual. Health Res.* **30**(9): 1314–1325.
9. Simon T.D. (2020). *Complex Care Has Arrived*. American Academy of Pediatrics Elk Grove Village, IL, USA, pp. 631–632.
10. Sudore R.L., Lum H.D., You J.J., Hanson L.C., Meier D.E., Pantilat S.Z., *et al.* (2017). Defining advance care planning for adults: A consensus

definition from a multidisciplinary Delphi panel. *J. Pain Symptom Manage.* **53**(5): 821–832. e1.

11. Rietjens J.A., Sudore R.L., Connolly M., van Delden J.J., Drickamer M.A., Droger M., *et al.* (2017). Definition and recommendations for advance care planning: An international consensus supported by the European association for palliative care. *Lancet Oncol.* **18**(9): e543–e551.

12. Back A.L., Arnold R.M., Baile W.F., Fryer-Edwards K.A., Alexander S.C., Barley G.E., *et al.* (2007). Efficacy of communication skills training for giving bad news and discussing transitions to palliative care. *Arch. Intern. Med.* **167**(5): 453–460.

13. Feudtner C. (2009). The breadth of hopes. *N. Engl. J. Med.* **361**(24): 2306–2307.

14. Orkin J., Beaune L., Moore C., Weiser N., Arje D., Rapoport A., *et al.* (2020). Toward an understanding of advance care planning in children with medical complexity. *Pediatrics* **145**(3): e1–11.

15. Carr K., Hasson F., McIlfatrick S., and Downing J. (2022). Parents' experiences of initiation of paediatric advance care planning discussions: A qualitative study. *Eur. J. Pediat.* **181**(3): 1185–1196.

16. Chong P.H., Walshe C., and Hughes S. (2019). Perceptions of a good death in children with life-shortening conditions: an integrative review. *J. Palliat. Med.* **22**(6): 714–723.

17. Gillam L. (2016). The zone of parental discretion: An ethical tool for dealing with disagreement between parents and doctors about medical treatment for a child. *Clin. Ethics* **11**(1): 1–8. March 2016.

Chapter 37

Advance Care Planning in Persons with Dementia

Philip Lin Kiat Yap

*Department of Geriatric Medicine,
Khoo Teck Puat Hospital, Singapore*

In tandem with the population ageing, the global rates of dementia are escalating exponentially. It was estimated that the 57 million persons living with dementia (PLWD) in 2019 will grow to more than 150 million by 2050.[1] The rising tide of dementia is even more significant in the Asia Pacific region where the number of PLWD is projected to increase three-fold from 23 million in 2015 to 71 million by 2050.[2]

Today, functional neuroimaging that detects amyloid and tau deposits in the brain as well as blood-based biomarkers can identify persons at risk of dementia at the pre-clinical and prodromal stages. These modalities for early detection are projected to be ready for clinical use in the coming years and will increase the prevalence of persons at risk of dementia many-fold. The advent of disease-modifying therapies such as monoclonal antibodies[3] that ameliorate disease progression will inevitably inflate the prevalence of PLWD and those in the pre-dementia stages who can all benefit from advance care planning (ACP). Therefore, an all-encompassing term, persons with cognitive concerns (PWCC), is used to refer to PLWD as well as those at risk of dementia at the pre-clinical and prodromal stages.

The Importance of ACP

As dementia gradually impairs intellectual abilities, there is only a limited period during the illness when the PLWD retains mental capacity to make informed decisions. Nevertheless, those with cognitive complaints but no clinical dementia yet will have a longer runway before eventual cognitive deficiencies limit decisional capacity. Despite living with a protracted duration of mental incapacity in the illness trajectory, PLWD can remain in a state of reasonable physical health for relatively long periods of time and may also live on for several years despite physical frailty in the advanced stages of dementia. Hence, planning their long-term health and social care needs as well as end-of-life care is pertinent.

Long-term care planning helps prepare family members, who are often burdened by the strain of caregiving and uncertainties in navigating the evolving disease, undertake decision-making with greater assurance that they are acting in the best interests and honouring the wishes of the PLWD. Knowing the wishes of the person could help reduce possible dilemmas faced by caregivers and reduce the potential for disputes among family members who may hold differing views on what is best for their loved one with dementia. For these reasons, ACP is advocated as a salient component of holistic care for dementia.

Challenges of ACP in Dementia

ACP involves conversations about one's future preferences and goals of care, communicating them to a loved one, proxy decision maker, or healthcare provider and may entail documenting these wishes. A recent review of ACP in dementia showed that patients with mild dementia can be engaged in ACP despite concerns about the utility of ACP conversations in this population.[4] Nonetheless, the rates of ACP completion in PWCC remain modest in most parts of the world. A study found that despite being cognisant of future decisional incapacity, only a minority of patients with cognitive impairment went on to complete ACP.[5] Another study of 150 PWCC conducted in a memory clinic in Singapore revealed that 36% were willing to engage in ACP conversations but only 10% documented their preferences in an advanced care directive.[6]

Several factors influence one's willingness to engage in ACP, including perspectives on life and death, perceived stability of end-of-life decisions, support from the family and enablers in the healthcare system, as well as an individual's coping style and personality.[7,8] There are also factors unique to the Asia Pacific region and to dementia.

Cultural beliefs and attitudes can be obstacles or enablers of ACP. Orientals who have a predilection for fatalistic beliefs, particularly that life events are predestined, tend to avoid taboo topics, such as death.[9,10] Moreover, as ACP is founded on upholding the autonomy of the person, more collectivist cultures such as those in the Asia-Pacific region which emphasize family-centred decision-making may render ACP less relevant. It is not uncommon for older persons to delegate family members to take over decision-making in medical issues, citing older age and low education. The primacy of filial piety in Oriental societies inclines children to step up on behalf of their parents to take on medical decision-making conceivably in their best interest.[11]

Dementia knowledge and awareness in the Asia Pacific, especially among older people, has been found to be poor which inevitably results in delays in seeking a diagnosis and intervention, including ACP.[12,13] Even for those who know that dementia is a medical illness, many fail to recognise that it is a progressive disease that eventually results in dependency and is ultimately fatal. Generally, involvement of PWCC in ACP decreases with poorer cognitive function as depicted by lower scores on the mini-mental state examination.[4] In particular, executive function, which is a function of education and general cognitive ability, mediates one's ability to engage in ACP and make informed decisions.[14,15]

Knowledge and awareness of one's medical condition are necessary prerequisites for meaningful conversations on care planning to take place. Furthermore, mental capacity — assessed by one's ability to retain information, reason, make informed decisions after weighing the options, and articulate one's decision — is germane to the ACP process. For PWCC, cognitive deficits that impair insight, capacity to reason, weigh options and make decisions, and articulate their preferences inevitably limit their ability to meaningfully participate in ACP.

Given the challenges of engaging PWCC directly in ACP, it is not surprising that most of the care planning is done with the surrogate decision maker who is usually a close family member, towards the more advanced stages of the illness. The conversations at that stage would revolve around end-of-life care on issues, such as tube feeding, cardiopulmonary resuscitation, and mechanical ventilation. This chapter, however, focuses on how to connect with and enable PWCC in order to better understand what matters to them. In so doing, we hope to engage them to plan for their care and safeguard their interests for the present as well as the future.

Person Centred Dementia Care and Its Relevance to ACP

Person-centred care (PCC) endeavours to secure the personhood of the PLWD by harnessing his innate potential despite dementia, maximise quality of life, and honour his care preferences for the present and future. It is noteworthy that the latter is well aligned with the goals of ACP to uphold individual autonomy. PCC emphasises knowing the PLWD in not only appreciating the nature of his disease but through exploring his past in his personality and life history, providing him with the necessary support to continue to thrive notwithstanding dementia.

The person-centred model of understanding dementia[16] can be expressed in this manner: PLWD = Neurological impairment + Health + Biography + Personality + Environment (Physical and Social). Under this rubric, by understanding the illness as well as the personal and historical aspects of the PLWD, we can provide a prosthetic environment that conduces him to thrive despite dementia. ACP can likewise draw on the ethos of re-enablement[17] by offering prosthetic handles to enable the PLWD to explicate the care he so desires in his own terms.

In PCC, particular emphasis is placed on understanding the person's life history; the past shines a light on what matters in the present. Through personal narratives expressed by the PLWD, one derives a deeper understanding of what matters to him, his life goals, values, and preferences and what may cause him worry and distress. These constitute precious nuggets of information that can help the healthcare professional guide the PLWD negotiate decision-making in care planning. It also empowers surrogate decision-makers to act in their best interest when faced with the moment health care decisions in the absence of a documented advanced care plan.

The Serious Illness Communication Framework[18] is a wieldy tool given its structured approach that not only elicits the person's understanding of his illness and its ramifications but also explores what is important to him and finally provides a recommendation having obtained a deeper appreciation of him and what he values. The ability to derive a comprehensive understanding of the PLWD and assist him, by way of proposing what might be most appropriate based on that understanding, is essential where care planning is concerned. As cognitive deficits may render difficulties for PLWD to articulate their thoughts, assisting them with prompts and suggestions can be helpful. At the same time, communication strategies such as motivational interviewing and negotiation[19] can be employed to facilitate the conversations to secure more positive outcomes.

In addition, deficits in short-term memory may constrain the ability of PLWD to hold information in their minds long enough to allow adequate processing and decision-making. Hence, enabling them with "memory prostheses" by way of repetitions and representations of the same information can be utilised as means to bolster their mental capacity so as to enable them to make and express a choice. If the person consistently makes the same choices and decisions with these cognitive aids, it may be construed that these choices are indeed what the person desires.

Similarly, if knowledge about dementia is lacking, especially in understanding its progressive nature and the state of total dependency in advanced dementia, the PLWD can be empowered with this information to provide the necessary impetus for making advance care plans. These practices are consistent with the Mental Capacity Act where medical professionals need to make every effort to communicate with the patient and undertake all practicable steps to help him make a decision.[20]

Willingness to Engage in ACP beyond Mental Capacity

Our team had previously explored why patients with early cognitive impairment (ECI), comprising those with mild cognitive impairment and early dementia but possessed adequate mental capacity, refused ACP.[21] The main themes that emerged from the qualitative study were as follows: (1) acceptance/acquiescence where the person was comfortable to leave future decision-making to family, friends, or associates whom they trusted, including healthcare professionals, as well as to providence/destiny, (2) irrelevant/unnecessary where the person saw no need for ACP because they had already undertaken informal planning by way of conveying their wishes to close family members or opined that they had nothing to plan for as they did not possess significant financial assets or had no one that they could entrust future decision-making to, and (3) avoidance/denial where the person was not ready to discuss future care planning, expressed uncertainty about the implications of ACP, or was in denial of his condition and still hopeful of a cure.

In another study[15] that employed an instrument to elicit the perceived barriers to ACP in a different sample of individuals with ECI, the three key factors that emerged were as follows: (1) avoidance coping — the person avoided ACP as he remained confident he would be able to continue to make decisions in the future or would get better, (2) passive coping — where the person did not think much about these issues and preferred to leave the future to his family or to destiny, and (3) procrastination — where the person did not see the urgency of making ACP, opined that plans might change in the future and attested that there were more important issues of immediate concern to attend to. The item in the perceived barriers tool that elicited the highest rating pertained to individuals acknowledging that prior to being introduced to ACP, they had not given much thought to it.

In a similar vein, persons with ECI were asked about the perceived benefits of making advance care plans, and the main elements that were endorsed include the following: ACP allows others to know my wishes and desires, my future can be more comfortable with ACP, and ACP makes it easier for the family when I have difficulties making decisions in the future. Understanding the persons' perceived barriers and benefits of ACP is useful to facilitate ACP engagement. It enables a personalised approach to reinforce the benefits and target the barriers perceived and is consistent with the person-centred approach that underpins good dementia care.

An Approach to ACP In Dementia

Assessment

First, it is necessary to assess the person's ability to understand dementia as a medical illness and its impact on daily life. He should be cognisant of the cognitive and functional deficits, and the increasing need for care as the person's ability to live independently becomes compromised. Importantly, he needs to recognise and acknowledge the late-stage manifestations of dementia such as recurrent infections, feeding issues with consequent malnutrition, and dehydration. Videos of persons living with advanced dementia[22,23] have been found to facilitate decision-making in randomised studies on ACP and can be used where acceptable and appropriate. The aim is to enable him to appreciate the relevance of ACP in end-of-life care and life-sustaining treatments, such as tube feeding, the use of antibiotics, cardiopulmonary resuscitation, and mechanical ventilation. A mental capacity assessment should also be conducted to ascertain whether the person is not only able to understand and retain the information presented but can reason and weigh the options at hand and articulate his decision by providing a clear rationale.

Second, it is salient to appraise the person's willingness to accept dementia or mild cognitive impairment diagnosis as the case may be and understand its consequences and the importance of conversations about future care plans. It is not uncommon that while some might appreciate that dementia compromises cognitive abilities such as short-term memory, they may not be ready to face up to its increasing severity with time and the ominous ramifications of advanced dementia. As such, they may not desire to enter into conversations about life-sustaining treatments in late-stage dementia.

Third, an understanding of the person's personal perspectives about ACP should be obtained and for this purpose the ACP perceived barriers and benefits tool[15] (refer to Table 1) can be useful. Knowing how the

Table 1.   Perceived barriers and benefits of advance care planning tool.

Question Prompt (Dementia ACP approach)

As you might already know, dementia is a progressive condition that renders a person increasingly incapable of caring for himself/herself. In advance dementia, the person may also develop problems with eating and swallowing and is prone to recurrent infections, such as pneumonia (chest infection) and urinary tract infection. Hence, while you are now well, it might be appropriate to start planning for the future. Planning for your future medical care is termed Advance Care Planning and I would like to know your opinion about this. I am going to read to you some statements, you might agree or disagree. Please rate if you agree or disagree with each statement. "1" is "strongly disagree", "2" is "disagree", "3" is "agree", and "4" is "strongly agree".

Question Prompt (General ACP approach)

As we would understand, life can be unpredictable and we might have known a friend or relative who was stricken unexpectedly by a serious illness, such as cancer or stroke. Hence, while we are now well, it might be appropriate to start planning for our future. For example, deciding how to manage our finances or our future care. Planning for our future medical care is termed Advance Care Planning and I would like to know your opinion on this. I am going to read to you some statements, you might agree or disagree. Please rate if you agree or disagree with each statement. "1" is "strongly disagree", "2" is "disagree", "3" is "agree", and "4" is "strongly agree".

(*Continued*)

Table 1.   (*Continued*)

Perceived barriers	Strongly disagree	Disagree	Agree	Strongly agree
1. It is difficult for me to do advance care planning because I don't think about such issues very much.	1	2	3	4
2. It is difficult for me to do advance care planning because I have many other important concerns	1	2	3	4
3. It is difficult for me to do advance care planning because I may change my plans in the future.	1	2	3	4
4. I do not need to engage in advance care planning because I believe that I can continue to make decisions for myself for a long time to come.	1	2	3	4
5. It is difficult for me to do advance care planning because my family will not support me in doing this.	1	2	3	4
6. I do not need to engage in advance care planning because I think I will get better.	1	2	3	4
7. I do not need to engage in advance care planning because my family will take care of me when I cannot decide for myself.	1	2	3	4
8. I do not need to engage in advance care planning because whatever happens in future is fated and cannot be changed.	1	2	3	4
9. I do not need to engage in advance care planning because I do not own a bank account or manage my own finances.	1	2	3	4

Perceived benefits	Strongly disagree	Disagree	Agree	Strongly agree
1. Advance care planning will benefit my family by making it easier for them when I have difficulties making decisions in the future	1	2	3	4

Table 1.   (*Continued*)

Perceived benefits	Strongly disagree	Disagree	Agree	Strongly agree
2. Advance care planning will help those around me to know what my wishes are for medical treatment.	1	2	3	4
3. My future can be more comfortable if I have advance care planning.	1	2	3	4
4. Advance care planning would help me receive the type of care I would like to have.	1	2	3	4
5. Advance care planning will help those around me know how I want my property and assets to be managed.	1	2	3	4

person perceives ACP will guide healthcare professionals in tailoring their approach to help clarify possible misunderstandings, negotiate, nudge, and encourage wherever and whenever appropriate to assist the person to secure care that is aligned with his goals, values, and preferences.

Tailoring to specific profiles

There are 4 possible profiles (refer to Table 2) that could emerge following the assessment outlined above. The subsequent approach to ACP can then be tailored to each profile specifically:

(a) *High ability, high desire*

This is the ideal scenario where the PWCC possesses a good understanding of dementia, has adequate mental capacity to make informed decisions, and appreciates the value and need for ACP. As such, one can delve into possible barriers the person may face and devise ways to circumvent them, reinforcing at the same time the benefits of ACP that the person already recognises.

Table 2.   An approach to ACP in Dementia.

1. **Assess**	

a. Ability
• understand dementia and its consequences (including dementia stages)
• appreciate the value of ACP
• assess mental capacity in decision-making
 	
   • understand dementia, its consequences, and the relevance of ACP
   • retain the information discussed and repeated it back
   • make a decision after weighing the pros and cons
   • communicate the decision and can provide a rationale for it
	b. Desire
	• know about dementia and its consequences
	• plan for the future through ACP conversation (can utilise the ACP perceived barriers and benefits tool)

2. **Action**	

a. High ability, high desire
• Explore any particular barriers to ACP and reinforce benefits
• Explore and plan for losses that will occur across the dementia continuum from mild to severe dementia, e.g., driving, finances, way-finding, custodial needs, and end-of-life issues, such as enteral nutrition and other life-sustaining treatments (offer to show a video of a person with advanced dementia[22,23])
• Proceed to formal ACP documentation and lasting power of attorney if ready
	b. High ability, low desire
	• Pace accordingly and provide information with nudges and reminders along the way. Explore PWCC's goals, values, preferences, and concerns/worries in general
	• Explore understanding of dementia and ACP, elicit barriers and facilitators to ACP
	• Tailor to specific barriers encountered, examples include the following:
	   ○ Passivity/Avoidance: provide example of conflictual situations among family members in the absence of ACP, inspire with stories of how ACP has helped others (offer to show videos, e.g., from the AIC ACP website[25])
	   ○ Reluctance to document ACP: position care planning as conversations, including family or trusted associates
	   ○ Opine ACP to be merely financial planning: educate and inform wider purpose of ACP beyond financial planning

Table 2.   (*Continued*)

c. Low ability, high or low desire
- Adopt a general rather than dementia-specific approach to ACP
- Explore their understanding of ACP, any barriers encountered, and if they appreciate the value of ACP
- Target specific barriers identified
- Elicit goals, values, preferences, and worries/concerns in general
- Involve family or trusted associate in conversations
- Pace accordingly with nudges and reminders

3.   Guiding Principles

a. Preferable to start early with the PWCC even before the onset of dementia if possible
b. Tailor approach and pace according to the readiness of the PWCC, move to next step in ACP only when he is ready
c. Position ACP as conversations rather than legally or medically binding forms or documents
d. Involve surrogate (family or trusted associates) as far as possible
e. Review ACP regularly
f. Derive a good understanding of PLWD's goals, values, priorities, worries, and concerns
g. Facilitate with cognitive aids, nudges, reminders, and stories of how others navigated ACP

It might be possible for ACP to be pursued with greater depth to encompass not only issues surrounding advanced dementia and end-of-life care but even adopt a stage-specific plan[24] that explores the deficits experienced at the different stages of dementia. For example, issues pertinent to mild to moderate dementia such as giving up driving, allowing the caregiver to manage medication and finances, and GPS trackers can be discussed. Formal documentation with medically binding advance care plans and legally binding lasting power of attorney would likely be acceptable to the person.

(b) *High ability, low desire*

PWCC with adequate mental capacity to comprehend the serious effects of dementia may have various reasons for being hesitant about ACP which can be examined with the ACP perceived barriers and benefits tool. For example, if a person has yet to give much thought to the matter or is not in the habit of making plans for the future, information on the benefits of ACP can be provided while at the same time pacing with the person with nudges and reminders along the way. For those who adopt a more passive stance in entrusting future decisions to loved ones or to destiny, one can provide examples of real-life scenarios where families find themselves in a quandary having to make difficult decisions on behalf of the person or conflicts arising from differing opinions may occur.[25]

Some might opine there is no need for making formal care plans as they have informally shared their preferences with those they trust or may express reservations about the need for formal documentation with ACP or LPA. Positioning care planning as conversations would be most appropriate in such instances as is the involvement of family members or other trusted relatives and friends. The emphasis should be on understanding the person's goals, values, priorities, and concerns and adopting a more general approach to future care planning.

Those who associate future planning with merely financial planning may also be helped by giving more attention to what matters to the person beyond financial matters. Finally, those who may be in denial of dementia or unable to come to terms with the dementia diagnosis and its dire consequences will need to be accompanied in navigating the illness with patience and gentleness. Through building rapport and trust, one can attempt to draw out their fears and concerns, while concurrently seeking out what is important to them with the goal of helping them live well in the present with a view to the future.

(c) *Low ability, high or low desire*

Persons under this category are usually more advanced in their cognitive deficits and characterised by their lack of mental capacity to engage in meaningful discussions about their health, illness, and care plans. Pursuing dementia as the reason to plan for the future is typically untenable but it may still be possible to decipher the person's thoughts and feelings about ACP from their responses in the ACP barriers and benefits tool. As described in (b), persons with high barriers to ACP will need further exploration and be accompanied over time with gentle persuasion and help clarify their doubts and misgivings.

Although intellect and mental capability are compromised, many PLWD still retain the ability to share their personal perspectives which are based more on subjective feelings and long-standing values and preferences. As such, adopting a general and non-dementia-specific approach to care planning might still be possible if they are assisted in the process.

As described in the above section on adopting a person-centred approach, through the personal narratives expressed by the PLWD, healthcare professionals can better appreciate what matters to him, his life goals, values, and concerns, and thereby assist the PLWD navigate care planning. With his consent, it would be appropriate to involve surrogate decision makers during ACP conversations so that they can be privy to his thoughts and preferences. Clearly, the PLWD can choose his surrogate and the latter needs to be willing to take on the responsibility. Having these conversations over time would help engender mutual trust and familiarity and ultimately allow healthcare professionals and surrogates to make shared decisions in the best interest of the PLWD regardless of the presence or absence of a documented advance care directive.

General Pointers on ACP of Relevance to the Asia-Pacific Population

It should be stressed that while these four profiles can be useful to guide our approach to ACP, PWCC may not fall neatly into these categories. A case in point may be a person with early dementia with adequate mental capacity but a less than accurate understanding of dementia arising not from his lack of cognitive ability but due largely to his long-held beliefs and ideas about the condition. In this instance, one may not construe his ability to understand dementia to be high despite possessing adequate mental capacity. Hence, it may be more appropriate to adopt a more general than dementia-specific approach to ACP. Next, it is worthwhile to reiterate some general pointers to ease both the PWCC and the healthcare professional into conversations about future care planning.

First, it is expedient to start early, perhaps even before dementia develops. Today, more people with subjective cognitive concerns are coming forward to be evaluated, and while some may already have dementia, many are in the pre-clinical or prodromal stages where cognitive abilities, in particular executive function, are still largely intact. Care planning involves complex thinking and decision-making mediated through executive function, which in large part determines the capacity in providing informed consent, appreciating the consequences of one's decision and reasoning.[26,27] Conversely, inverse relationships have been found between executive functioning and apathy[28] which could be contributory to passivity towards ACP. Given the high levels of passivity in our patients,[15] it is essential to start education and discussions on ACP early to increase awareness and understanding of its importance.

Second, ACP should be process-oriented rather than a one-off transaction with forms and check-boxes. Research has evidenced increased rates of ACP completion through efforts at education and conversations over time.[29,30] Interventions which involve completion of ACP through direct patient-healthcare professional interactions over multiple visits[31] have been found to be beneficial. As ACP is a multi-stage process,[32] one should move to the next stage only when the person is ready. Interactive interventions have secured better ACP completion rates[9,28] as sharing information through regular one-to-one engagement promotes receptiveness while nurturing rapport and trust in pacing alongside the person.

Third, family members generally play a pivotal role in ACP discussions unless the PWCC thinks otherwise. Some PWCC decline ACP because they do not have the support and agreement of loved ones while others cede decision-making to family members. This exemplifies the Asian mindset of familial and collective decision-making, and a predilection towards external control beliefs such as the influence of others and fate. Under this rubric, the presence of trusted family members during advance care conversations will enable them to hear and appreciate what matters to the person which would in turn incline them to honour his preferences and make decisions in his best interest in the future.

Fourth, studies on the elderly in Asia have found that while they generally recognise the value of ACP, most are diffident about formal documentation.[9,33] As the ACP process involves several stages, patients could remain in stages where they are exploring their own values, priorities, and future treatment wishes and discussing with their loved ones without eventually documenting their plans formally. We should therefore be open to frame ACP as conversations rather than completing legally or medically binding forms or documents. It is equally important to stress that continued discussions and reviews over time are appropriate. To this end, it is most valuable to include trusted surrogates in family and friends who know the person well and will do their utmost to honour their values and preferences amid changing circumstances in the future.

However, even as we involve families, surrogate decision makers, and healthcare professionals to assist the PLWD in decision-making, the ethical imperative demands that we elicit what matters to him, uphold the primacy of his wishes, and make every effort to respect them. We will do well to avoid being paternalistic in imposing our opinions and wishes on the PLWD who is ultimately vulnerable.

Conclusion

ACP is a crucial aspect of holistic care for people with dementia and cognitive impairment given its emphasis on upholding agency and personhood. The advent of biomarkers which identify people at risk of dementia at the pre-symptomatic or prodromal stages, and disease-modifying therapies that ameliorate disease progression, render ACP ever more relevant and necessary.

Even as mental capacity may diminish with progressive cognitive decline, several factors that influence ACP engagement are beyond cognitive competence and may pertain to personal, socio-cultural, and circumstantial issues. Therefore, an in-depth assessment to better elucidate the underlying issues can facilitate a tailored approach to improve ACP engagement and outcomes. Moreover, the ethos of person-centred care calls for greater efforts and ingenuity in devising strategies to foster better buy-in and participation from the person.

The noteworthy considerations in ACP for PWCC include starting the process early, even before the onset of dementia, as that is when mental capacity is still preserved. It is also salient to involve surrogates in family members and trusted associates as far as possible to be privy to the conversations. This would allow them to have first-hand knowledge of the wishes of the person and be in a position to honour them when the situation demands.

Finally, for those who hold the notion of ACP being a transactional form completion affair, efforts at continued conversations and assurances that decisions can be reviewed in the spirit of upholding their life goals, values, and preferences, and securing their best interests amid changing circumstances should be reaffirmed. Above all, ACP endeavours to better prepare the PLWD and their surrogates for current and future medical decision-making and goes beyond documenting life-sustaining treatment decisions.

Case Study

John, a 67-year-old Chinese male who was married with a son, had retired from his long-held position as an accountant at a food and beverage company 2 years ago. He had medical problems of hypertension, hyperlipidaemia, and a family history of dementia in his mother. He experienced short-term memory and cognitive decline for a year which had become more consistent. The cognitive deficits had begun to impact his ability to navigate less familiar places and manage his financial portfolio. After much persuasion from his wife, he sought medical attention for his cognitive symptoms and was eventually diagnosed with mild dementia of Alzheimer's type. As he had cared for his mother previously, he was aware of the long-term implications of dementia. However, he was sceptical of the diagnosis as he felt he was still well and independent and "very far from what his mom used to be". He acknowledged his short-term memory was "not as good as before" but attributed it to "senior moments" and remarked he "would get better if he improved his post-retirement lifestyle by exercising more, eating more healthily and getting to bed earlier instead of watching television late into the night". At the point of diagnosis, he was assessed to possess adequate mental capacity to manage his personal and financial affairs.

The multidisciplinary team in the memory clinic explored the ramifications of the dementia diagnosis with him and introduced the notion of care planning for the present and future with the intention of helping him receive the care he would desire. Although he did not reconcile his understanding of dementia, which was steeped in the more advanced stages of the illness given his experience with his mother, with the diagnosis of early and mild dementia that he was informed of, he was receptive to suggestions to start pharmacological and non-pharmacological therapies to retard cognitive decline. Framing the treatments offered as interventions to maintain brain health and forestall decline was more acceptable to him than prescribing treatments for dementia *per se* — an example was using the term cognitive enhancers instead of anti-dementia drugs for the medications prescribed.

With this understanding, the team decided not to approach ACP for dementia in a disease-centred manner but adopted the perspective of general planning for the future given the uncertainties anyone would face in illness and death. He became more open to conversations of this nature and even shared that the unpredictability of life had crossed his mind when an old friend, who similarly had risk factors of hypertension and hyperlipidaemia, recently suffered a stroke with severe dysphagia that necessitated enteral tube feeding. This opened the avenue for the team to initiate conversations around ACP by drawing some questions from the ACP perceived barriers and benefits tool without administering the tool in its entirety.

It became clear from these discussions that he understood that ACP could help him be more comfortable if he should become seriously ill and receive the care he desired. He acknowledged ACP could ease the burden and uncertainty of decision-making his loved ones may face and shared his personal experience in making those hard decisions for his mother in the past. However, at the same time, he was not fully accepting the diagnosis of dementia. He opined that he would still be able to make decisions for a significant period of time and remained positive his cognitive symptoms will improve. Besides, he was confident that his family would make decisions in his best interest and did not see the need to document formal advance care plans.

Empowered with these insights gains, the team tailored their approach to care planning conversations by reassuring John that the goal was not to sign off ACP forms but to better understand his care goals, values, preferences, and possible worries or concerns. With his agreement, his wife and son accompanied him during these sessions, and as they discussed the issues as a family, all members subsequently expressed their deep appreciation to the care team for the opportunity to share their deep and honest thoughts and feelings as until then they had never delved into these issues.

It also came to light during one of the sessions that John's reluctance to accept the dementia diagnosis stemmed in large part from him seeing "how dementia decimated my mom" and hence "my fear of facing the same prospect" and "imposing a burden on my beloved family". However, the conversations allowed him and his family to confront the fear together as it dawned on them the reality of ageing, illness, and losses would befall anyone. So, if it was not dementia, then at some point in time another life-limiting disease would inevitably befall John. It was at this juncture, which was about 6 months from his initial diagnosis, that John decided on his own accord to formally document his wishes in an advance care directive. He indicated his wishes for limited measures when confronted with the prospect of a life-limiting condition but asserted his desire for his wife and son to be consulted in decision-making and gave them the prerogative to be the final arbiter.

John is characterised by his low desire to accept the dementia diagnosis and engage in ACP initially even as his mental capacity was assessed to be adequate. The care team patiently accompanied him over time to attempt to understand him and his concerns while at the same time adopted a general rather than dementia-centred approach to care planning which he was open to. As they built more rapport with him and came to appreciate what he valued and his fears, they made it a point to include his family and provided a safe space for them to express their thoughts and feelings. With increased mutual understanding and trust built between John, his family, and the care team, John eventually came to terms with the diagnosis of dementia and realised the value of documenting his care plans formally on his own.

Learning Objectives
- Dementia is a progressive and incurable illness that will increasingly render the PLWD incapable of independent living. There are also salient implications for life-sustaining treatments in advanced dementia. Hence, ACP is an essential component of holistic dementia care.
- Dementia results in diminishing mental capacity for decision-making. There is only a narrow window period, typically during mild dementia, when the PLWD may still be capable of making informed decisions. Thus, it is preferable that ACP be initiated even before dementia is formally diagnosed when the person first presents with subjective cognitive complaints.
- It is possible to assist the PLWD in ACP with a careful assessment of their ability to appreciate the impact and prognosis of dementia, their mental capacity, as well as willingness to make advance care plans. The latter can be evaluated with the ACP perceived barriers and benefits tool, and the barriers identified can be addressed accordingly.
- Care planning can be done over several sessions with the need to derive a good understanding of PLWD's goals, values, priorities, and concerns. ACP aims to prepare the PLWD and their surrogates for current and future medical decision-making and goes beyond documenting life-sustaining treatment decisions. Effective communication skills, including the use of negotiation, nudges, and cognitive aids, can be helpful.
- Involve the surrogate decision maker if the PLWD is agreeable. This can allow the surrogates to have first-hand knowledge of the wishes of the PLWD and be in a position to honour them when the situation demands.

References

1. GBD 2019 Dementia Forecasting Collaborators. (2022). Estimation of the global prevalence of dementia in 2019 and forecasted prevalence in 2050: An analysis for the Global Burden of Disease Study 2019. *Lancet Public Health* **7**(2): e105–e125.
2. Alzheimer's Disease International, and Alzheimer's Australia. (2014). Dementia in the Asia Pacific Region. Alzheimer's Disease International (ADI). Retrieved January 4, 2023, from https://www.alzint.org/resource/dementia-in-the-asia-pacific-region/.
3. Van Dyck C.H., Swanson C.J., Aisen P., Bateman R.J., Chen C., Gee M., Kanekiyo M., Li D., Reyderman L., Cohen S., Froelich L., Katayama S., Sabbagh M., Vellas B., Watson D., Dhadda S., Irizarry M., Kramer L.D., and Iwatsubo T. (2022). Lecanemab in early Alzheimer's disease. *N. Engl. J. Med.* 10.1056/NEJMoa2212948.
4. Dening K.H., Jones L., and Sampson E. (2011). Advance care planning for people with dementia: A review. *Int. Psychogeriatr.* **26**: 1–17.
5. Garand L., Dew M.A., Lingler J.H., and DeKosky S.T. (2011). Incidence and predictors of advance care planning among persons with cognitive impairment. *Am. J. Geriatr. Psychiatry* **19**: 712–720.
6. Lo T., Ha N., Ng C., Tan G., Koh H., and Yap P. (2017). Unmarried patients with early cognitive impairment are more likely than their married counterparts to complete advance care plans. *Int. Psychogeriatr.* **29**(3): 509–516.
7. Ng H.L.R. (2009). Advance care planning: Let's talk about your preferences for care at the end of life. *Singapore Fam. Physician* **35**: 93–99.
8. Levi B.H., Dellasega C., Whitehead M., and Green M.J. (2010). What influences individuals to engage in advance care planning? *Am. J. Hosp. Palliat. Med.* **27**: 306–312.
9. Htut Y., Shahrul K., and Poi P.J.H. (2007). The view of older Malaysians on advanced directive and advanced care planning: A qualitative study. *Asia Pac. J. Public Health* **19**: 58–66.
10. Bowman K.W., and Singer P.A. (2001). Chinese senior's perspectives on end of life decisions. *Soc. Sci. Med.* **53**: 455–464.
11. Ho Z.J.M., Krishna L.K.R., and Yee C.P.A. (2010). Chinese familial tradition and Western influence: A case study in Singapore on decision making at the end of life. *J. Pain Symptom Manage.* **40**: 932–937.
12. Purandare N., Luthra V., Swarbrick C., and Burns A. (2007). Knowledge of dementia among South Asian (Indian) older people in Manchester, UK. *Int. J. Geriatr. Psychiatry* **22**: 777–781.
13. Tan W.J., Hong S., Luo N., Lo T.J., and Yap P. (2012). The lay's public understanding and perception of dementia in a developed Asian nation. *Dement. Geriatr. Cogn. Disord.* **2**: 433–444.

14. Del Missier F., Mantyla T., and de Bruin W.B. (2010). Executive functioning in decision making: An individual differences approach. *Think. Reason.* **16**: 69–79.

15. Tay S.Y., Davison J., Jin N.C., and Yap P.L. (2015). Education and executive function mediate engagement in advance care planning in early cognitive impairment. *J. Am. Med. Dir. Assoc.* **16**(11): 957–962.

16. Kitwood T.M. (1997). *Dementia Reconsidered: The Person Comes First.* Open University Press, Buckingham.

17. Poulos C.J., Bayer A., Beaupre L., Clare L., Poulos R.G., Wang R.H., Zuidema S., and McGilton K.S. (2017). A comprehensive approach to reablement in dementia. *Alzheimer's Dement. Transl. Res. Clin. Interv.* **3**: 450–458.

18. Jacobsen J., Bernacki R., and Paladino J. (2022). Shifting to serious illness communication. *JAMA* **327**(4): 321–322.

19. Campbell M., Seltzer A., Ramirez-Zohfeld V., and Lindquist L.A. (2021). Negotiation training for case managers to improve older adult acceptance of services. *Prof. Case Manag.* **26**(4): 194–199.

20. Thirumoorthy T. (2016). The mental capacity act — understanding the legal concepts in providing medical care for persons lacking capacity. *SMA CMEP — Resources.* Retrieved from https://www.smacmep.org.sg/resource/ The-Mental-Capacity-Act--Understanding-the-Legal-Concepts-in-Providing- Medical-Care-for-Persons-Lacking-Capacity.

21. Cheong K., Fisher P., Goh J., Ng L., Koh H.M., and Yap P. (2014). Advance care planning in people with early cognitive impairment. *BMJ Support. Palliat. Care* **5**(1): 63–69.

22. Mitchell S.L., Shaffer M.L., Cohen S., Hanson L.C., Habtemariam D., and Volandes A.E. (2018). An advance care planning video decision support tool for nursing home residents with advanced dementia: A cluster randomized clinical trial. *JAMA Intern. Med.* **178**(7): 961–969.

23. Volandes A.E., Paasche-Orlow M.K., Barry M.J., Gillick M.R., Minaker K.L., Chang Y., Cook E.F., Abbo E.D., El-Jawahri A., and Mitchell S.L. (2009). Video decision support tool for advance care planning in dementia: Randomised controlled trial. *Br. Med. J. (Clin. Res. Ed.)* **338**: b2159.

24. Gaster B., Larson E.B., and Curtis J.R. (2017). Advance directives for dementia: Meeting a unique challenge. *JAMA* **318**(22): 2175–2176.

25. AIC Singapore. (2022, January 18). Advance Care Planning (ACP) Awareness — Dementia. YouTube. https://www.youtube.com/ watch?v=TI5V5TcOWnc.

26. Jefferson A.L., Lambe S., Moser D.J., Byerly L.K., Ozonoff A., and Karlawish J.H. (2008). Decisional capacity for research participation in individuals with mild cognitive impairment. *J. Am. Geriatr. Soc.* **56**(7): 1236–1243.

27. Schillerstrom J.E., Rickenbacker D., Joshi K.G., *et al.* (2007). Executive function and capacity to consent to a noninvasive research protocol. *Am. J. Geriatr. Psychiatry* **15**: 159–162.

28. George M., Whitfield T., and Walker Z. (2013). Association of apathy with frontal lobe dysfunction in amnestic mild cognitive impairment and Alzheimer's disease. *J. Neurol. Neurosurg. Psychiatry* **84**: e1

29. Chu L.W., Luk J.K., Hui E., Chiu P.K., Chan C.S., Kwan F., Kwok, T., Lee D., and Woo J. (2011). Advance directive and end-of-life care preferences among Chinese nursing home residents in Hong Kong. *J. Am. Med. Dir. Assoc.* **12**: 143–152.

30. Wong S.Y., Lo S.H., Chan C.H., Chui, H.S., Sze, W.K., and Tung Y. (2012). Is it feasible to discuss an advanced directive with a Chinese patient with advanced malignancy? A prospective cohort study. *Hong Kong Med. J.* **18**: 178–185.

31. Ramsaroop S.D., Reid M.C., and Adelman R.D. (2007). Completing an advanced directive in the primary care setting: What do we need for success? *J. Am. Geriatr. Soc.* **55**: 277–283.

32. Sudore R.L., Schickedanz A.D., Landefeld C.S., Williams B.A., Lindquist K., Pantilat S.Z., and Schillinger D. (2008). Engagement in multiple steps of the advance care planning process: A descriptive study of diverse older adults. *J. Am. Geriatr. Soc.* **56**: 1006–1013.

33. Akabayashi A., Brian T.S., and Ichiro K. (2003). Perspectives on advance directives in Japanese society: A population-based questionnaire survey. *BMC Med. Ethics* **4**: 5–14.

Chapter 38

Advance Care Planning in Long-term Care

Helen Y. L. Chan[*] and Edward M. F. Leung[†]

[*]*The Nethersole School of Nursing, Faculty of Medicine,
The Chinese University of Hong Kong, Hong Kong*
[†]*Hong Kong Association of Gerontology, Hong Kong*

Introduction

Long-term care facilities are usually the last resort for older adults with frailty and comorbidities. They are more susceptible to infection, complications, and death.[1] Despite their palliative care needs, efforts for integrating palliative care approach into geriatric care only gained attention in recent decades. The preferences of care home residents towards end-of-life care are seldom explored.[2–4] Their family members are generally unaware of the anticipated health deterioration and end-of-life care preferences of their older relatives.[5]

In this chapter, we will share the experience of introducing advance care planning (ACP) into care home services in Hong Kong over these 10 years. Given that the healthcare services are predominantly curative-oriented, most of the deaths occurred in hospitals. This raises concern about the end-of-life care preferences of older adults with frailty living in care homes.

End-of-life Care Preferences Among Older Adults

We were among the first to examine the end-of-life care concerns of older adults living in care homes in Hong Kong. Dated back to 15 years ago, most of the respondents in our study were uncertain about their treatment preferences for end-of-life care, regardless of their frailty level, and did not realise their roles in treatment decision-making.[6] Over half of them delegated their decisions to doctors and their family members.[6] Yet, they tended to avoid the discussion and rarely shared their preferences with their family members or healthcare providers.[7]

Introducing ACP in Long-term Care Setting

A nurse-facilitated ACP programme, namely Let Me Talk, was specifically developed for older adults with frailty.[8] It comprises three components (Figure 1):

- My Stories: to build rapport between facilitator and clients through a brief life review,
- My Views: to promote reflection on values and goals of care, and
- My Wishes: to discuss end-of-life care preferences and unfinished business.

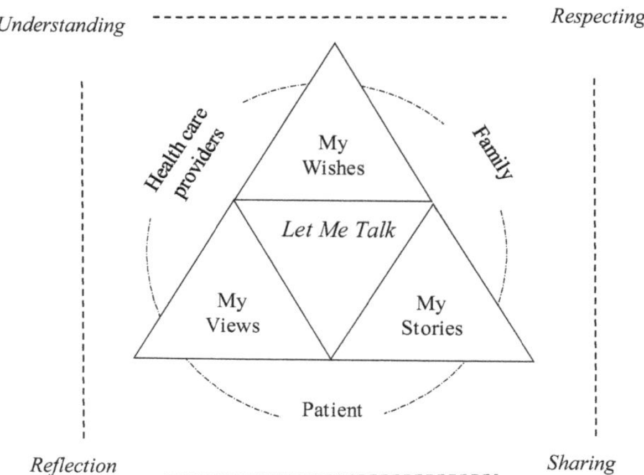

Figure 1.   Conceptual framework of the ACP programme.

More than two-thirds of the participants shared with their families that they preferred comfort care at the end of life. They generally felt relieved after sharing their thoughts and they hoped that this can prevent them from lingering on with a burdensome death. This ACP programme has been adopted in long-term care facilities in mainland China with good acceptance.[9]

Staff Preparedness

Integrating palliative and end-of-life care, including ACP, into the care home services involves a substantial change of culture and practices. However, staff members in long-term care settings are unprepared for their roles and responsibilities in ACP.[3] Apart from skill training, the psychological preparation for staff members is a cornerstone for success. Hence, we have developed an instrument to measure their preparedness in terms of willingness, perceived competence, and resilience. Perhaps with a more comprehensive pre-registration education, staff members of professional grades were significantly more willing and confident than the care assistants in providing palliative and end-of-lfie care.[10] The findings revealed the importance of adopting an all-inclusive approach in staff training because the service provision requires the involvement and support of all staff members in different capacities.

Capacity Building

To fill this service gap, Hong Kong Association of Gerontology has pioneered a "Palliative and End of Life Care in Residential Care Homes for the Elderly (RCHE) in Hong Kong" project since 2016, with funding support from the Hong Kong Jockey Club Charities Trust. The project comprises staff training, environmental restructuring, protocol development, and public education to support the paradigm shift in care. A professional coaching team provides both theoretical and practical on-the-job training and supervision for care home staff to facilitate them in attempting the new model of care. In the project, the care home staff are encouraged to initiate ACP with residents and their family members proactively. These are in line with the core components identified in the literature for the delivery of palliative and end-of-life care in care home setting.[11]

Besides, the Association played a pivotal role in negotiating with community geriatric outreach healthcare teams, hospital departments, ambulance services, and funeral services to facilitate the implementation of this novel care model. In addition, each care home is also being sponsored to renovate a single room for providing care and privacy to residents being diagnosed as nearing the end of life. With this personalised space, their relatives and friends are allowed to accompany the resident to walk through the last journey without visiting hour restriction.

Up till 2023, 50 subvented care homes participated in the project. The project has served more than 3,200 terminally ill patients and 8,400 family caregivers, trained more than 30,000 professionals and 3,400 volunteers, and more than 220,000 citizens gained knowledge of palliative care through planned public education activities.

Case Sharing

The merits of ACP are particularly outstanding during the COVID-19 pandemic when hospital admission is not preferred.

Uncle Nie moved to a care home due to hearing impairment and poor mobility. Later, he was diagnosed with colon cancer. During the COVID-19 pandemic, Uncle Nie's health condition was unstable and he had been admitted to hospital several times. Due to visitation restrictions, his family members could not visit him, leading to worries that they would not be able to see him again if he died during this period.

Eventually, through the ACP process, Uncle Nie and his family decided to forgo all kinds of life-sustaining treatments at the end of life and stay in the care home to receive care for as long as possible. "We understand that it is impossible to cure my father's condition. Maintaining a sense of security and providing holistic and timely care is the most important issue for him at that point of time." His daughter believed that it was the best arrangement for her father to take his final journey in a familiar environment with trusted caregivers and nurses.

In 2022, Uncle Nie's family members and the care home staff had held a party to let him and his wife celebrate their 73rd wedding anniversary. They gathered at a day care centre next to the nursing home on a Sunday. Knowing that Uncle Nie was a bartender when he was young, the staff members decorated the centre as a pub using a banner as a backdrop and let his grandchildren try to make a cocktail drink that Uncle Nie was proud of designing. "On the day of the party, it was as if everyone had forgotten their sadness," his daughter told. That day, his children also arranged for their parents, who had only gone through marriage rituals but had not signed a "marriage certificate", to sign their marriage vows in front of everyone. "He was very weak, but he could still hold a pen and sign his name on the marriage certificate." His son-in-law recalled and believed that it was the atmosphere that gave him strength. Finally, the couple kissed each other and said, "I love you" to each other. His daughter continued: "We also took this opportunity to thank our parents for raising us and also said 'I love you' to our father and mother." A week after the party ended, Uncle Nie passed away in the care home. The wedding anniversary party unintentionally became a farewell party.

Conclusion

Uncle Nie's family experience highlighted that the meaning of ACP is not only limited to making medical decision, but, more importantly, empowering older adults and their family members to live well in the remaining time. Open discussion allows elicitation of values and preferences and encourages a person-centred ethos. Conversations need to be part of a systems approach to care. Our works have cultivated an open culture among older adults and their family members to discuss end-of-life care. These provide strong ground for the government to expand ACP services across the territory for the benefit of more residents in long-term care facilities.

Acknowledgements

This is part of the Jockey Club End-of-life Community Care (JCECC) project is funded by The Hong Kong Jockey Club Charities Trust.

References

1. Dent, E., *et al.* (2019). Management of frailty: Opportunities, challenges, and future directions. *Lancet* **394**(10206): 1376–1386.
2. Kawakami, A., *et al.* (2021). Advance care planning and advance directive awareness among East Asian older adults: Japan, Hong Kong and South Korea. *Geriatr. Gerontol. Int.* **21**(1): 71–76.

3. Stewart, F., *et al.* (2011). Advanced care planning in care homes for older people: A qualitative study of the views of care staff and families. *Age Ageing* **40**(3): 330–335.

4. Towsley, G.L., Hirschman, K.B., and Madden, C. (2015). Conversations about end of life: Perspectives of nursing home residents, family, and staff. *J. Palliat. Med.* **18**(5): 421–428.

5. Xu, X., *et al.* (2023). Preferences for end-of-life care: A cross-sectional survey of Chinese frail nursing home residents. *J. Clin. Nurs.* **32**(7–8): 1455–1465.

6. Chan, H.Y.L., and Pang, S.M.C. (2007). Quality of life concerns and end-of-life care preferences of aged persons in long-term care facilities. *J. Clin. Nur.* **16**(11): 2158–2166.

7. Chan, H.Y.L., and Pang, S.M.C. (2011). Readiness of Chinese frail old age home residents towards end-of-life care decision making. *J. Clin. Nur.* **20**(9–10): 1454–1461.

8. Chan, H.Y.L., and Pang, S.M.C. (2010). Let me talk — An advance care planning programme for frail nursing home residents. *J. Clin. Nur.* **19**(21–22): 3073–3084.

9. Deng, R., *et al.* (2020). The effectiveness of a modified advance care planning programme. *Nur. Ethics* **27**(7): 1569–1586.

10. Chan, H.Y., *et al.* (2018). Staff preparedness for providing palliative and end-of-life care in long-term care homes: Instrument development and validation. *Geriatr. Gerontol. Int.* **18**(5): 745–749.

11. Chan, H.Y., *et al.* (2022). Key components for the delivery of palliative and end-of-life care in care homes in Hong Kong: A modified delphi study. *Int. J. Environ. Res. Public Health* **19**(2): 667. https://doi.org/10.3390/ijerph19020667.

Section 4

Stories from People, Caregivers and Professionals

Chapter 39

"Patient Voice" Bridging the Gap between Patients and Healthcare Providers

Naomi Sakurai

Cancer Solutions, Tokyo, Japan

If I do the best I can now, I leave the rest to the world.

The world is made to work.

Focus on what needs to be done now.

~Words from a friend living in Stage IV are noted~.

What Advance Care Planning (ACP) Conveys

(1) Japan's ACP, which has been conducted by "A-Un"

According to the "White Paper on Aging Society (2022 edition)" by the Cabinet Office, Japan's population aged 65 and over was less than 5% of the total population in 1950, but it exceeded 7% in 1970 and 14% in 1994, and the aging rate reached 28.9% as of October 1, 2021. On the other hand, the total population is in the process of long-term decline and is expected to continue to decline even after the population drops below 120 million in 2029, falling below 100 million to 99.24 million in 2053 and 88.08 million in 2065. It is estimated that the Japanese society will come to where one out of every 2.6 people will be over the age of 65. In addition, the average life expectancy of both men and women is increasing, and by 2065, it will reach 84.95 years for men and 91.35 years for women (medium mortality assumption). Thus, the national government has promoted various projects under the slogan of "extending health life expectancy", among which are the initiatives on public awareness and dissemination of advance care planning (ACP). The Ministry of Health, Labour and Welfare (MHLW) website introduces a variety of tools, including leaflets, the nickname and logo, the ACP learning site, ACP videos, and roundtable discussions on ACP. The government has taken the initiative in promoting ACP.

In Japanese culture, there is a phrase called "A-Un breathing". This means to skillfully grasp the subtle tones and feelings of one another and synchronize their breathing without expressing it in words or attitudes. After the high economic growth period following World War II, the way of the family and the medical care system in Japan have changed drastically. In other words, from the days when families took care of their loved ones in their homes and held funerals, people now continue medical treatment, die in medical institutions or senior citizen facilities, and have their funerals held in ceremonial halls. Thus, in our country, which has become estranged from the dying process and subsequent rituals, the reality is that the "ACP of A-Un" has been "somehow" conducted with the family. The government-led ACP awareness campaign was an important effort to address this unique Japanese view of family and culture, but it has resulted in a disconnect between patients and their families and the feelings of the parties involved. Even the phrase "obtaining ACP" has been used in association with the addition of medical reimbursement evaluations in 2022. I have the impression that ACP of "A-Un breathing" has been replaced by a discussion of how and where the patient should die: (1) stay at home until the end of life, (2) go to a hospice or palliative care unit, or (3) continue to seek medical treatment. I would like to consider these misunderstandings and failures surrounding ACP.

(2) Different ACPs according to national cultures and legal systems

Table 1 summarizes the definitions of ACP in various countries as provided by academic societies and other groups. In Japan, ACP is defined as "an individual's thinking about and discussing with their family and other people close to them, with the support as necessary of healthcare providers who have established a trusting relationship with them, preparations

Table 1.   Various definitions of ACP (based on Sagara *et al.*[1]).

National Academy of Medicine (IOM) (2015)[2]	The whole process of discussion of end-of-life care, clarification of related values and goals, and embodiment of preferences through written documents and medical orders (e.g., advance directive, physicians' orders for life-sustaining treatment).
Sudore *et al.* (USA and other countries) (2017)[3]	A process that supports adults at any age or stage of health in understanding and sharing their personal values, life goals, and preferences regarding future medical care.
European Association for Palliative Care (2017)[4]	ACP enables individuals to define goals and preferences for future medical treatment and care, to discuss these goals and preferences with family and healthcare providers, and to record and review these preferences if appropriate.
Miyashita *et al.* (2022)[5]	An individual's thinking about and discussing with his or her family and other people close to them, with the support as necessary of healthcare providers who have established a trusting relationship with the individual concerning preparations for the future: his or her current state of health and future way of life and medical treatment and care that the individual wishes to receive in the future.

for the future, including the way of life and medical treatment and care that they wish to have in the future." In Japan, where funerals are rarely held at home due to the growing trend toward nuclear families and the housing situation in Japan, death and illness tend to be viewed negatively as an "abomination". Even if such "negative" images are replaced by "positive" or "fear-mongering" images through celebrities or videos, the essential meaning and significance of the ACP are not easily conveyed. I have the impression that the ACP has become an entity that is far removed from the original definition of the ACP in Japan.

Different Needs for ACP

The Japan Federation of Cancer Patient Groups, of which I am a board member, conducted a patient survey in 2021 titled "Our Views on Cancer

Survivorship" (first survey: March to May 2021, second survey: February 2022). In this survey, 642 participants responded (141 males, 498 females, and 3 did not respond), of which 558 were those who experienced cancer, family members and bereaved family members in total, and 84 were healthcare providers and others.

The survey was based on the items covered in the US NCCN's "Survivorship Guidelines," with the addition of topics that patients thought were necessary, and rated 27 topics on "how important" and "how troubling" they were to the patient, each on a 6-point scale of importance (Table 2).

Table 2.   27 topics covered in the survey.

1. Periodic monitoring for second cancers and cancer recurrence	10. Evaluation, care, and treatment of emotional distress	19. Information on cancer treatment and systems
2. Collaboration and coordination of care between primary physicians and oncologists	11. Evaluation, care, and treatment of fatigue	20. Treatment decisions and decision-making support
3. Maintaining a high level of physical activity	12. Evaluation, care, and treatment of sexual dysfunction	21. Second opinion
4. Food and nutritional considerations	13. Evaluation, care, and treatment of menopause	22. Money
5. Smoking cessation	14. Evaluation, care, and treatment of sleep disorders	23. Schooling and employment
6. Sobriety	15. Evaluation, care, and treatment of pain	24. Communication
7. Vaccination	16. Oral care	25. Genetic counseling and genome information
8. Cardiotoxicity caused by anticancer drugs	17. Evaluation, care, and treatment of sequelae and side effects of cancer treatment	26. ACP
9. Evaluation, care, and treatment of cognitive dysfunction	18. Appearance care* (e.g., for the treatment of skin conditions)	27. Family care and grief care

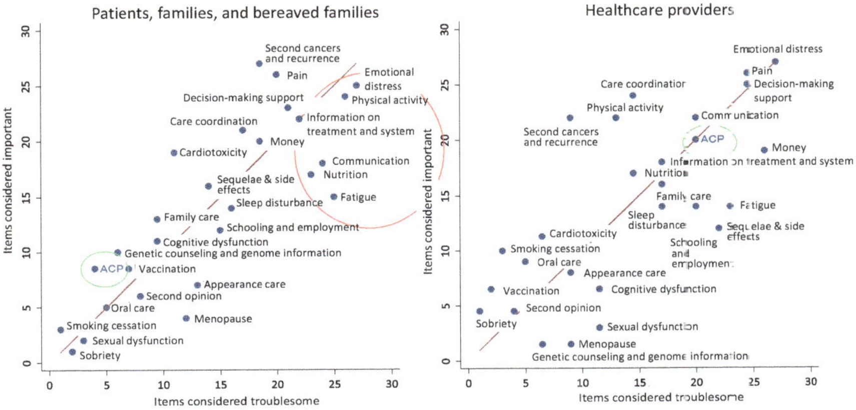

Figure 1. Cancer survivorship survey.

Figure 1 summarizes the results. The items placed in the upper right area of the figure are those that were "important" and "troublesome," while those placed in the lower left are those that were "not important" and "not troublesome". The results revealed that there is a large discrepancy between the two groups. In other words, the results show that healthcare providers consider ACP important and troublesome, while patients and their families do not consider ACP to be so important or troublesome.

These divergences are easy to sort out when considered in terms of behavioral economics prospect theory.

Prospect theory states that "people do not judge things in proportion to their expected values from given information, but rather distort those expected values depending on the situation and conditions" and that biases are introduced into human behavior depending on how information is passed. The theory also states that "people have a habit of trying to avoid losses" and that they think in terms of "reference points (standards of value)" when considering what constitutes a loss and what constitutes a gain. In the current situation where ACP is performed at an advanced stage of the disease, differences in reactions to information concerning "loss or waste" are thought to be caused by differences in the "reference point" viewed by the healthcare provider, the patient, and the family (see Figure 2).

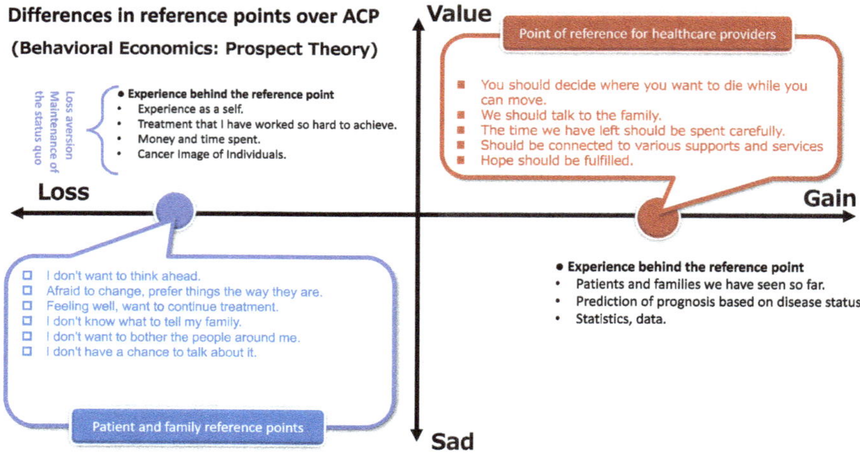

Figure 2.   Difference in reference points.

Healthcare providers have experience in end-of-life care for many patients. Based on such clinical experience, they know "what lies ahead" and believe that "we must do ACP for the patient's sake" because "if we don't discuss what will happen to the patient soon, his/her strength will be taken away and he/she will not be able to do what he/she wants to do". In other words, they consider ACP to be a "gain" and recommend it. However, the "reference point" of such healthcare providers is "the future" for patients and their families, and it is a "world they have not yet experienced". If a patient is suddenly told one day that there will be no more treatment, without taking into account the patient's feelings of not being able or not wanting to think about what will happen in the future, it is natural that the patient will feel a desire to "avoid losing something". A question such as "What is important to you?" or "Where do you want to spend your last days?" does not seem to be a "gain" but rather keeps patient away from thinking. In a confused state, it is difficult for people to make "rational choices" as healthcare providers think. The healthcare provider may wonder, "Why doesn't this patient understand me (the healthcare provider) who is trying to do the right thing (gain)?" In order to avoid such misunderstandings, I understand ACP to be a process of clarifying the "gap in reference points" between the healthcare provider and the patient, and between the patient and the family, and providing information and empathy over time in order to narrow the gap.

The Importance of Visualizing What Can Be Achieved with ACP

(1) Changes that were good or bad after ACP

So, what changes by performing ACP? When we surveyed patients and family members who have actually performed ACP, they pointed out the "good points" and "bad points" as shown in Table 3.

For changes that seem to be getting worse, one can move the reference point by clearly showing the availability of long-term care insurance services and collaboration with community healthcare, i.e., providing a new viewpoint. For example, for "fear of change," we can improve the way we think of losses as gains by sharing information about what life will be like, how to respond to sudden changes, emergency contact systems, and so on (Figure 3). It is important to visualize and communicate these "tough" discussions, rather than just handing out pamphlets or leaving it to the patient and family to "go think about it". It is also necessary for healthcare providers to provide and visualize information among themselves, with healthcare providers as experts standing in between, especially for those involving medical conditions. Thus, in ACP, healthcare providers will need to work as a team to disseminate training that also takes into consideration how to pass on information, when to pass it on, and where to pass it on.

Table 3.   Changes that were good or bad after ACP.
(Conducted in September 2022, web-based survey/100 bereaved families, 100 patients)

Changes that seem to have gotten better	Changes that seem to have gotten worse
• I've been able to receive appropriate treatment.	• Fear of a sudden change in condition has increased.
• I've been able to get the information I wanted about treatment, care, etc.	• There was a change in the caregiver's life (increased burden); I don't want changes in life of myself and the caregiver.
• The explanation of the treatment was easy to understand, and the story was easy to accept.	• I don't know what to say to my family.
• I've been able to build a trusting relationship with my healthcare provider.	• I did not have enough time with patients.
• More supporters around me.	• Timing was fast and I felt like I was being told I couldn't be treated.
• It gave me a chance to talk to my family.	• I've lost faith in the relationship.

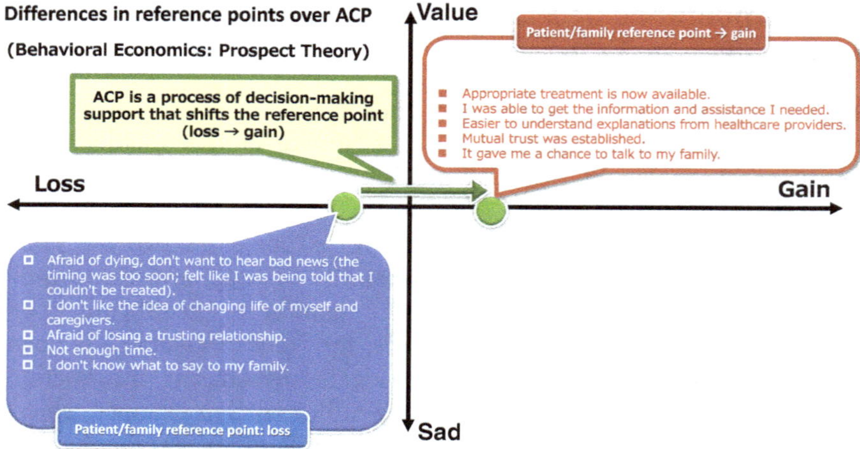

Figure 3.   ACP reference points.

(2) To bring the reference point displacement closer

The results of a survey of bereaved families conducted in Japan are summarized in the "Survey on the Actual Conditions of Medical Care and Recuperation Life Used by Patients before Their Death" (National Cancer Center[6]). This "summary" contains the following statement:

- Among bereaved family members of cancer patients, 35.7% reported that there was a discussion between the patient and the doctor regarding the patient's wishes for the final place of care and medical treatment. In order to realize the provision of medical care in accordance with patients' wishes and desires, decision-making by the patients themselves based on information provided by their attending physicians and other medical personnel is fundamental and therefore needs to be improved. Specific measures need to be studied after investigating the impact caused by inadequate discussions.

Whereas healthcare providers think "ACP should be done", patients wish to "receive information according to their medical conditions and the severity of their illnesses". Instead of starting ACP with "discussion of the place of final place of care," one should prioritize "discussion of medical care".

Many patients have never been asked or thought about their end-of-life intentions when they are healthy. Even if they were patients, they would not be able to answer the question, "What do you want to do?" We would like to request that healthcare providers, as a healthcare consultant team, provide "decision-making support (a process to visualize and bring patients closer to their reference points)" based on the assumption that they are aware of and involved with patients' values and reference points and that they can provide a new viewpoint or correct misunderstanding.

The impact of COVID-19, which began in December 2019, has had a major impact on the medical field. The closure of palliative care units, the reduction of hospital beds, restrictions on visitation, and, moreover, the reduction of funerals and other rituals, "death without goodbye" is causing families who live afterwards to carry a great deal of regret in their hearts. And opportunities to think about "death" are becoming increasingly rare. People will die someday, regardless of whether they are ill or not. Dying is something that no one has ever experienced and cannot predict. However, I hope that there will be a place and time where people can look back on their anxieties and loneliness, and on their lives to date, and talk about them.

Summary: Grief Care in Which Departing Patients Can Participate

One method of care for the bereaved is grief care. In general, grief care often starts from the time of the loss of a loved one. However, I believe that there is "grief care in which patients can participate" and ACP has such a role.

When treatment becomes difficult, differences in reference points arise not only between patient and healthcare provider but also between patient and family. It is good if the patient's medical condition is shared between the healthcare provider and the family, for example, if the family accompanies the patient to outpatient visits, but in cases where this is not possible, the patient himself or herself has to tell his family about his or her condition, which is likely to lead to bias. By sharing their own medical needs, how they want to live their lives, what they value, and what they don't want to do, the family can also gain support, participate in the treatment process, reflect on their lives, and make time to be close to the patient. We should cherish the present moment, remembering that there is grief care that we can participate in even before our death for the sake of our families and loved ones who will have to live after our departure.

Learning Objectives

- Be aware that there is a gap between the "reference point (standard of value)" that healthcare providers and patients consider as "gain" or "loss" and that they see different landscapes.
- The information provided needs to be visualized so that what patients consider a "loss" becomes a "gain," and healthcare providers should work as a consultant team.
- The ACP is a process that considers the patient's way of life and should be done according to the "reference point" and according to the disease status and the severity of cancer.

Acknowledgement

With special thanks to Dr. Masanori Mori for his work in translating this chapter from Japanese to English.

References

1. Sagara Y., Mori M., Yamamoto S., *et al.* (2021). *Oncologist* **26**: e686–e693.
2. Institute of Medicine. (2015). *Dying in America; Improving Quality and Honoring Individual Preferences Near the End of Life.* Washington DC: The National Academies Press.
3. Sudore R.L., Lum H.D., You J.J., *et al.* (2017). Defining advance care planning for adults: A consensus definition from a multidisciplinary Delphi panel. *J. Pain Symptom Manage.* **53**: 821–832.
4. Rietjens J.A.C., Sudore R.L., Connolly M., *et al.* (2017). Definition and recommendations for advance care planning: An international consensus supported by the European association for palliative care. *Lancet Oncol.* **18**: e543–e551.
5. Miyashita J., Shimizu S., Shiraishi R., *et al.* (2022). Culturally adapted consensus definition and action guideline: Japan's advance care planning. *J. Pain Symptom Manage.* **64**: 602–613.
6. Report on a survey of bereaved family members regarding medical treatment received by patients, Ministry of Health, Labour and Welfare-commissioned project to understand the actual conditions of cancer patients in the final stage of their recuperation, National Cancer Center Cancer Control Research Institute, March 2022.
7. Hirai K. (2017). Healthcare x Behavioral Economics Serial 1. Igaku Kai Shinbun. August 28.

Chapter 40

Observations and Reflections on the Promotion of Advance Care Planning in Taiwan

Sam Rong Hwang

Formosa Transnational Attorneys-At-Law, Taipei, Taiwan

- Taiwan has dedicated legislation known as the Patient Right to Autonomy Act (PRAA) that stipulates the right to autonomy, the power to make advance decision/directives, and the requirement of advance care consultation.
- The PRAA raises public awareness of enjoyment of the right to autonomy but also limits the exercise of this right.
- Current PRAA/ACP practice in Taiwan focuses on the achievement of the preferred outcome that an advance decision/directive be signed while neglecting the process of dialogue and discussion. This is a key problem in the promotion of the PRAA and ACP in Taiwan.
- ACP is a procedural right in exercising the right to autonomy in law, rather than simply being a communication process in clinical practice.
- From a person-centred perspective, it is necessary to advocate not only Advance care Planning (ACP) but also Advance Total Planning (ATP).

Introduction

In January 2019, Taiwan's Patient Right to Autonomy Act (PRAA) officially entered into force. The PRAA explicitly stipulates that patients have the right to autonomy including but not limited to rights to know, choose, and make decisions. At the same time, it also explicitly regulates advance care consultation (ACC)[1] and requires patients to undergo a mandatory ACC process provided by a medical institution before signing an advance medical decision (AMD).

Since the implementation of the PRAA, government agencies, hospitals, and civil society have actively promoted the exercise of the patient right to autonomy by encouraging members of the public to receive ACC and sign AMDs. However, there are in fact many limitations on the exercise of the patient right to autonomy based on the PRAA as well as problems with the promotion of the exercise of this right. These problems include the following: (1) placing more emphasis on medical-based approaches than the person-centred approaches, (2) giving more attention to the outcome than the process, and (3) favoring pursuit of a good death and making intentional interventions in personal value judgments. These problems will be explored in more detail in Sections 3.1–3.4.

From a person-centred perspective, I believe that it is appropriate to consider planning in advance not only healthcare but also finances and life at the same time. In addition to advance care planning (ACP) for healthcare, advance financial planning (AFP) for finances and good life planning (GLP) for life should be integrated and deployed in advance to form what can be called advance total planning (ATP) (as shown in Figure 1). ATP is discussed in more detail in Section 4.

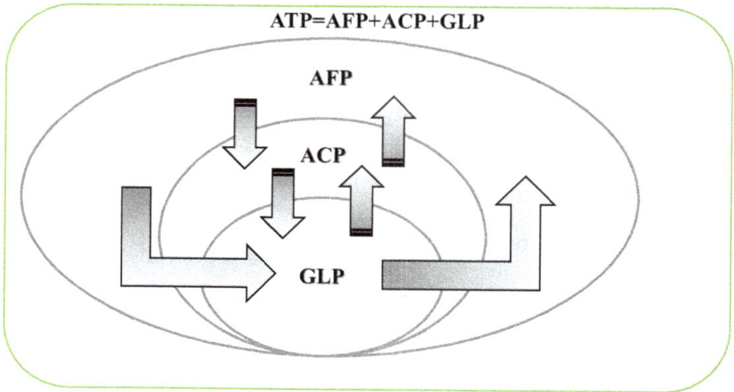

Figure 1.   Framework for ATP.

This chapter begins by first reviewing how Taiwan currently promotes ACC and ACP. Second, observations of the current situation of Taiwan's promotion of ACP/ACC are explained. Third, ATP is briefly elucidated with the call for promotion of not just ACP/ACC but also ATP. Fourth, and finally, a follow-up agenda for Taiwan's promotion of ACP/ACC is proposed in the conclusions.

Current Promotion of the Patient Right to Autonomy in Taiwan

Provisions of the PRAA

The PRAA stipulates the patient right to autonomy including, but not limited to, the right to know, the right to choose, and the right to decide. It also requires ACC and stipulates the content of AMDs. In particular, the PRAA provides that an AMD must include the acceptance or refusal of all or part of life-sustaining treatment (LST) or artificial nutrition and fluid feeding (ANH) in specific clinical conditions:

1. terminal illness,
2. irreversible coma,
3. permanent vegetative state, and
4. severe dementia.

The PRAA further authorizes the Ministry of Health and Welfare of the Executive Yuan (MOHW) to announce other clinical conditions to which an AMD is applicable if the clinical condition meets the following requirements:

1. the patient's condition or pain is unbearable,
2. the disease is incurable, and
3. there are no other appropriate treatment options available given medical standards at the time of the disease's occurrence.

To make an AMD with the legal effect under the PRAA,[2] the patient must:

1. undergo ACC provided by a consulting team before signing the AMD,[3]
2. have the medical institution affix its seal on the AMD,

3. have two or more persons with full disposing capacity (i.e., with the capacity to make legal decisions, such as entering into a contract) witness the patient sign the AMD or sign the AMD before a public notary,
4. register the AMD in the patient's National Health Insurance IC card after signature.

The consulting team is composed of physicians who are generally palliative care/family medicine specialists, nurses, psychologists, and social workers who work at a medical institution and meet the conditions stipulated in the PRAA and other regulations.

Moreover, when a patient receives an ACC, the counseling team must explain certain matters (Matters) to the patient. The principle Matters are as follows:

1. the right to autonomy, such as the right to make decisions,
2. the specific clinical conditions for terminating, withdrawing, or not administering LST and ANH,
3. the format of the AMD, and
4. the right to designate a healthcare agent (HCA).

PRAA's main legal structure can be expressed with the following propositions:

First, the patient has the right to autonomy including but not limited to the right to know and the right to choose and decide. Additionally, medical institutions and physicians have obligations to inform the patient of the diagnosis of his or her disease, treatment options, proposed procedures, medications, prognosis, possible negative reactions, and other related issues. This obligation to inform may be met at an appropriate time and in an appropriate manner as judged by the medical institution or physicians.

Second, a patient with disposing capacity exercises their right to autonomy by signing an AMD and designating an HCA but only after receiving mandatory ACC. The PRAA stipulates the ACC procedure as well as the format and contents of the AMD.

Third, medical institutions and physicians can implement an AMD provided that one of the specific clinical conditions defined by the PRAA or lawfully designated by the MOHW has occurred. When a medical institution or physician implements an AMD by terminating, withdrawing, or withholding LST/ANH, the patient must be provided with or referred to palliative care and other appropriate measures.

Fourth, a medical institution or physician cannot be subjected to criminal or administrative liability when it, he, or she terminates, withdraws, or withholds LST/ANH in accordance with the regulations of the PRAA. They are furthermore exempted from compensatory damages arising from harm to the patient unless their conduct is intentionally or grossly negligent and violates the patient's AMD.

Current Efforts to Promote Patient Autonomy

Taiwanese government agencies, hospitals, and civil society actively promote the right to autonomy under the PRAA.[4] These efforts are however mainly aimed at the general public who are not hospitalized or do not live in facilities. Medical institutions set up ACC clinics where the fee for each ACC session by the consulting team may not exceed NT3,500 (approximately US$115). During the ACC process, the consulting team mainly focuses on explaining the right to autonomy, HCA, the applicable specific clinical conditions, as well as the content and procedures stipulated in the PRAA for refusing (terminating, withdrawing, or not administering) LST/ANH. Depending on the consulting team though, values and preferences may not be fully discussed with the person who is considering making an AMD.

People can receive ACC individually or with their families. Some medical institutions have used what they call "explanatory sessions" to conduct ACC for multiple members of the public simultaneously. After these group ACC sessions, the consulting team encourages the participants to sign the AMDs on site.[5] This suggests that medical institutions and consulting teams regard the purpose of ACC to be to increase the number of AMDs. Government agencies have also offered monetary incentives based on the number of signed and registered AMDs to encourage medical institutions to actively encourage the public to sign AMDs.[6]

In addition, when promoting the exercise of the right to autonomy, hospitals and civil society organizations are often prone to put forward the proposition that "it is better to have a good death than to live with suffer and without dignity" and that one should seek a "good death". That is, it is argued that an AMD should be signed in advance and that the choice to refuse LST/ANH can avoid a state of life without dignity (such as being in an irreversible coma, a permanent vegetative state, or having severe dementia). This is said to be desirable because the person making the AMD can thereby have a good death. The media also often publishes stories that equate the exercise of the right to autonomy with a good death. In particular, these stories tend to associate refusal of LST/ANH and voluntarily stopping eating and drinking (VESD) with good deaths.

As of April 13, 2021, the MOHW has announced specific clinical conditions for a total of 14 rare diseases[7] including amyotrophic lateral sclerosis. This means that patients with a rare disease who meets the specific announced clinical conditions for that disease may also sign an AMD in accordance with the PRAA and have it implemented even if they are not terminally ill, in an irreversible coma, in a permanent vegetative state, or have very severe dementia. Some civil society organizations serving special groups such as patients with rare diseases encourage these patients to sign AMDs.[8]

Observations

On the one hand, some positive comments regarding the PRAA and Taiwan's promotion of ACP may be made. First, the PRAA is dedicated legislation with the policy objective of ensuring that individuals enjoy the right to autonomy. It can be expected that the PRAA will continue to raise public awareness that individuals can exercise the right to autonomy. Moreover, ACC, which is clearly stipulated by the PRAA, can be regarded as a very meaningful way to emphasize the importance of the decision-making procedure rather than merely the legal outcome. Second, the public is able to legally and formally use AMDs to exercise their right to autonomy by refusing or accepting LAT/ANH, avoiding treatments that they do not want or that are non-compliant with their will and preferences. Third, the PRAA provides immunities to medical institutions and physicians if they terminate, withdraw, or withhold LST/ANH in accordance with Article 14(5) of the PRAA (no criminal or administrative liability in most cases). This provision makes medical institutions and physicians less hesitant to encourage and assist patients in exercising the right to autonomy.

But on the other hand, the following criticisms of how Taiwan currently promotes ACP can be put forward.

Unduly Restricting the Exercise of Right to Autonomy

Although Taiwan prides itself on having officially implemented Asia's first patient autonomy law in 2019, the PRAA improperly or even unconstitutionally restricts the exercise of the right to autonomy in the following ways:

1. The PRAA confuses the difference between disposing capacity and mental capacity by requiring patients to have the disposing capacity in order to receive ACC or make an AMD. This restricts persons who do not have disposing capacity but have mental capacity (such as those who have been declared under guardianship) from exercising their right to autonomy.

   In reality, the concepts of mental capacity and disposing capacity are not equivalent. Mental capacity is psychological ability in the sense of the ability to understand, retain, use/weigh information, and express a decision or the ability to understand, appreciate, reason about the information provided, and make a choice. In contrast, disposing capacity is not a psychological concept at all but a legal status or standing. A person with disposing capacity is a 'player in civil society' who can enter into financial and other contractual relationships with others. In short, the concept of mental capacity should not be confused with the notion of disposing capacity.

2. The PRAA limits the voluntariness of the exercise of right to autonomy by requiring patients to undergo ACC at a medical institution before signing an AMD and compelling them to attend ACC in person. ACP should be a voluntary process based on respecting the person's right to autonomy. The compulsory nature of the ACC process in Taiwan is inconsistent with the voluntary nature of ACP and harms the exercise of the right to autonomy.

3. The PRAA restricts the content of an AMD to acceptance or rejection of LST/ANH under specific clinical conditions, such as terminally ill patients. This limits not only the clinical conditions to which the AMD can apply but also the scope of which treatments the patient can accept or refuse. Even though AMDs by their nature are intrinsically limited because the full range of future clinical conditions and all of the future treatments contained in an advance decision/directive (AD) cannot be anticipated completely, limiting AMDs to accepting or rejecting LST/ANH under specific clinical conditions can be regarded as over-restricting the right to autonomy.

4. Another restriction on the exercise of the right to autonomy is the rule that a person must have disposing capacity to designate an HCA. As mentioned above, AMDs intrinsically limit the right to autonomy. To overcome this limitation, designation of an HCA is highly recommended in order to fully exercise the right to autonomy. By requiring a person to have disposing capacity as a precondition to designating an HCA, the PRAA inappropriately restricts the right to autonomy.
5. The PRRA requires a patient to amend any existing AMD in writing and complete a process to change the corresponding annotation on the patient's National Health Insurance IC card in order to modify the existing AMD to refuse LST/ANH. This is yet another restriction on the exercise of the right to autonomy.

These undue restrictions on the exercise of the right to autonomy have the negative effect of causing the provisions of the PRAA to become *pro forma* protection. In order to ensure that protection of the right to autonomy is more than a mere mantra, advocates and policymakers should work conscientiously to loosen these inappropriate restrictions on the right to autonomy.

Medicine-Based Approach Emphasized More than Person-Based Approach

Although the PRAA explicitly guarantees the autonomy of patients, there are nonetheless a number of situations in which the medicine-based approach is emphasized than the person-based approach:

1. It is expressly stipulated that a person must undergo ACC provided by a medical institution's consulting team before signing an AMD regardless of the individual's independent willingness to receive ACC.
2. When medical personnel explain the Matters such as the right to autonomy as required in ACC, they are in the unequal and superior position of an informer or consultant who provides a description of the right to autonomy, HCA, and specific clinical conditions and LST/ANH. They are not engaging in dialogue and discussion with the person as an equal.
3. The PRAA requires that medical personnel provide ACC to assist the person in signing an AMD that complies with the requirements of the

PRAA. This results in ignoring the possibility that a person may wish to voluntarily choose to seek ACC from a person who is not a medical professional.

Focusing on the Achievement of Outcomes but Neglecting the Process of Dialogue and Discussion

In reality, there are two constituent components to the right of autonomy in law: a substantive right and a procedural right. The first component encompasses the substantive rights to know, to choose, and to make decisions. The second component is the procedural right in the form of ACP and necessary support to exercise the substantive right of autonomy. It follows that ACP is more than a process of communication in clinical practice. More accurately, it is the procedural means through which the right to the substantive aspects of the right to autonomy is exercised in a legal sense. In other words, ACP is the process that realizes the right of autonomy. It should not be conceived as simply a tool or process aimed at the signing of an AMD.

In addition, the ACP process should be expected to achieve not only a decision-making outcome (such as signing an AMD) but also a changed relationship between the individual and their families and the healthcare providers who participate in ACP. It should also achieve the transformation of the individual's will and preferences during the process of decision formation. In particular, when we focus on the will and preferences of the person, we can even say that the continuous process of ACP is more important and necessary than a one-time AMD.

Nonetheless, promotional materials such as videos and media reports emphasize the importance of signing an AMD and rejecting LST/ANH in advance on grounds that these decisions and choices can ensure that a person avoids losing dignity due to loss of mental capacity, long-term bed rest, and deteriorating quality of life. In other words, the emphasis is on the outcome of advance planning. For example, some hospitals hold what they call "explanatory sessions" of about two to three hours for a large number of people (such as 50 people). After the explanatory session, the participants are invited to sign AMDs. These large sessions do not seriously engage in a process of dialogue and discussion before the participants sign the AMDs. Moreover, the public's values, will, and preferences about LST/ANH are usually ignored and dismissed. This creates a situation in which the achievement of outcome, such as counting the number of AMDs completed, is weighted more heavily than how the process of dialogue is conducted.

Promoting the Pursuit of a Good Death and Intentionally Intervening in Value Judgments

"It is better to die well than to live in suffer" and "pursuing a good death" are two common ways of expressing one of Taiwan's main goals in promoting patient autonomy. In particular, it is not uncommon for some members of civil society, and even medical professionals and the media, to actively advocate for the exercise of right to autonomy and signing AMDs that register rejections of LST/ANH in order to obtain a good death.

However, whether or not a death is a good death subjectively involves one's values, will, and preferences. There is no absolute objective standard for a good death, and the possibility of a good death is affected by one's physical, mental, and external environment at the time of death. A good death cannot be generalized and handled by simply signing an AMD and choosing to reject LST/ANH. In particular, the strong impetus to promote the signing of AMDs that choose to reject LST/ANH to obtain a good death results in the dominance of certain values. Those who do not agree with this choice but intend to sign an AMD in which they choose to accept LST/ANH will be subjected to the pressure of imposed values from the collective community and endure undue influence in ways that harm the exercise of right to autonomy.

In particular, does the practice of actively advocating that patients with rare diseases sign AMDs while encouraging these patients to choose the option of refusing LST/ANH to obtain a good death deny the right to life of patients with rare diseases? This way of advocating for patients with rare diseases to exercise their right to autonomy paradoxically seems to single them out as a distinct cohort with a different kind of human dignity or even subject them to indirect discrimination. At the same time, does it also cause rare disease patients to choose to refuse LST/ANH against their true will and preferences in order to avoid or reduce financial burden and physical burdens on family members and other caregivers? The current promotion of ACP for patients with rare diseases is guilty of oversimplification for the cause the good death.

From ACP to ATP

ACP is a process of communication in which future healthcare matters are discussed and may be decided in advance. However, from a person-centred perspective, it can be seen that life and death are not simply just healthcare matters that must be planned in advance. In parallel with healthcare matters, there are financial matters as well as life matters that should be dealt with and even decided and prepared in advance. At the same time, the planning of healthcare matters is often based on the values, preferences, and intentions of the person in life. This planning will be related to financial/life matters such that advance healthcare planning and the planning of health and life matters will affect one another. In other words, the planning of health, financial, and life matters are not separate and independent planning processes. Instead, they should be planned comprehensively and integrally. For this reason, it is necessary to advocate not just for ACP but also for advance total planning (ATP).

In an effort to develop ATP further, I advocate not only ACP for healthcare but also advance financial planning (AFP) for finances (such as insurance, trusts, attorney for property, intentional guardianship, and wills) and good life planning (GLP) for life. GLP is based on health literacy and management, financial literacy and management, life and death literacy and management, plus a positive health attitude. Properly implemented, GLP strengthens the individual's capability of health (i.e., maintaining one's health), financial ability (to manage finances), learning ability (to continue learning), and service ability (to engage in volunteer services) and then enhances the ability for a good life (integration of the first four abilities). Figure 1 illustrates the way that GLP flows out into ACP and AFP and how ACP and AFP affect one another as well as flow into GLP. In other words, the purpose of the diagram is to show how GLP, ACP, and AFP are interdependent and interactive. Therefore, ATP provides an appropriate model for holistic and integrated planning based on the person-centre perspective.

A grassroots movement has been formed to promote ATP in Taiwan. For instance, in order to promote ATP, the Taiwan Chengyun Association for Death and Life Education has launched an ATP Kit (as shown in Figure 2) that includes the Chengyun Q Card, Chengyun NOTE, and Chengyun MEMO.[9] The Chengyun Q Card contains various questions with respect to life outlook, healthcare, and finances that help the individual easily discuss and engage in dialogue about the relevant questions

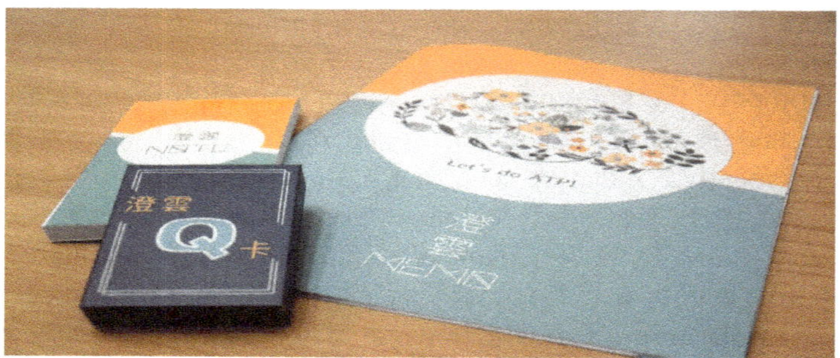

Figure 2.   ATP Kit.

with the individual's family and healthcare providers. Next, the individual can use the Chengyun NOTE to note the main points of the dialogue. Finally, decisions can be recorded in the Chengyun MEMO. In addition, in November 2022, Chengyun cooperated with other non-governmental organizations to hold an ATP Promoter training program to continue to actively promote ATP.

Conclusion — Go Forward

Since January 2019, Taiwan's government agencies, medical institutions, and civil society have promoted the exercise of the right to autonomy based on the provisions of the PRAA. The main practice is to encourage people to complete a one-time ACC and sign an AMD in which the person opts to refuse LST/ANH for the purpose of seeking a good death. In other words, Taiwan does not focus so much on promoting ACP. Its promotional work instead encourages people to exercise their substantive right to autonomy and sign an AMD for a good death. That is, the current mainstream practice in Taiwan is not to focus on the processes of dialogue and discussion in the course of ACP but rather to seek the signing of AMDs. Namely, the purpose of promoting ACP is not to enhance or improve the relationship between the person and his family through the dialogue and discussion process of ACP or to grasp and understand the values, will, and preferences of the person involved in the healthcare decision but rather to try to secure a good death by signing an AMD that records refusal of LST/ANH.

This mainstream approach in Taiwan can be said to have the following problems: (1) unduly restricting the exercise of the right to autonomy,

(2) giving priority to a medical-based approach over a person-based approach, (3) emphasizing the achievement of outcomes but neglecting the process of dialogue and discussion, and (4) promoting the pursuit of a good death and interfering in value judgments. In particular, there are profound ethical issues with how Taiwan (1) encourages the pursuit of standardized end-of-life and (2) actively advocates that patients with rare diseases sign AMDs and encourages these patients to choose to reject LST/ANH. Here, the state or civil society induces or even imposes a view of life and death on people and then manages their view of life and death. These practices should be changed. Therefore, it is hoped that efforts will be made in Taiwan to ensure that ACP (1) protects autonomy and does not unduly restrict autonomy under the PRAA, (2) implements the person-based approach over the medicine-based approach, (3) practices a process of dialogue and discussion between the person and the persons family and healthcare providers without a bias toward the achievement of particular outcomes, and (4) does not standardize the quality of what constitutes dignity and a good death.

Furthermore, since the person should be centred and healthcare is only a part of one's life, it is necessary that in addition to ACP for health-care matters, ATP for financial and life matters should be promoted.

Personally, I believe that Taiwan should continue to promote ACP based on the following six directions:

(1) From Act to Person-centred,
(2) From AMD to ACP,
(3) From Outcome to Process,
(4) From Hospital to Home,
(5) From Healthcare to Total Domains (including finances and life domains),
(6) From Good Death to Good Life.

All in all, ACP is a procedural right in the exercise of the substantive right to autonomy in law, rather than being simply a process for communication in clinical practice. ACP should be expected to effect change in the relationship between the person and their family and healthcare providers as well as the transformation of the person's will and preferences during the process of decision formulation. It should not be reduced to just signing an AMD. It is hoped that these six directions can be helpful in providing potentially valuable ways for the continuous promotion and improvements of ACP in Taiwan that encompasses the full range of respecting, protecting, and exercising the right to autonomy in law and practice.

Acknowledgements

The author is indebted to Dr. Masanori Mori of Seirei Mikatahara General Hospital for much of his thinking related to ACP and thanks him for his kind invitation to have this opportunity to introduce the author's observations of and reflections on ACP promotion in Taiwan.

References

1.   In Taiwan, Advance Care Consultation is commonly equated with Advance Care Planning (ACP). However, it is based on the differences (1) the former focuses on explanation and consultation while the latter focuses on communication and dialogue; (2) the former focuses on obtaining the result of AD signing, while the latter focuses on the process of communication and dialogue, and (3) the former is expressly enforced by law, while the latter is voluntary. Therefore, I do not think it is appropriate to regard Advance Care Consultation as ACP.

2.   The legal effect of making an AMD is mainly set out in Article 14, Item 5 of the PRAA, "A medical institution or physician shall not be subject to criminal or administrative liability when it, he or she terminates, withdraws or withholds life-sustaining treatment and/or artificial nutrition and hydration in accordance with the regulations in this article; they shall bear no responsibility of compensation for the damage incurred, unless intentional or grossly negligent conduct and violation of the advance decision of patients are involved."

3.   For example, specialists or nurses who have practiced for more than 2 years and completed a prescribed ACC training course.

4.   In 2010, the Palliative Care Foundation of the Republic of China (Taiwan) began to promote ACP several years before the Taiwan Legislature enacted the PRAA. See https://www.hospice.org.tw/content/918?page=1. Last accessed 21 December 2022.

5.   An important reason for adopting group consultations is to lower the cost of ACC. The fee for a group consultation is less than what must be paid for individual ACC. In some cases, group ACC is free. Lower ACC cost encourages more people to receive ACC and sign AMDs.

6.   For example, at a press conference on the 4th anniversary of the implementation of the PRAA on January 6, 2023, MOHW and civil society organizations

disclosed and emphasized that the number of signed AMDs reached 43,466 in 2022. In 2023, the number of AMDs is expected to reach 60,000. See https://health.ltn.com.tw/article/breakingnews/4176490. Last accessed on 9 January 2022.

7. As of April 13, 2021, MOHW has announced specific clinical conditions for a total of 14 rare diseases, including ALS. See https://hpcod.mohw.gov.tw/HospWeb/RWD/PageType/acp/autonomy.aspx. Last accessed 26 December 2022.

8. Such as the Patient Autonomy Research Center. See https://parc.tw/news/center/article/468. Last accessed 26 December 2022.

9. A Chengyun Q Card video and introductions to Chengyun NOTE and Chengyun MEMO are available on the Association's website. See https://www.twchengyun.org. Last accessed 21 December 2022.

Chapter 41

Advance Care Planning's Legacy to Families

Wakako Kaneko

End-of-Life Issues
Life Terminal Network, Tokyo, Japan

Introduction

I am a bereaved family member who bereaved my husband in 2012.

And now, I am working to give shape to the various things my husband entrusted to me. The starting point for my current activities is the experience of running alongside my husband during his battle with illness and death and watching him live his life right up to the end.

Today, the term "end-of-life issues" ("*shukatsu*") is widely accepted in Japan. According to a survey conducted by a private company, the recognition rate is as high as 96%.[1] The term "end-of-life issues," which first appeared in a weekly magazine series in 2009, refers to various preparations for the end of one's life. In Japan, where the population aging rate is 29.1% (in 2022),[2] many people are interested in this topic, but the reality is that few people practice it yet.

My husband's death played a role in spreading the concept of "end-of-life issues" throughout the country. Before his death, he prepared a will to prepare for his inheritance, planned and arranged for his wake, funeral, and other post-death ceremonies, prepared a grave for him and me, and even wrote the funeral appreciation letter himself. He also decided to write a book summarizing the various events leading up to his death and publish it on the 49th day after his death (a memorial service held on the 49th day after death, one of the Buddhist rites) and persuaded those around him to make this happen.

All of this, as well as the fact that he was reported in the press as a person who embodied "end-of-life issues," provided an opportunity for people to expand their understanding of what exactly "end-of-life issues" is all about.

At the time, however, I felt a strong sense of discomfort. I wondered if making preparations for one's own afterlife, such as writing a will, was really "end-of-life issues". From my perspective as someone who was with my husband, this was only a small part of what he did, and the essence of what he did was not there. I even had a feeling akin to impatience, thinking that this was not what my husband had entrusted to me, given the situation in which "end-of-life issues" were spreading throughout the world using what he had done as an example.

So, what was it that the husband did? This was exactly what ACP is. I came to know that what my husband practiced was ACP many years after his bereavement.

In this chapter, I would like to introduce what my husband did and what I am doing now in response to what he did, and what meaning and value ACP has for the families of those who have practiced ACP and died.

Limited Life Suddenly Made Known

In May 2011, a doctor at a local clinic told him that he probably had terminal lung cancer, and he immediately visited a specialist hospital. The definitive diagnosis was lung carcinoid, and it was terminal. The 9 cm tumor was pressing on his airway, and the doctor at the specialist hospital said, "I wouldn't be surprised at all if you died in front of me right now."

What pushed us further into a corner was the reality that there was no cure. We were told that anticancer drugs were ineffective, that radiation would be useless, and that surgery was impossible given the size of the tumor. In other words, there was virtually nothing we could do. The doctor recommended that a stent be placed in the throat to reduce asphyxiation, but we did nothing. Or, perhaps I should say, we couldn't do any. We were told that he was going to die, but nothing had changed in his condition or situation, let alone his physical status. We did not understand the reality accurately.

In addition, my husband is a public speaker, appearing on television and other media and giving lectures. We asked the doctor what would happen if he had a stent in his throat, and the doctor said that there would probably be some discomfort in his throat. Hearing this, my husband insisted right then and there that he would have a problem with that. I still remember well how the doctor in front of him looked at him for a moment and said, "Is your job more important than your life?" I remember that I felt the same way as the doctor at that moment.

However, what should we do? Is there nothing to do but to continue to do nothing and just wait to die? ...... I was desperately trying to suppress my feelings of wanting to do whatever I could. I had lost my father to stomach cancer two and a half years earlier, and I had regretted forcing him to take anticancer drugs, even though he did not want to, without regard to his own will.

"I Want to Work until the Moment I Die"

We asked for a second and even a third opinion, but the results remained the same. Aggressive treatment was not indicated. We were simply told that if he wanted to be admitted to the hospice ward in the hospital, it would not be possible right away and that we should see an outpatient palliative care specialist as soon as possible anyway.

While attending the thoracic surgery department of the first hospital where he received the definite diagnosis (I think the doctor was puzzled by the patient who kept making appointments even though he could not treat the disease...), we also attended the palliative care outpatient clinic as we were told and then, as recommended by the palliative care doctor, decided to go to the radiology department next.

Throughout this process, the husband clearly verbalized his intentions.

"I want to work until the moment I die. If I'm on TV, I want to breathe my last the moment the broadcast is over, and if I'm giving a lecture, I want to breathe my last the moment I return to the wings of the stage."

Perhaps it was because he truly accepted the reality that there was no cure through his interactions not only with the thoracic doctor but also with doctors in other medical departments. At the same time, perhaps it was also because he was fortunate to have carcinoid disease, which allowed him to move even though he was in a very advanced stage of the disease. At a very early stage after the disease was discovered, he came to clearly state, "I want to work until the moment of my death, so I want to delay my death even one day". He did not say vaguely, "I want to live," but rather, "I want to die 'as a distribution journalist,'" which was his job.

Thus, it was decided to start discussions, at least with those involved in the work, centred on the idea of allowing him to continue working as long as he wanted, even if only for a day.

Treatment Selected According to What Is Important

On the other hand, no progress was made regarding treatment. However, although he had a severe cough, he was hardly aware of any pain or breathlessness, and he continued his relationship with the hospital without any actual treatment. One day, an acquaintance recommended a certain treatment. It was an endovascular treatment. It was a treatment that aimed to reduce the size of the tumor while minimizing organ damage by injecting medication through a catheter into the arteries that nourished the cancer.

At the time, we thought it was a little-known treatment, but the fact that it was covered by health insurance and, above all, that it had few side effects, short hospitalization, and quick return to work, matched my husband's wish to "work until the moment of death."

The endovascular treatment was successful, and about four months after the start of treatment, the tumor in the lung shrank from 9 cm to 3 cm. However, while we were both relieved that the risk of asphyxiation had been significantly reduced, around the middle of January 2012, the pain caused by bone metastasis, which had been pointed out at the time of the definitive diagnosis, began to appear. Well, perhaps he was so preoccupied with the thought that he might die that he was simply unaware of the pain from the bone metastasis until that time.

Later, the pain from the bone metastasis was resolved with intensity-modulated radiation therapy, but in March, he was hospitalized due to fluid in his lungs. It became increasingly difficult to balance work and fighting the disease. Nevertheless, my husband's desire to "work until the moment of death" was clear, and each time, the parties involved would continue to discuss both work and treatment, based on how they could realize this intention. By this time, he had already cut ties with the first hospital where he received his definitive diagnosis (not surprisingly, since aggressive treatment was already off the table) and was being supported by the doctors and nurses at a clinic in town that also provided home medical care.

He tried various treatments and said, "I want to work until the moment of my death. So I want to delay my death even one day longer." The medical staff worked with him to fulfill his life goal, but in mid-July, he finally contracted pneumonia, which we had feared. He was approached about hospitalization, but again, my husband refused, claiming that he could not spend his time freely. He decided to receive medical care at home, and as a result, he passed away in October of that year while continuing to receive home medical care.

Business Associates Got Together to Discuss It

Even though he could no longer travel by air due to his lung condition, and even though he could no longer appear on TV or radio because he could no longer use his oxygen concentrator, he still discussed with medical and business associates how he could fulfill his wish to "work until the moment of his death". Of course, my husband himself joined us.

For example, the dosage of opioids was delicately adjusted, so much so that medical staff said, "It is possible to completely take away the pain, but if you do that, you cannot think clearly and cannot work. It is difficult to find a balance between pain relief and the ability to work, but I think I can make use of this for future patients. I am really learning a lot." In the end, the dose was even adjusted in 1 mg increments while the Fentos tape was cut under my husband's direction.

Thus, my husband **worked until the moment of his death**, as he wished. He was interviewed by a magazine until a few hours before his death, called the funeral home he had discussed with in advance to confirm the arrangements immediately following his own death, and while doing so, proofread an interview article, thanked the doctor who came to make house calls, and said goodbye and thank you to the manager who supported his work.

My husband had another wish. He wanted to spend his final days alone with me. He showed me more than enough of how people die, what is in between life and death, how we should live and die, and the death that came after a dialogue with my husband, who was clearly aware of death but kept challenging himself to think about how he should live. I myself believe that we shared it together.

Immediately after my husband's death, what follows is the start of my current activities. It all started when the doctor asked me to confirm the cause of death to be written on the death certificate. He said, "I want it to be pulmonary carcinoid. The existence of this disease will be known to the world if my death is reported even a little". The doctor wrote down "pulmonary carcinoid" as the cause of death in accordance with my husband's wish, and as a result, it was reported and the disease was explained in many media outlets.

The same is true for funerals. I won't bore you with the length of the story, but my husband's own death also sent a message to the world about the state of funerals, his attitude toward religion, and his wishes for religion.

Through this process, I started to put into practice what my husband entrusted to me.

Life Terminal Network

About a year after bereavement, I started an activity called Life Terminal Network. The following diagram represents what death looks like for the individual or his/her family, and the three important points are (1) not biased anywhere, (2) party-oriented, and (3) practical. This is because we have experienced that for the individual and his/her family, the division of professionals around death is a rather harsh reality that confronts them at that moment in front of death.

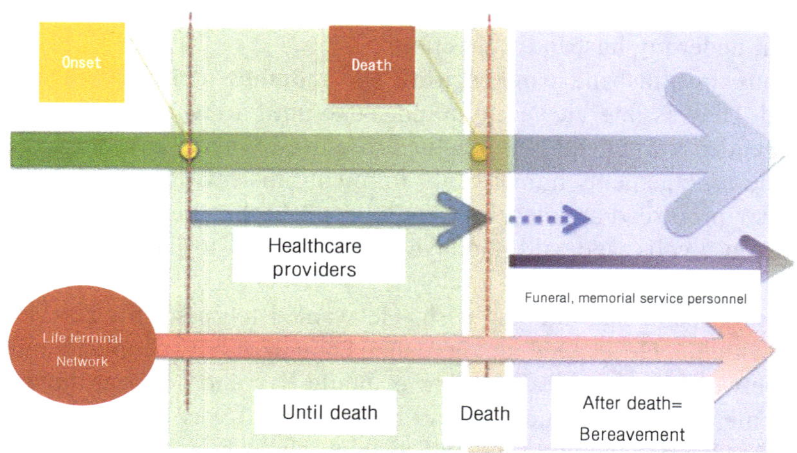

For example, when a person wants to discuss the medical care and care he or she will receive in the final stages of life, the person must, so to speak, assume that he or she will die. No matter how much they are told that they can change their minds and that it is natural for them to do so, the hurdle for making such a choice or decision is extremely high. However, in the medical field, the medical staff wants to decide on the direction of medical treatment and care "for the person". This is because medical and nursing care professionals have a mission to support the "life," or "quality of life," of the person until the time of his or her death.

However, thinking about death head-on is extremely painful for the person concerned. And for some people, it is a great shock to have the topic of death broached by a medical professional who has fought the disease with them until now.

At such times, words such as "I am worried about my grave" or "I have a wish about my memorial service" may be uttered by the person concerned. This is also the case with some of the consultations I receive. In many cases, the person is not talking about death but rather wants to discuss death and talk about it in the form of a consultation, using the topic of his/her own afterlife as an opportunity.

In the medical and nursing care fields, however, most people are not able to discuss graves and memorial services because they are not "experts". The same can be said of the funeral and memorial service industry. While they may be able to discuss graves and memorial services, they are not able to discuss the medical and care issues that they are facing.

The Life Terminal Network suggests dividing death into three stages, as shown in the diagram, and considering them as a set of three. This is because for the individual and family facing the special life event of death, they do not even know that the professionals are divided. Therefore, some people may feel hurt that the experts they relied on at the time did not meet their expectations.

Supporting "Parties"

My husband and I were the first to realize this when we learned of his condition, that he could have died of asphyxiation at any time. Different experts have different values. Above all, we did not have the "words" to explain ourselves in a way that would be understood by professionals who were used to dealing with death on a daily basis (i.e., people who were used to it only happening a few times in an individual's lives).

It took me a long time to understand his values, even as a family member myself. I guess it was so difficult for me to accept my husband's death that I had a hard time admitting how important "being a distribution journalist" was to him, to the extent that people around me would take it as "is work more important than life?" I can explain this now.

That is why at Life Terminal Network, we emphasize the verbalization of thoughts. Sometimes we first verbalize what we cannot speak well in front of professionals or even among the parties involved and then work together to figure out how to communicate this to the professionals.

When we consulted with a daughter who was having difficulty communicating with the medical and nursing staff at a nursing home regarding her mother with dementia, we helped the daughter verbalize her feelings toward her mother, what her mother would want, and her distrust of the staff in advance. Later, at the daughter's request, we also attended a meeting with the staff. While both the daughter and the staff avoided the topic of death and were unable to get to the heart of the matter, we were able to spark an opening and lead to a concrete discussion.

I will never forget the look of relief on the faces of the medical and nursing staff at that moment when I turned the subject of death around, knowing that we could now finally discuss the important things. I believe that in the face of death, not only the individual and his/her family but also the medical and nursing care professionals involved are "parties concerned."

Practice of Dialogue Presided over by Citizens

Even if we talk about verbalization, it is not easy to do so at the stage of near death. For this reason, the group has been holding a dialogue on a single question, with a theme related to life and death as the starting point (the group was suspended due to the Corona Disaster but will be resumed in 2023). The group was started by volunteer members of a study group led by a philosopher, which was held to study dialogue between researchers and citizens together, in an attempt to practice dialogue by citizens.

The key point of this initiative is that it is presided over by a citizen. In a place presided over by a medical professional, whose knowledge and experience are asymmetrical in relation to patients, and who can easily be relied upon, it is difficult to create an equal relationship, which is the most important aspect of dialogue. This is why we decided to create a "dialogue meeting by citizens."

In the meetings we conduct, we do not force the disclosure or concealment of names, occupations, family structures, etc. (we strongly request that they not be divulged to outside parties). As a result, there were some participants who, after the meeting was over, revealed that they were healthcare professionals, saying, "Actually...," and there were others whom we knew but who did not tell us at the meeting that they were healthcare professionals. These people also commented that they "wanted a place like this" (where we could be equal).

Through the practice of dialogue meetings, we aim to increase the number of opportunities for people to think about topics related to life and death that are usually difficult to talk about, to help people verbalize what they are unable or unwilling to verbalize (this may include values and life goals), and to promote understanding that people have values that differ from their own. (Sometimes, before or after death, conflicts of values can cause things to happen that the person does not want to happen.)

Resolving Problems Also Starts with Verbalization Support

The Life Terminal Network also assists individuals, their families, and bereaved families in resolving their problems. Many people have various problems, but they often do not understand (or are unable to verbalize) what is troubling them. In most cases, the first step is to help them verbalize their problems.

One day, I was introduced by an acquaintance to meet a 31-year-old man. He had just gotten married and had been diagnosed with stage IV colon cancer and had just started anticancer treatment after surgery when we met. At first, he was to be with his wife, but later his parents were to be present as well. I still remember it well. He, his wife, and his parents lined up side by side in front of me, and he quickly explained to me that he was practicing the kind of "end-of-life issues" that I described at the beginning of this manuscript.

The "end-of-life issues" that are spreading around the world as an example of what my husband did are, so to speak, preparations for death. Despite the fact that he, like my husband, was excitedly talking about doing this and that, his parents' faces were dark and faded, and his wife seemed to have no idea what was going on. The family was not aligned in the face of the illness. ... No, it was nearly impossible for them to be aligned, but it was clear that their feelings were very different from each other.

So I called out to him. Of course, I thought that this person would understand the meaning of my words.

"Are you preparing to die? My husband was not 'preparing to die' in any way."

Until that moment, I don't think he understood what my husband really did, i.e., practiced ACP. I told him that the will and grave preparations were only a small and superficial part of what my husband did, that what he really did was share his view of life, his values, and what he valued, and that the results of what he did were only what they seemed.

Incidentally, his father is a physician and himself involved in hospital management. Although he has a policy on "medical choice" and makes tough and difficult choices each time, when I first met him, he had not yet reached the point of understanding the significance of ACP for the parties involved, especially the family.

After this visit, he immediately contacted me, saying that this time he and his wife were going alone and wanted to discuss the cemetery. At first, he said that he wanted to get information about the grave, but as I asked him why he wanted the information, he said, "My intentions are set regarding the treatment, but I really wonder if my wife will be okay with it." He wondered if the wife would shield her husband's will in front of his relatives and if this would put her in a difficult position after his death. Since the issue of the grave is one that requires keeping close relations with the relatives for memorial services, etc., he did not want to add more anguish to his wife's future by his own death.

Of course, his wife, who was listening to the conversation beside him, said to him, "Don't worry about that! Don't worry about it." What is important is the sharing of these thoughts and feeling that they will continue even after his death. I could feel that what he cherished was his family, especially his wife, and that he wished her to continue to live cheerfully and vigorously after his death, just as she would.

People Around the Person (1) — Judicial Scrivener

Now, I have another activity as an end-of-life issues journalist. I cover the fields related to the pre- and post-death period (including medical care and nursing care) and disseminate information in connection with the ACP through lectures and other means.

Why do we do this? Because ACP, in particular, is based on the person's views of life, values, and life goals, and I wonder if it is really possible to deeply understand the deepest aspects of a person's life in a medical setting with limited time and personnel. There are various entry points for a person to become aware of his or her views on life, values, and goals in life. I want people to know that.

In terms of decision-making, the adult guardianship system is one of the systems in Japan to support individuals. This system provides legal protection and support for people with dementia and other conditions that make them anxious or concerned about making decisions on their own. Currently, judicial scriveners are responsible for most cases, and the number of cases of adult guardianship is increasing every year. It has also been noted that the number of single-person households is increasing in Japan, with a high percentage of women aged 75–84, as well as the aging of single-person households for both men and women.[3]

In other words, we can expect even more support from legal experts in the future. Information on the adult guardianship system is provided by the Ministry of Health, Labor and Welfare for medical, nursing care, and other related organizations, and training on decision-making support is also provided for judicial scriveners and other adult guardians.[4]

However, as far as judicial scriveners are concerned, there are still many people who "have heard about ACP but do not know what it is" or "have never even heard of the name." As the legal guardians of the person, they are the ones who look after the person in a different way from the professionals in the medical and nursing care fields, though it is highly likely that they are in touch with the person's values and outlook on life from the stage before the person receives full medical and nursing care services.

Despite this, the reality is that adult guardians are not aware of the ACP, and even medical and care professionals do not yet have a full understanding of the role of adult guardians and other related issues.

Even in the "until death" phase of the diagram shown earlier, professionals are divided. Even if a person is unable to talk about his or her views of life and values in a medical setting, these may be verbalized through such avenues as property management. In order to connect the person's story told outside the hospital to ACP, it may be necessary to expand the boundaries of "other professions," as it is often called in the medical and nursing care fields.

People Around the Person (2) — Life Insurance Solicitors

One area of pre- and post-death involvement that I have been focusing on is life insurance solicitors. Because they are involved with the individual even before he or she becomes ill (one cannot purchase life insurance if he or she is not healthy), and because they sell life insurance to prepare for the eventualities of a long life, they often take the time to listen to their clients about their life plans. Otherwise, they would not be able to guide the customer to the appropriate insurance product for that person. This is why they undergo a variety of training to be able to listen to what is deepest in a person, such as what is important to them in life, their goals, and even their views on life and values.

One of our recruiters shared the following story with us. A client whose cancer had progressed to the point where the end of his life was in sight told us that the anticancer drug treatment was so painful that he feared he would just die in the pain. But there was something he wanted to do before death. The solicitor then introduced a living needs rider (a rider that allows the insured to receive part or all of the death benefit or other benefits before death if the insured is given six months or less to live), which the customer wanted to do.

However, the application for the living needs rider required a clear statement of life expectancy and cessation of anticancer drug treatment by the doctor, but the doctor refused to do so. A life insurance solicitor intervened to support the customer's wish to discontinue the anticancer drug treatment and worked with the customer to persuade the doctor, thereby protecting the customer's wishes.

The doctor may have felt that there was still room to challenge the treatment and why to stop now. However, the solicitor also received financial advice from the patient and his family (few people would ask a healthcare professional for financial advice). Furthermore, the individual had things he wanted to do in anticipation of his death, including the company he was running and his family. Considering these various factors, he decided to discontinue the anticancer drugs.

I do not know to what extent the healthcare professional was aware of the person's important concerns and life goals at that time. Although ACP was probably not that widespread at the time, I was impressed by this life insurance solicitor who acted as if he had a mission to protect the rights of his clients.

When verbalizing their views on life and values, some people think in terms of money. My husband, an economics journalist, used to say, "How you spend your money shows how you live your life." This is one of the reasons why I see the potential for ACP support in insurance recruiters, who provide information on insurance for life's contingencies.

People Around the Person (3) — Private Companies

I also pay attention to the private sector. Tokyu Corporation ("Tokyu") was established in 1922. The company has been expanding its business to solve social issues by promoting both its railroad business and urban development along its railroad lines, as well as lifestyle services targeting the people who live there, and even into the hotel and resort sector. Under such circumstances, the company anticipated that the aforementioned increase in the number of single-person households and the further progression of the super-aging of society would lead to increased social unrest. Targeting people living along the railway line and their families, the company launched a one-stop business offering a variety of pre- and post-death services.

What was interesting was the art event titled "END Exhibition — Your Life Story Asking from Death," which was held in the early summer of 2022 under the theme of "death" and "aging".[5] The exhibition on this theme was bumped up to a venue in an area where many young families live, especially in the towns along the railroad lines where Tokyu operates its railroad business.

The approach was through manga. "Do you want to be born again?" "Do you know how you want your family to mourn?" "Have you ever talked about it?" "What is life?" and many other questions, sometimes even philosophical, are accompanied by questionnaire data and a frame from a manga related to the question, as well as artworks, such as "Type Trace / Last Words" (10-minute testament) (dividual inc. (Dominique Chen + Takumi Endo)).

Tokyu also has a group company that is responsible for the production of various cultural arts, such as art and music. There was some concern about how many people would be attracted by this theme, but as a result, the number of visitors was double the number expected by the specialized group companies, with about 10,000 people coming to the exhibition over the 13-day period.

As for satisfaction with the exhibition, most of the respondents answered "very good" or "good" in their questionnaires. "The exhibition was light and did not make me feel sad in front of the theme of death" (a man in his 30s) and "I was able to have various dialogues with my family. I hope they do it again, it was really good!" (40s female), "It was very stimulating to answer questions that I have never thought about. It was interesting because I don't usually see other people's views on life and death. I realized how diverse it is" (a woman in her 40s), "I feel like my view of life and death changes as I get older, so I want to touch on this topic regularly" (a man in his 20s), and many other free responses were also received.

I also went to the exhibition and saw how many people commented on the comment board that adorned the end of the exhibit (the board read, "Is there anything you would like to do before you die? What is it?" and visitors were able to leave their comments), I was moved. I had been working in the field of pre- and post-death for 10 years since my husband's bereavement, but I had never seen so many "ordinary people" sincerely thinking about death and expressing their own words about it. Many people **are willing to talk** about life and death, as long as there is an opportunity that suits them. I even felt that what I had vaguely felt through my practice up to this point had been proven.

One of the challenges in promoting ACP is the lack of a sense of life and death in Japan, and the values and outlook on life that ACP is based on should be based on a sense of life and death. In Japan, however, the tendency to avoid talking about death has persisted for a long time. In fact, I think this tendency still remains among the elderly.

The exhibition was crowded mainly by people in their 20s and 30s. The children and grandchildren of the generation that Tokyu considers to be the main target of this project visited the exhibition, and we could sense a good possibility that discussions could be initiated among the families through the encouragement of their children and grandchildren.

At the End

My problem with the ACP can be summed up in one statement:

A person's view of life, values, and goals in life, which we want to assume in the practice of ACP, are not found in the hospital, but in life itself.

So I believe the challenge lies in the fact that the ACP appears to be medically driven. Few people are able to speak their deepest thoughts and feelings in a hospital, an unusual space for the general public, when asked a series of questions by a doctor to whom they might say they have entrusted their lives. Nor do they necessarily mean what they say. In fact, there are probably not that many Japanese people who live their lives with this in mind.

In the medical field, it is also a reality that medical professionals and patients are asymmetrical in terms of the amount of information, experience, and knowledge they have. In Japan, there are many patients who are dependent on healthcare professionals, saying that they will "leave everything," including treatment, to them even though it is their own bodies that are being treated. In such a relationship, is it possible to share views of life, values, and goals in life?

Furthermore, it takes time to verbalize these unspoken and hard to put into words. Under the Japanese healthcare system, can we really spend that much time on patients? ......

- **Support for verbalization**

The aforementioned practice of dialogue meetings, support in resolving problems, plus the promotion of understanding of ACP to industries other than medical and nursing care that are involved in the pre- and post-death period, is based on the idea that one's view of life, values, and goals in life are within life itself.

Life is not only about old age and illness. People's daily lives are colored by a variety of factors, and it is only natural that priorities will change from time to time. Also, life is much longer than we think. It is important to educate the general public, including the individual and family members, but we can also increase the number of words that the public can speak in the medical and nursing care fields by deepening the understanding of ACP, which is practiced in the final stages of life, among those who watch over that length of time from a distance (for example, life insurance solicitors and services by private companies would also fall under this category). This would also increase the number of general people who can speak the language in the medical and care fields.

- **The Power of the Community**

In Japan, with its declining birthrate and super-aging society, it is impossible for professionals to continue to take on all the responsibilities.

However, it is not possible for people to "help each other out" as much as they would like to in today's society. In this sense, we are paying attention to the activities of private companies. In some cases, business development targeting residents living along railway lines, such as Tokyu, has formed a "community" that is different from the region. There is also the education industry, which started with children's education and expanded into services for their families, for example, the senior market, and even the ending industry. In each case, a "community" may be created by customers who trust the company.

When considering sustainability, Japan's declining birthrate and aging population make it unsafe to rely on tax revenue-based government services. We have heard that the corporate side is also still groping its way through the process, but we would like to keep an eye on their challenges.

Now, what I have written so far is based on various dialogues and sharing with my husband who, before his death, made his life purpose clear: "I want to die as a distribution journalist." You may clearly see the fact that what I gained through ACP has supported me after bereavement.

Herein lies the greatest value of ACP for the individual and his/her family. It is not just about making medical and care decisions; what is gained in the process of practicing ACP supports the survivor and has the potential to spread its impact further into the community and society. ACP should not be practiced "to make medical and care decisions" but rather with **an eye toward what lies beyond medical and care decisions.** As a family member of a patient, I strongly hope so from my personal experience.

The aforementioned man was diagnosed with stage IV colorectal cancer at the age of 31. He is now 35 years old, and a baby boy was born to him last fall. After the cancer was discovered, he underwent fertility treatment and after many challenges, the couple gave birth to a new life. What were their thoughts when they decided to give birth, and what views on life and values were shared? Needless to say, there was the understanding and support of obstetricians and other healthcare professionals.

It should not end with the person's death. "For what lies beyond the medical and care decisions," the ACP is there.

Acknowledgements

First of all, I would like to express my heartfelt thanks to the core members of Life Terminal Network: Naomi Kuroda and Michiko Uchimiya.

They have always worked together cheerfully without being impatient with our activities, which proceed slowly at my pace.

I would also like to add my thanks to a recent member Soichiro Ishigaki. He is the "35-year-old father and stage IV colon cancer patient" featured in this chapter. With his addition, Life Terminal Network will be heading to a different stage.

This chapter also has a number of interview contributors. We interviewed judicial scriveners Mr. Toshioki Suzuki and Ms. Noriko Ando about the current situation of judicial scriveners. Regarding the experiences of life insurance solicitors, we interviewed Mr. Koji Makino of Prudential Life Insurance Company. Ltd. and Mr. Takahisa Suzuki and Mr. Satoshi Ishidera of Tokyu Corporation about their business creation as well as an exhibition on the theme of death.

The understanding and cooperation of many medical and care professionals are essential for such activities in my position. In this chapter, I would not have had this opportunity if Dr. Masanori Mori had not approached me.

I would like to express my deepest and most sincere thanks to all of you. Thank you very much.

And finally, I would like to express my gratitude and love to my late husband, who still supports me as always. He taught me how people live and die. All of this has been my driving force.

Acknowledgement

With special thanks to Dr. Masanori Mori for his work in translating this chapter from Japanese to English.

References

1. https://souzoku.asahi.com/article/14326436.
2. https://www.stat.go.jp/data/topics/topi1321.html#:~:text=%E7%B7%8F%E4
   %BA%BA%E5%8F%A3%E3%81%AB%E5%8D%A0%E3%82%81%E3%
   82%8B%E9%AB%98 E9%BD%A2,29.1%EF%BC%85%E3%81%A8%E3
   %81%AA%E3%82%8A%E3%81%BE%E3%81%97%E3%81%9
   F%E3%80%82.
3. https://www.stat.go.jp/data/kokusei/2020/kekka/pdf/outline_01.pdf.
4. https://guardianship.mhlw.go.jp/.
5. https://hiraql.tokyu-laviere.co.jp/end-exhibition/.

Chapter 42

Advance Care Planning for Dying with Dignity: A Physician's Perspective*

Sang-Yeon Suh

*Department of Family Medicine, Dongguk University,
Ilsan Hospital, Goyang, Republic of Korea*

*Department of Medicine, Medical College,
Dongguk University, Seoul, Republic of Korea*

Introduction

Two Decades as a Palliative Physician in Korea, before and after the Legislation

When I was a university student, I've came across a paragraph in a novel. The description was simple. "People all have common delusion, it is that they believe they would live forever". I thought it was hilarious at that time. However, after becoming a family physician in the 1990s, I realized how the delusion was widely spread among ordinary people. Even patients having serious illness and their families seemed to ignore or avoid talking about death. My journey as a palliative physician started in 2003 at a public hospital. Koreans had neither legislation nor social consensus of stopping life-sustaining treatment (LST) then. Thus, palliative physicians had no way but to rely on do not resuscitate orders, but I could sense silent

---

* Voices of healthcare providers.

consensus about the withdrawal of futile LST at a hospice ward. If they were not admitted to the hospice ward, they had no choice but to be surrounded by ventilators and monitoring machines in intensive care units. More than hundreds of deaths occurred there a year. Every patient died differently. I still remember the clear contrast between two dying men patients. One was in his nineties while the other was in his early thirties. Unexpectedly, the younger patient showed calm attitude but the older patient was not able to let go of hope to live more. The young man told me that "My father, and uncles all passed away from rectal cancer. So it was no wonder to me that I got diagnosed of the same disease. I even felt inner peace when I knew my disease, because it was something to be destined to happen... Even I became free from fear of the disease ironically." It may be an extreme case. However, two cases showed how dying patients can be different according to their experiences, thoughts, feelings, and views of death.

During my sabbatical stay at Duke, United States, in 2010, I met Dr. Deborah T. Gold there. She is a professor of medical sociology, Duke University, and she has been giving a lecture about "Death and Dying" to freshmen students. It was a six-month course and students were mostly in their early twenties. During the lecture, students postulated what if they had to face death within six months, and what they would like to do. They were also asked to write diaries or letters to their families and close friends under the assumption of a limited short life span. After the lecture course, many students sent thank cards to the professor. Because young students' views of life changed seriously just by thinking of their own end-of-lives as a possible scenario. I've been also delivering a lecture on palliative care to medical students. Most of them are in their mid-twenties. So I wondered how realistic young students could think about dying and death. Dr. Gold shared a story. A 20-year-old male student attended her lecture course in the first semester, and unfortunately, he got diagnosed with lethal brain tumor at the end of the year. He wrote a letter to the professor to tell how much he appreciated the lecture. He felt like he could prepare himself and he expressed gratitude to his family and friends in advance, attributed the homework from the lecture. Dr. Gold explained that traffic accidents and gunshot accidents could happen in the United States. Thus, young adults are not free from risks of sudden death. She and I totally agreed the process — thinking about their end-of-lives and discussions with families — would be absolutely needed for patients with serious illness or elderly people.

I encountered an outpatient at my clinic, the patient was in his sixties and pondered about the end-of-life care for his mother in her nineties. All knew if the elderly was admitted to an intensive care unit, it would hinder peaceful dying. However, healthcare professionals hesitated due to lack of legislation to protect themselves to stop LST. Since then, more than a decade has passed. We Koreans have had legislation related to advance care planning (ACP) and promoting palliative care since 2018.[1] Obviously, the legislation greatly helped public awareness of ACP and promotion of palliative care in Korea. At the same time, there are pros and cons of legislation. Let me share the Korean situation based on statistics, voices from stakeholders, guidelines, and researches.

Legislation of Advance Care Planning in Korea: What We Learned

1. Legislation Brought Dramatic Changes

Korean population is about 52 million and its gross domestic product ranked 10th in countries belonging to the Organization for Economic Cooperation and Development (OECD) in 2021.[2] The average life expectancy is 83.6 years in Korea based on statistics in 2021. Around 373,000 people died in 2022, and 74.8% died in hospitals.[2] Quality of death (QOD) index of Korea ranked 4th among 81 countries in 2021. Korea took 2nd place in Asia for QOD.[3] Korea ranked 18th QOD in the whole OECD countries, and it had 4th QOD in Asia in 2015. QOD index consisted of five categories as ① palliative and healthcare environment, ② human resources, ③ affordability of care, ④ quality of care, and ⑤ community engagement. Legislations enhanced all indicators across the above categories. Another clear contrast was shown from a national survey. In 2014, home was the most preferred place of death in Korean adults. In 2021, hospice & palliative care institutes replaced the most preferred place of death.[4] Evidently, it shows widespread trust in hospice & palliative care. Figure 1 shows the propagation of palliative care services after legislation in Korea. Increment in the number of institutes and beds was noticed in 2016, which meant the trend started just by the announcement of the law.[4]

Public awareness of ACP greatly increased after legislation. Hospitals, the Ministry of Health and Welfare, and agencies for advance directive (AD) promote public awareness through posters, leaflets, online seminars, and activities in online communities.

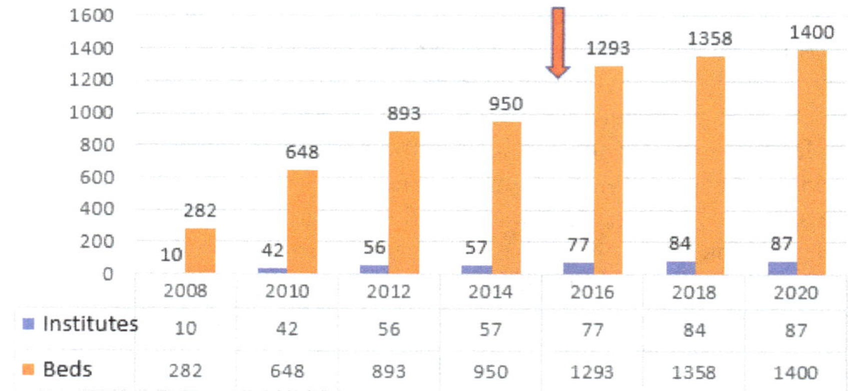

Figure 1.   Increments of numbers of institutes and beds of palliative care services after legislation in Korea.

Note: Red arrows indicated the year 2016, the announcement of the law about advance directives was performed.

2. Voices from Clinicians through Years' Experiences

A. Uncertainty of Prognostication

Medical diagnosis is the most important thing to determine the dying phase according to the law related to ACP in Korea. However, prognostication always carries uncertainty. Nowadays, novel targeted therapy appears rapidly attributed to the advancement of pharmaceuticals. Therefore, medical oncologists confess that it is very hard to predict who will benefit from novel therapy or not. It is especially difficult when doctors and families hold a little bit of hope.[5] There is no universal answer for these cases; the golden rule in palliative care "Hope for the best, plan for the worst" would be an alternative solution.

B. Individual as a Member of Family

Legislation empowered an individual's power of self-determination by the law. "Self-determination" and "First-degree family members as legal representative" are two key points of legislation of ACP in Korea. Evidently, the legislation made discussion of end-of-life scenarios have a way of coming to the surface in Korea. In practice, Korean clinicians face families mainly for ACP discussion of elderly patients, similar to other Asian countries.[6] Thus, it is not easy for clinicians to be against families' opinions when families' opinions are different from those of patients. Some clinicians wonder why ACP law emphasizes too much about the right to know of patients. For self-determination, one must know about his/her own health status such as death is expected within a few months. According to individual characters and family backgrounds, "leaving it to family" can be patients' preferences.[5] It is commonly seen for elderly, rural, less educated, and women patients. Under the law, patients are not able to have the right of not knowing unless they are uncommunicable.

If there are no expressed will of patients, and patients are uncommunicable, then total 1st-degree family members must agree to stop LST. There are two common pitfalls of the process of gathering consent of legal representatives in Korea. First, families can live abroad or get sick seriously (rarely in jails), then it may not be easy to reach total consent quickly. Patients with serious illness should think about their end-of-lives and clarify their will by ADs while they can express their preferences. The second situation is that 1st-degree family members can have inconsistent views for stopping LST. Then, LST has to be maintained till total consent is achieved. Therefore, clinicians recommend that seriously ill patients need to clarify their wills of LST to their families. It would be desirable for families to think about end-of -life care of patients altogether before too late.[6]

A previous national survey showed that "being not burden to others" is the biggest component of good death in Koreans.[7] Many elderly people choose ACP because they consider their children. The ACP law protects personal autonomy for dying with dignity explicitly. In frontline, healthcare professionals engaged ACP feel that one of the strongest motivations for patients with serious illness to choose AD is to lessen the emotional burden on their families. Healthcare professionals still meet some families embarrassed by knowing patients' self-determination of AD later. We cannot deny that AD is still considered as a taboo, news related to death to some people. Hopefully, people can approach ACP more openly, by full discussion with loved ones, through all walks of life.[8]

C. Official Guidelines for "Shared Decision-Making"
The Ministry of Health and Welfare and the Korea National Institute for Bioethics Policy announced the official guideline for "shared decision-making".[9] Government empowers a clinician as a moderator in ACP conversations. It is a clinician who assesses end-of-life/dying phases based on patients' medical status. Thus, clinicians should encourage all participants to express their hopes, concerns, and fears. When conflicts arise, clinicians should investigate the reasons behind the views of the family. Meanwhile, it is necessary to remind gently for the family using phrases

such as "The patient wished to be respected by the family" or "We're here to support the patient's self-determination".

The Ministry of Health and Welfare and the Korea National Institute for Bioethics Policy also recommended "shared decision-making" in stepwise approaches.[9] First, clinicians should ask the patient about his/her family involvement in the process of ACP discussion. In the case which the patient does not want the family to participate, the choice should be respected. Because patients' values and wishes are top priorities under this law currently. Clinicians should communicate with patients and families together about patients' medical status and their own preferences to reach the best goal of satisfying all. At the same time, clinicians need to inform clearly that the final decision should be patient-centred. If conflicts arise among patients and families, then a step-by-step approach is needed. Sharing information should be understandable manner, and patients and families need time to reconsider. By attentive listening and attitude of acceptance, empathy can solve many conflicts. If there are still unsolved conflicts, ethics committees in medical institutes are the last resort to intervene.

3. Future Considerations Based on Researches and Personal Ideas

A. Flexibility of Legal Representatives

Legislation brought many advantages for ACP in Korea. Dying patients have legal rights to stop LST through two processes. Namely, one is registered AD which is decided by patients themselves, and the other is family consent in case of AD is not prepared. Raised public awareness and promotion of palliative care are also favorable aspects of legislation. However, some people are concerned that legislation emphasized individual's right to determine one's end-of-life care too much. Korea has a long tradition of "relational autonomy", which means family-based decision-making style, similar to other Asian countries. Family consent is a complementary pathway when patients' ADs are not available. However, only 1st-degree family members have the right in Korea under current law. Western countries allow legal proxies for ACP including significant others, close friends. In the rapidly changing society, nowadays, the Korean traditional view of families is also facing challenges. For example, birth rate decreases by 0.78 in 2022 and single-person households increase by 33.4% in 2021 in Korea.[2] For instance, I had heard about a case conference in a palliative care centre. A dying patient lived in a temple almost for her lifetime. Thus, a Buddhist priest there observed her closely and the priest was considered as someone who knew what was best for the patient. The patient had cognitive dysfunction; it made the ACP discussion more complicated. There was no expressed the patient's will for ACP. The priest requested to stop LST. However, the patient's sister appeared suddenly from abroad and insisted not to stop LST. In this case, her sister solely had the legal right to stop LST. The sister might want to spend time more with the patient. However, long cycles of chemotherapies seemed to be too much more than the patient could handle. Under current law, we Koreans have no opportunity to listen to other closely related persons of the patient. Thus, the designation of a legal representative should be extended and modified to reflect societal change through social consensus in the near future.

B. Consideration for the Underprivileged Groups in the Society
Underprivileged people need special support to use ACP system. In Korea, there are nationwide AD agencies. However, access may be limited in special groups. For example, a group of people having cerebral palsy was eager to participate ACP discussion. In reality, they were not able to go to AD agency without others' help for mobility. Thus, visiting counseling services may facilitate ACP discussion for the handicapped people.[10] Clinicians and counselors have difficulties to explain the terms of ACP to frail, elderly patients with cognitive dysfunction. Unless they are totally uncommunicable, clinicians and counselors have to explain to the individuals first, then healthcare professionals wonder how much patients understand actually. Officially promoting video clips for ACP are available now for cognitively intact people. It is needed to develop easier guidelines (e.g., flashcard and animation) for counseling to people with cognitive dysfunctions in the near future. Meanwhile, minor (children/ adolescents) groups with limited life expectancies have also rights to know accompanied by their parents as legal representatives. It is still a very sensitive matter how to deliver the bad news to minor groups.

C. Education and Training for Clinicians to Practice ACP
Clinicians wish specific education for counseling and secured time to prevent burnout. Nurses and medical social workers are working frontline for ACP discussions in big hospitals in Korea. Physicians involved in palliative care and ACP are family physicians, medical oncologists, pulmonologists, nephrologists, and psycho-oncologists in Korea. There are no standardized education or supporting systems for clinicians. Other

important lay health workers are counselors working at non-medical AD registry agencies. They have difficulties to explain LST and palliative care services exactly since non-medical AD agencies are separated from palliative services.[10] Counselors may have a wide variation in their competencies and experiences. Adequate reimbursement for ACP counseling will enhance both quality and quantity of ACP discussions. Burnout of clinicians and counselors would be important issues since ACP discussions can bring enormous emotional burden and require substantial time for repeated processes.

Focus group discussions, peer reviews, and online meetings are currently performed in nationally designated palliative centres in Korea to support continuous education of health care professionals. Webinars and online gatherings are helpful and convenient in this era of COVID-19.

Conclusion

Advance Care Planning as a Gentle Reminder of "Memento Mori"

ACP requires scenarios of one's end-of-life care. Talking about death was such a taboo in Asia; it's still a challenging topic. As a palliative physician and a professor in a medical school, I realized the value of addressing death through my journey for two decades. The more prepared toward death, the more passionate and responsible attitude to life was shown. Thus, I believe "good death education" are lessons for life having less regrets. It brings so special feelings to me when young medical students express great interest in palliative care and ACP during my lecture. Students told me that they were impressed by a quote "As a well spent day brings happy sleep, so life well used brings happy death -Leonardo da Vinci". It is inspiring that many youngsters show interest in ACP worldwide. I think ACP discussions give two opportunities. Thinking about the hidden aspects of life and communicating with families and closely related persons about critical scenarios. Just by thinking of death and dying, it can reframe our thoughts and value system about life. It is the same context that "Memento Mori (Remember death is inevitable)" is a thought experiment for "Carpe Diem (Seizing the moment)". My experiences as a palliative physician are truly a privilege to understand life and death better. Actually, our lives are surrounded by others' deaths and it is literally true in palliative care units. I also had hard times when families refused to reveal the truth to patients. Or patients denied dying and did not give up hope to live more. Nevertheless, at the end, or during palliative care, my team and I could sense most patients and families adapted to realistic expectations according to disease trajectory and passage of time. It is impressive to see almost all dying patients and families appreciate palliative care team no matter what happened. Such great interactions and memories are motivations for us to move forward.

Acknowledgments

I appreciate all patients at the hospice ward and the palliative care centre in my workplace. Some of them were role models to show how brave and graceful dying people can be. Others reminded me of the importance of preparedness for one's end of life as well as communication with family members.

I would like to thank Dr. Chang Hwan Yeom who led me on the journey of palliative physician. Many thanks go to Dr. Yoshiyuki Kizawa, Dr. Masanori Mori, and our amazing Asian ACP project team. Our project kept me updated and aware of more of the Korean situation through well-organized meetings.

Lastly, my sincere gratitude goes to my family, who inspire and encourage me to do my best for the next generation.

Learning Objectives
- Diverse perspectives from Korean healthcare professionals after legislation of advance care planning in Korea.
- Official guidelines recommend "shared decision-making" among clinicians, patients, and families.
- Flexibility for legal representatives and consideration for underprivileged groups are future tasks in Korea.

References

1. The website of National Agency for Management of Life-Sustaining Treatment in Korea. https://www.lst.go.kr/decn/establish.do.
2. Statistics Korea. (2021). Population indices in Korea. https://kosis.kr/visual/populationKorea/populationIndex.do.
3. Finkelstein E.A., Bhadelia A., Goh C., *et al.* (2022). Cross country comparison of expert assessments of the quality of death and dying 2021. *J. Pain Symptom Manage.* **63**: e419–429.

4. The ministry of health and welfare and the national hospice center in Korea. (2021). The annual report of national hospice palliative care status.

5. "The gap between the law and the reality". A podcast about the law related to advance directive and physician orders for life sustaining treatments from the official homepage of Seoul National University Hospital. http://www.snuh.org/health/tv/view.do?seq_no=126.

6. Yamaguchi T., Maeda I., Hatano Y., *et al.* (2021). Communication and behavior of palliative care physicians of patients with cancer near end of life in three East Asian countries. *J. Pain Symptom Manage.* **62**(2): 315–322.

7. Yun Y.H., Rhee Y.S., Nam S.Y., *et al.* (2004). Public attitudes toward dying with dignity and hospice palliative care. *Korean J. Hosp. Palliat. Care* **1**(3): 17–28.

8. Kim M., and Lee J. (2020). Effects of advance care planning on end-of-life decision making: A systematic review and meta-analysis. *Korean J. Hosp. Palliat. Care* **23**(2): 71–84.

9. The ministry of health and welfare in Korea and the Korea national institute for bioethics policy. (2020). Manual for healthcare professionals about advance care planning.

10. Kim Y., Yoo S.H., Choi W., *et al.* (2020). Barriers to counseling on advance directives based on counselors' experiences: Focus group interviews. *Korean J. Hosp. Palliat. Care* **23**(3): 126–138.

Chapter 43

Advance Care Planning to Bring Peace of Mind to Patients: A Nurse's Perspective*

Sayaka Takenouchi

Department of Nursing Ethics, Division of Human Health Sciences, Graduate School of Medicine, Kyoto University, Kyoto, Japan

Introduction

The End of Life's Journey

How would you like to spend the last days of your life?

As people get older, they quietly and secretly develop ideal visions about the end of their lives. One may wish to be taken to heaven in joy and gratitude, surrounded by loving family, without suffering from painful symptoms. Others may hope to die peacefully and naturally, like a tree returning to the earth after it has decayed. Another may prefer to die in a familiar home, surrounded by the usual pleasant sounds and the flow of time. In short, what one wishes for the end of one's life journey is based on one's own values and is, therefore, unique to each individual.

While it would be ideal if everyone could have the end of life the way they wanted it, for people with serious illnesses, the end of life is often not the way they want it. To remedy this situation, compassionate healthcare professionals (HCPs) have been searching for years for the best strategy

---

* Voices of healthcare providers.

to help patients spend their final days in a fulfilling way. Could advance care planning (ACP) really be a solution? If so, how can we make ACP work? In this chapter, I would like to explore the answer to these questions based on my experience as a nurse and researcher supporting patient decision-making.

Challenges of ACP in Asia

(1) Discussion that Often Involves Mental Distress

I have been a nurse for 24 years in Japan and the US and have had the honor of assisting many patients with ACP. Yet, I have always regretted that I was not able to provide adequate ACP support to my father-in-law, who died of a serious illness. Why is ACP a difficult subject for many HSPs in Asia?

One of the main contributing factors may be that even with traditional Asian spiritual beliefs and religious guidance, many Asians fear "death" and avoid talking about it.[1,2] Few patients, especially those with serious illnesses, are willing to actively discuss with their families and HCPs their preferences for future treatment/care should their condition deteriorates. Unfortunately, in many cases, patients are reminded of their grim future during the ACP discussion process. ACP can be emotionally draining and painful not only for the patient and family but also for the HCPs.[3]

(2) HCPs' ACP Initiatives and Outcomes

In countries with advanced palliative care services, studies on effective ACP strategies began around 2000, and many trials have been conducted to verify the efficacy of ACP.[4,5] Many Asian HCPs are learning from the evidence reported in these Western countries and are making efforts to implement ACP in their clinical practice. However, to what extent are these efforts contributing to the benefit of patients in Asia?

Although I have had the opportunity to practice ACP support for many advanced cancer patients, there are not many instances where I got clear feedback from the patients about the benefits and burdens of ACP. One of the main reasons for this may be that patients who no longer respond to curative treatment at the university hospital lose the opportunity to visit me as they are transferred to local palliative/hospice care services. Or perhaps the patients did not fully understand the purpose and meaning of ACP, so thus did not have the chance to think about their future or discuss it with loved ones, and therefore did not benefit from or bear the burden of ACP. Furthermore, even if the patients did benefit from ACP, they may not have realized that it was a positive influence of ACP.

Therefore, we interviewed patients with advanced cancer for whom we provided ACP support about their impressions of the ACP discussions and their impact on their lives. Patients expressed that ACP "brought peace of mind," "I felt relieved that my family understood my feeling," and "It was reassuring to know that there was someone who cared about me and that I could talk to that person." We believe that these patients' impressions obtained from interviews are part of the positive outcomes of ACP, reflecting the unique Asian cultural background. In addition, many of the comments from patients regarding the effectiveness of ACPs indicated that their relationships with their loved ones were strengthened and that they felt more secure as a result of the ACPs. This could be considered part of the positive outcomes of ACPs with an emphasis on the Asian context.

(3) Need for Evaluation Based on Asian Patient-Centred Approach
ACP programs and systems that are currently considered effective were developed based on Western culture, and the evidence obtained from numerous clinical studies is also based on outcomes recognized in Western countries.[5] Many Asians tend to value harmony with family and loved ones more than asserting their own opinions, and they need support in ACP from a different perspective than in a Western context.[6,7] For this reason, we need to develop ACP support programs that work best for them, and these are currently in the process of being developed and tested. At the same time, outcome measures from the perspective of Asian patients are still undeveloped. So to validate the true outcomes of ACP programs for Asians that are now being developed, we also need to identify optimal patient-centred outcome measures from the lived experiences of Asian patients. I look forward to the day when the latest Asian research reports will enable more HCPs to learn and implement ACP strategies appropriate for Asians in their clinical practice, thereby helping patients and families.

Lessons Learned from My ACP Practice and Research in Japan

In the following sections, I introduce creative solutions for ACP support that I have learned from my ACP practice and research in Japan.

(1) Do Utilize a Method to Explore What Matters Most to the Patient
It is essential for HCPs to explore patients' values in ACP discussions,[8] but for Asians, who rarely speak openly about their own values in public,[7] exploring ways to do so is often a great challenge for us. In exploring various approaches, we realized that we could explore what was most important to patients through a life review.[9]

We, therefore, conducted a qualitative study to determine whether the Lifeline Interview Method (LIM) could be used to explore the value in the process of ACP.[9] The LIM was developed in the Netherlands as part of a psychological study and has been used worldwide. The LIM is a creative and integrative method for eliciting detailed autobiographical information about the life history and future expectations related to the emotions of each significant life event in an individual's life as shown in Figure 1.[10] The LIM, by its very nature, requires active self-involvement and a description of the reasons for emotional ups and downs. Thus, using the LIM, a self-focused recounting of life story events, will likely encourage people of Asian descent, who value family-centred decision-making, to talk about what matters most to them.

The results of our study suggest that the LIM is an excellent means for HCPs to elicit patients' values and priorities. Furthermore, using the

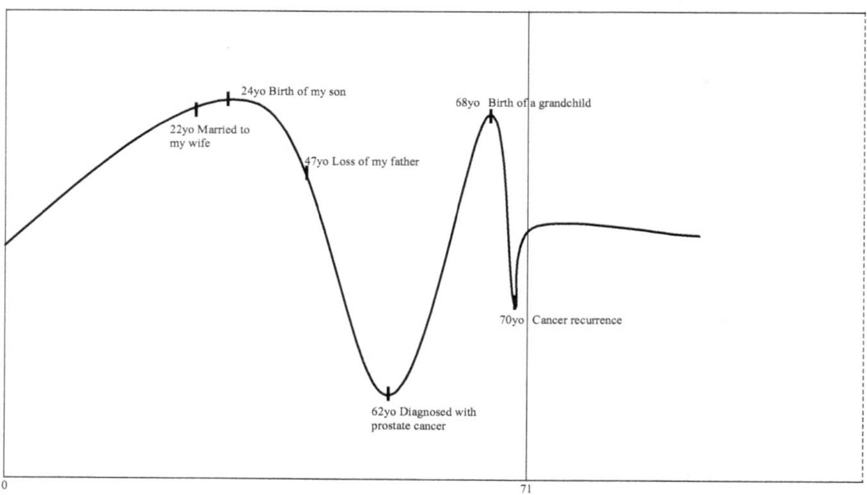

Figure 1.   An example of the life-line.

LIM may help HCPs successfully bridge ACP discussions, consider what matters most to the patient, and provide optimal palliative care.

(2) Do Build a Framework for Compassionate ACP Support

In practicing ACP for patients with serious illnesses, we employ a team approach as shown in Figure 2. Each region or sector should have a framework that works well. First, I would recommend that you form a team of nurses and physicians whom you trust with each other, which will be the minimum unit of ACP practice. Then, you may gradually expand the team of ACP support and build an optimal framework.

The attending physician should introduce the nurse in charge of ACP to the patient before beginning the discussion so that a trusting relationship can be established first. Then, as the patient's condition progresses, the nurse and physician work together to facilitate compassionate discussions with the patient. We often proceed with ACP discussions using the flow shown in Figure 3. Depending on the patient's needs and situation, the physician and nurse may also take a multidisciplinary team approach in collaboration with other professions, as shown in circle B in Figure 2.

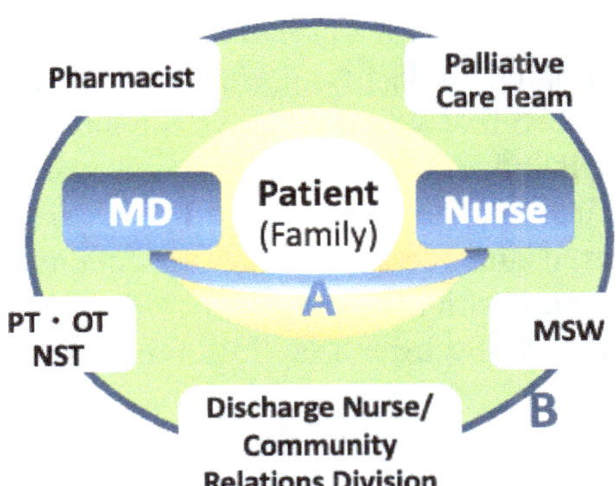

Figure 2.   Multidisciplinary ACP approach.

Abbreviations: MD, medical doctor; PT, physical therapist; OT, occupational therapist; NST, nutrition support team; MSW, medical social worker.

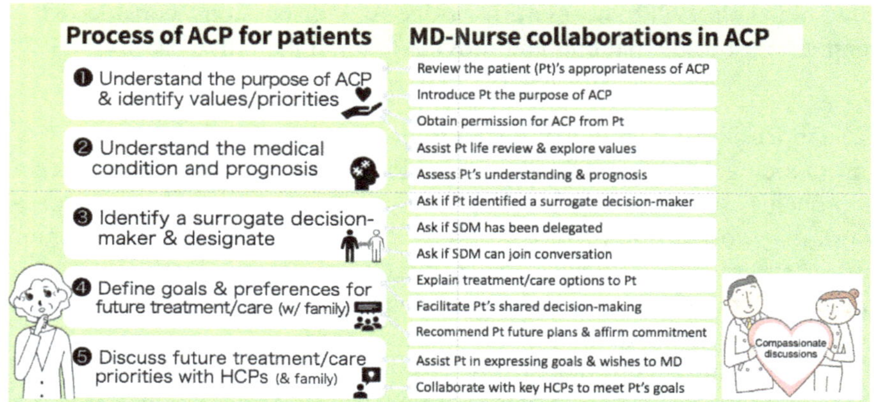

Figure 3. Process of ACP support for patients through collaboration between physicians and nurses.

Abbreviations: ACP, advance care planning; w/, with; HCPs, health care professionals; Pt, patient; SDM, shared decision-making; MD, medical doctor.

(3) Don't Make ACP Discussions the Patient's Homework

Asian patients prefer family-centred shared decision-making and want to avoid the emotional burden on their families.[11,12] Patients, especially those with serious illnesses, choose to be able to discuss their treatment/care preferences at the end of life with a clinician they trust and do not want to take the discussion home and discuss it with their families.[11]

We had experienced that when we gave advanced cancer patients a letter following ACP induction with topics, we wanted them to think about at home regarding their future health and care, about half were more or less prepared and ready for the subsequent discussion at the hospital. But not many patients continued to further the conversation with their families at home after that following discussion with their HCPs at the hospital.

As previously mentioned, many Asian patients are reluctant to discuss the topic of ACP with their families at home. Therefore, it would benefit everyone if HCPs recognized that ACP discussions rarely occurred in patients' homes and facilitated these discussions in hospitals or other clinical settings. We have learned from experience that assigning homework to patients and their families to discuss ACPs is unlikely to be effective, especially if patients do not clearly understand the purpose and significance of ACPs.

(4) Don't Get Caught Up in Cultural Stereotypes

Although we often view Asian cultural norms as barriers to ACP, we should not be stereotyped and see them as positive possibilities to build upon.[13] Rather, cultural and regional norms should be considered to be assets and powerful facilitators of the natural decision-making process.[11]

For example, future publications of research outcomes on the benefits of ACP to Asian patients' families and other significant others, such as the evidence delivered from Western countries,[14,15] would provide a boost to clinical practice that can offer family-centred decision support as a matter of course, upon patient request.

A Message to Nurses Who Commit to ACP

(1) Nurses Play a Vital Role in ACP

It has been reported that the HCPs in Asia do not adequately support ACP.[3] However, nurses have been eager to learn ACP knowledge and skills and accumulate practical expertise. I am particularly excited about the development and advancement of ACP practice among nurses. Originally, nursing is a process of interpersonal relationships and aims to achieve its goal based on establishing trust. Nurses spend the most time at the bedside with patients among HCPs, as they are the closest to the patient. Because nurses are patient advocates, they can tailor each step of the ACP process to the individual patient. Furthermore, nurses should be able to successfully support ACPs by utilizing trusting relationships built through daily care delivery and the basic nursing skills of listening and empathy. In the future, it is expected that nurses in Asia will have more opportunities to acquire the knowledge and skills necessary for ACP and that evidence for nurse-led ACP will be established.

(2) Address Small Concerns in Patients' Daily Lives

Nurses need to be sensitive enough to notice small concerns in patients' daily lives. Detecting patients' concerns and reflecting them in in-the-moment decision-making is a consideration that can only be made by nurses who provide comprehensive care for patients from the perspective of whole-person care. This consideration builds and further strengthens trust and rapport between nurse and patient.[12]

For example, the nurse can address appearance issues such as hair loss and skin conditions, dietary concerns, and financial challenges on time by recognizing them in casual conversation. In addition, if the relationship is nurtured to the point where the patient can talk about their values and goals, the nurse can encourage the early realization of events that the patient looks forward to, such as family vacations and family photo shoots. The accumulation of each such trust-building relationship directly leads to successful discussions of future medical/care decisions. The nurse can use this trusting relationship to act as the patient's advocate and attempt to make adjustments to make the best decision for the patient, even if the patient is reserved to family members or reserved to the physician.

ACP is not a one-time conversation but a series of these compassionate communications. Nurses and HCPs who can listen to the small concerns in a patient's life are able to value together what matters most to the patient. An ACP led by such HCPs will surely enhance the patient's well-being and bring peace of mind to the patient.

(3) All the Little Happiness in Patients' Daily Lives Is the Energy Source of Nursing

Walking the dog, driving his wife to the grocery store, high-fiving the grandchildren, and growing organic vegetables for the family. These are all ordinary but essential daily routines for the patients I have cared for. Our goal as nurses is to help our patients live peacefully for as long as possible, with days when they are autonomous and able to do the things they love.

ACP may be difficult and not often rewarding for HCPs. Still, when a patient passes by in the clinic and says, "Same old, same old" (no particular change in his/her physical condition or life) or smiles and tells us about a happy little event, perhaps that is the outcome we are looking for. Successful decision-making support that comes from a good and trusting relationship with the patient and the peace of mind it gives the patient is what supports us nurses and gives us the energy to continue taking on challenges.

Conclusion

ACP Brings Hope in the Face of Despair

Patients in despair in the face of serious illness and its suffering can eventually find meaning and rediscover their own strength through appropriate shared decision-making and ACP support from HCPs with whom they have built a trusting relationship. It is no exaggeration to say that ACP is the support that enables patients to think about what is best for them and to "live" their remaining time with pride that they have done their best in steering their own lives. What is expected of us as HCPs is that the target of our care is a person before being a patient and that we take the perspective of a holistic approach to enhance their well-being. And through careful and compassionate involvement, we must bring out their ability to be "autonomous."

You may be pessimistic, thinking that you lack the knowledge, skills, or time to carry out ACP or that ACP is difficult because you are afraid of putting the patient through a painful experience. However, effectively supporting ACP for patients with life-threatening illnesses is a topic that continues to challenge HCPs worldwide, and you are not alone. I hope that the ACP tips described in this article will be of some help to you in your clinical practice. I believe that improved patient well-being through optimal ACP will have a synergistic effect on the well-being of HCPs.

May compassionate care in your daily clinical practice give you more opportunities to listen to what matters most to your patients, and may the circle of ACP support, which connects patients' hope, gradually expand around you. I wish you all the best in your endeavors from Kyoto, Japan.

Acknowledgments

I would like to thank all my patients who gave me the most important wisdom and taught me the honor of being a nurse. I would also like to thank my mentors, Mihoko Nishimori, Dr. Kazuko Nin, Dr. Betty Ferrell, Pam Malloy, Dr. Keiko Tamura, Dr. Yoshiyuki Kizawa, Dr. Polly Mazenec, Dr. Masanori Mori, and Dr. Ai Chikada, the best project team who continues to explore better ACP approaches with me, and my family, who is my source of strength.

Learning Objectives
- To explore new perspectives on advance care planning (ACP) that Asian healthcare professionals (HCPs) should have by discussing strategies to support patient-specific ACP.
- To consider measures to help HCPs know what matters most to their patients in the Asian context.
- To engage in activities that foster a different perspective on the patient, "caring for the 'person' behind the patient."

References

1. Chan H.Y., Kwok A.O., Yuen K.K., Au D.K., and Yuen J.K. (2020). Association between training experience and readiness for advance care planning among healthcare professionals: A cross-sectional study. *BMC Med. Educ.* **20**(1): 451.
2. Tang M.L., Goh H.S., Zhang H., and Lee C.N. (2021). An exploratory study on death anxiety and its impact on community palliative nurses in Singapore. *J. Hosp. Palliat. Nurs.* **23**(5): 469–477.
3. Martina D., Lin C.P., Kristanti M.S., *et al.* (2021). Advance care planning in Asia: A systematic narrative review of healthcare professionals' knowledge, attitude, and experience. *J. Am. Med. Dir. Assoc.* **22**(2): 349.e341–349.e328.
4. Jimenez G., Tan W.S., Virk A.K., Low C.K., Car J., and Ho A.H.Y. (2018). Overview of systematic reviews of advance care planning: Summary of evidence and global lessons. *J. Pain Symptom Manage.* **56**(3): 436–459.e425.
5. McMahan R.D., Tellez I., and Sudore R.L. (2020). Deconstructing the complexities of advance care planning outcomes: What do we know and where do we go? A scoping review. *J. Am. Geriatr. Soc.* **69**(1): 234–244.
6. Kirmayer L.J. (2007). Psychotherapy and the cultural concept of the person. *Transcult. Psychiatry.* **44**(2): 232–257.
7. Cheng S.Y., Lin C.P., Chan H.Y., *et al.* (2020). Advance care planning in Asian culture. *Jpn. J. Clin. Oncol.* **50**(9): 976–989.
8. Rietjens J.A.C., Sudore R.L., Connolly M., *et al.* (2017). Definition and recommendations for advance care planning: An international consensus supported by the European association for palliative care. *Lancet Oncol.* **18**(9): e543–e551.
9. Takenouchi S., Chikada A., Mori M., Tamura K., and Nin K. (2022). Strategies to understand what matters to advanced cancer patients in advance care planning: A qualitative study using the lifeline interview method. *J. Hosp. Palliat. Nurs.* E135–E143.
10. Schroots J.J., van Dijkum C., and Assink M.H. (2004). Autobiographical memory from a life span perspective. *Int. J. Aging Hum. Dev.* **58**(1): 69–85.
11. Biondo P.D., Kalia R., Khan R.A., *et al.* (2017). Understanding advance care planning within the South Asian community. *Health Expect.* **20**(5): 911–919.
12. Rosa W.E., Izumi S., Sullivan D., *et al.* (2023). Advance care planning in serious illness: A narrative review. *J. Pain Symptom Manage.* **65**(1): e63–e78.
13. Chikada A., Takenouchi S., Nin K., and Mori M. (2021). Definition and recommended cultural considerations for advance care planning in Japan: A systematic review. *Asia-Pac. J. Oncol. Nurs.* **8**(6): 628–638.

14. Lorenz K.A., Lynn J., and Dy S.M. (2008). Evidence for improving palliative care at the end of life- a systematic review. *Ann. Intern. Med.* **148**(2):
147–159.
15. Chiarchiaro J., Buddadhumaruk P., Arnold R.M., and White D.B. (2015).
Prior advance care planning is associated with less decisional conflict
among surrogates for critically ill patients. *Ann. Am. Thorac. Soc.* **12**(10):
1528–1533.

Chapter 44

I am an End-of-life Doula in Singapore

Tay Jia Ying

End-of-life Doula, Happy Ever After, Singapore

One afternoon in February 2018, I texted Mummy on WhatsApp to ask her if we could find a time to discuss her and Papa's end-of-life (EOL) plans and matters. She blue-ticked me. My grandmother-in-law had just passed away a few days before, my brother's heart condition caused some worry in the family around the same time, and on the same day I texted her, my uncle fell off a chair, hit his head, and broke his arm when retrieving an object from a tall cupboard (he has recovered fully since). After three long days of silence, I decided to text her again, this time to tell her that given the series of unfortunate events that have taken place recently, I think I understood why she did not respond to me, but that whenever she was ready to chat, I would be here. She blue-ticked me again, and we never spoke about it since.

By that time, I had already been involved in *Both Sides, Now*[a] for 5 years. I had also just experienced what I thought was a very well-prepared end-of-life journey with my husband's family. My grandmother-in-law lived with Parkinson's disease for years before her death, and her husband, children, and grandchildren have been with her every step of the way, providing emotional, physical, and spiritual support, and ticking

---

[a]An Singapore arts-based community engagement project to open up end-of-life conversations in the community by ArtsWok Collaborative and Drama Box from 2013 to present (www.bothsidesnow.sg).

every checkbox in the end-of-life planning "toolkit" (if there was such a thing). Her funeral was beautifully executed according to plan — everyone knew where to be, what to do and played their part lovingly. It had motivated me to finally initiate a conversation with Mummy after 5 years of hesitation — I had hoped that she would have engaged me at some point earlier having attended *Both Sides, Now.*

My EOL Doula journey began one November morning in 2020. I had woken up and the thought of becoming one just struck me. From somewhere deep inside, I felt a desire to accompany people as they transitioned from this life, so that they may feel less afraid and alone in the process. I must have come across the idea of EOL Doulas at some point in my life before this, but I could not pinpoint where and when. I did not know what being a "professional" EOL Doula entailed, and I was unsure if my heart was going to be strong enough to come so close to death. However, it was the first time I felt so much hunger and curiosity about something that I decided I had to follow it to see where it would take me. That day, it took me down a Google rabbit hole researching EOL Doula courses, related articles, and videos, as well as hospice volunteer opportunities. Over the next few months, I took an EOL Doula course, got certified as an EOL Doula and Advance Care Planning facilitator, volunteered with hospices, hosted regular Death Cafe sessions, and facilitated EOL planning conversations with my friends and family.

I approached G to be my first "case study", to help me with scoping the services I could offer as an EOL Doula. I told myself then that even if this EOL Doula work did not pan out in the long run, I would consider myself to be successful as long as I helped get his EOL affairs in order. For the 7 years before this, every time a new iteration of *Both Sides, Now* came along, I would invite him to the programme, which would prompt conversations about his desire to prepare for his EOL affairs. I had provided him with links to the various resources, but so many years later, he was still at square one.

I met with him and his partner soon after, where I outlined the areas they might want to think about and make decisions for. We then set out dates for when we expect each item to be completed — their doctor's appointment to sign their Advance Medical Directives[b] (AMD), their

---

[b] An Advance Medical Directive is a legal document in Singapore that one signs in advance to inform the doctor treating you (in the event you become terminally ill and unconscious) that you do not want any extraordinary life-sustaining treatment to be used to prolong your life.

lawyer's appointment to affect their Lasting Power of Attorneys[c] (LPA) and wills, their plan to review their Central Provident Fund[d] (CPF) nominations and insurance plans at their own time, and a next meeting with me to discuss their Advance Care Plans. Subsequently, I checked in with them on their progress every few weeks or nearing each deadline — I was their project manager, cheerleader, and "professional nagger". It took us more than a year to get everything together.

I had expected this process to be much faster, for I know both of them to be super efficient people, who seemed to already have a clear idea of what they wanted. But as the process unravelled, I found that "life" often gets in the way, with more tangible urgencies taking priority, and one really needs to intentionally set aside space and time from everyday living to contemplate and administrate our ends. Thinking about our EOL requires us to go into a heavy emotional space we do not naturally want to enter, and when you do get there, you sometimes realise that you are actually facing some harsh realities of life.

"Who should I name my Donee/Nominated Healthcare Spokesperson?" can translate to "Who around me can I bring myself to place this burden of decision making on my behalf?"

"How should I distribute my assets after I die?" can translate to "How do I distribute my assets so that my children do not deem it unfair and fight amongst themselves after my death?"

After G, I had a handful of EOL planning conversations with friends and family who were willing to volunteer their time with me. When that pool dried up, I started a website with the hope of connecting with strangers who were ready to have a conversation. I quickly learnt that it takes proper strategising and marketing to get one's presence out there, which I still do not have to date, so that did not take off yet. Every once in a while, I will get an email or text from someone asking for support, or a referral from a friend because they know I was doing this work. For now,

---

[c]The Lasting Power of Attorney is a legal document in Singapore which allows a person who is at least 21 years of age ("Donor"), to voluntarily appoint one or more persons ("Donee(s)") to make decisions and act on his/her behalf if he/she loses mental capacity one day. A Donee can be appointed to act in the two broad areas of personal welfare and property & affairs matters.

[d]The Central Provident Fund is a compulsory comprehensive savings and pension plan for working Singaporeans and permanent residents primarily to fund their retirement, healthcare, education, and housing needs in Singapore.

I am content beaming off my readiness to engage with anyone within my reach. When they become ready to chat, I will be there.

Last September, my uncle asked in our family group chat for anyone interested to attend a free LPA and AMD webinar organised by his company. I was pleasantly surprised that the first to sign up was Mummy. I thought that the time might finally be ripe for me to initiate a conversation, and this time I took it really slowly. The week after the webinar, I asked her how it went, and if she had any questions coming out of the session ("You can ask me, you know!"). She briefly responded to say that Papa and her are thinking of making their LPAs, but are still discussing, and will let us know when they are clearer of their plans. I did not push further. It was a huge step from the blue-tick days, and I decided that I should take her lead.

Just a few weeks ago, Mummy shared with me about a friend who recently had a bad fall. She lived alone and did not have anybody she could depend on to take care of her. She had been admitted to a community rehabilitation facility after her operation, but could not go back to living alone. Mummy worked with her social worker to find her a nursing home to go to after her discharge, but she had additional worries on her mind. She asked the social worker to assist with her friend's LPA and will, given her old age and propensity to fall, but did not manage to get immediate support because it was not within the social worker's work scope. "I can help! That's exactly the work I am doing, Mummy!" I exclaimed enthusiastically. "Yah, that's why I'm telling you this," she responded. I was quite touched at that moment, not just for her recognition of my work but also to see her be such a strong advocate for someone else's EOL matters.

I always think about why the thought of becoming an EOL Doula hit me that morning. I've identified many reasons since, and think that one of them may have come from my anxiety of not having had EOL conversations with my parents — this may be a really elaborate gesture to get my parents to talk to me. It seems to have worked finally, maybe. I am worried that the day may come before we are prepared, and that we would not be able to take care of them as they would have wanted. I have to keep reminding myself that everyone moves at their own pace, and while others can support and cheer them on, it was ultimately their journey.

While we cannot force anyone against their wishes, I believe we can create better conditions around us so that we can become ready sooner to engage than we would on our own. My hope is for better death literacy in the community, where we are open to talk about death, prepare for our EOL matters, and where we have a good number of EOL workers and advocates around, ready to take EOL conversations further as they come up and support each other on our EOL journey. And that is a reason for the EOL Doula journey of mine to continue.

Chapter 45

Advance Care Planning: Making Conversations Count

Kerrie Noonan

Death Literacy Institute, Australia
Western NSW Local Health District, Dubbo,
NSW, Australia
School of Social Sciences, WSU,
Kingswood, Australia

When I was invited to write a personal reflection on Advance Care Planning (ACP) as a health care provider, many stories and experiences came to mind. My views on ACP are simple. More often than not, planning for the end of life is a helpful experience for everyone involved. The person dying is comforted by knowing there is a plan in place, carers are reassured, and health systems function better when health professionals have a clear treatment plan to follow. My experience of advance care planning is far more complicated. I've seen how good care planning can help patients and families, and I've worked with families after traumatic experiences when advance care plans and directives were disregarded and ignored.

I have also conducted many ACP workshops with community members and for health professionals. Over the past 15 years in Australia, there has been a collaborative effort to improve ACP rates in aged care, primary health care, and hospitals. In 2019, a national prevalence study examining advance care directives (ACD) in older people found that 25% of aged care residents had a health directive identified on their hospital file.[1] Of these, only 6% of participants had a statutory advance care directive outlining their preferences for care. Aged care facilities performed better, with 38% of residents having an ACD.[1]

In a recent community survey, the Council on the Aging NSW (COTA NSW) found that 24% of people over 55 had an Advance Care Directive (ACD). The Council on the Ageing (COTA) NSW is the peak organisation for people over 50 in the state of New South Wales and is an independent, consumer-based, non-government organisation. COTA members were invited to participate in a survey using the Death Literacy Index[2] to understand more about the education needs of this community.[3] Of the 830 people who responded, 80% reported having an ACP, and 36% said they had written down their end-of-life plans and made an ACD. Despite this, only 20% had "talked to a doctor about my end-of-life plans/wishes." We were curious about this finding because this group had higher Death Literacy than the Australian population, especially in factual knowledge about end-of-life care. I am used to hearing workshop participants talk about having their end-of-life documents completed with a solicitor only to find out it was sitting in the solicitor's office or in the safe at home. Frequently, community members said they were reluctant to share their plans with family members or general practitioners because they feared being "talked out of it" or because they had been discouraged — "You're too young" or "You're too healthy to worry about that yet."

I've often reflected on how different the experience of ACP can be. For some, the "paperwork" is the easiest part, while for other patients and families, the emotions can feel too overwhelming. I recall a family member telling me that the aged care team had given them a "big pile of papers to fill in about what treatments they she did or didn't want." She thought it was consent forms, but instead, it was a long-form ACD. It had at least 30 pages and she stopped after a few pages. It was simply too much to do on her own.

I've also seen families who enthusiastically embrace end-of-life planning. I remember working with a man who wanted a home funeral. The family lived in a rural setting, and transporting the person back and forth between the hospital and home after his death was going to be a significant barrier. The family decided they would need to plan well and support each other by setting up rosters, organising medical and nursing care, and utilising the support of family and neighbour. They also had many conversations with their general practitioner and made sure they had an adequate supply of medication to manage any symptoms. In this unique situation, the conversations about after-death care and home funerals sparked the plan for home-based end-of-life care.

In other situations, barriers to communication interfered with EOL planning. Joyce was fearful about "being sedated" at EOL and not being able to talk and interact with her family.

Joyce was 65. She told me the story of her mother's experience of dying 10 years ago. Joyce believed her mother was given "too much" medication, preventing her from communicating with her family. She felt her mother was "fighting against the medication." The nurses tried to reassure her, but Joyce felt that "she had something more to say. I could feel it, I just knew that about her. She didn't look in pain to me, she looked upset about not being able to communicate."

Joyce then told me, "I don't want to be in the hospital when I die, I'd rather be at home in pain if it came down to it."

We talked about her fears, about her family, about how she imagined the last few days and hours of her life. It wasn't the place that was as important, it was having her family with her and she rated being able to communicate with her family as more important than being "knocked out" by pain relief.

When I asked Joyce about her relationship with the palliative care team, she said she felt safe and that they had respected her choices and decisions so far. I wondered if she had told them about her fear of being sedated. She laughed, noting that she was nervous about "telling the doctors how to suck eggs." I admired her spirit. Our interactions always made me laugh. She was a great communicator, often inviting me to sit on the bed with her with a cup of tea.

There were more conversations over a few days on the ward.

The next time I saw Joyce, she told me she had talked to her husband. They both had a bit of a cry when she talked about her fears. She then had a similar conversation with her adult children and updated them on her prognosis and her care preferences for end of life. Joyce told me that her children reassured her that they supported her decisions.

She asked me to be present while she talked to the medical team about her fears about being sedated. They sat with Joyce and her husband and asked questions to clarify her concerns. Joyce even asked questions about how the team might tell other doctors in the hospital about her plans. Her family also asked questions about non-sedating and non-medical pain relief.

Joyce had multiple admissions over the next few months, and each time she reminded us about her preferences regarding pain management. Each admission seemed to provide added reassurance about her care, she trusted us more, and when her time for dying came, she decided to stay in the ward. Her husband was with her throughout her dying, and her children too. They smiled when they told me she was talking about her mother just before she died. She wasn't completely symptom-free, but her family felt the balance between pain and symptoms management and sedation had been achieved.

In this situation, an ACP was also important for the healthcare team. We talked about Joyce's wishes, and as Joyce got clearer, she would also communicate directly with the nursing and medical team about her medication. It took many conversations to get here. The unpacking of fears and Joyce finding the words to express her fears about past experiences helped.

The nursing team advocated for Joyce's wishes, despite concerns that Joyce may have been carrying too much symptom load.

I shared Joyce's story at an ACP training workshop with first-year medical residents a few years later. One of the doctors was wide-eyed. She was considering the information, grappling with Joyce's decisions. She said she felt uncomfortable because she had always seen her job as taking away the symptoms — that "no one should die in pain."

Another doctor spoke up. She said "I think she had pain, but she wasn't suffering. She got to die in a way that was right for her."

We contemplated the difference between pain and suffering and the doctors started to share stories about how their own experiences of dying and death were all medicalised — in hospital, people in cardiac arrest, in the ICU, in surgery, sedated. Distressing and traumatic experiences that included pain AND suffering.

"Why would anyone choose to have pain or symptoms?" they wondered.

Many talked about having never considered exploring pain beyond the SUDS scale; they started to share stories about past experiences when pain and distressing symptoms had surfaced. They talked about times when distress and agitation were never fully relieved.

Another time, I was working on a palliative care team as a clinical psychologist in a hospital when a family requested a meeting with me and our social worker. We checked with the team if there was an ACD on file because we knew the family was requesting information about body donation. In Australia, it is possible to donate your body under some circumstances to science via several university programs. We knew that there was an application process and that it might take up to 6 months for the application to be processed. There was no ACD, but there had been some planning, however the cancer had progressed more quickly than everyone had expected.

We found Fiona and Phillip sitting quietly together. Phillip had lung cancer, his organs failing, his energy now low, he sat propped up head slightly back making each breath count. Fiona sitting on the bed was facing him, holding Phillip's hand, her body tight as if she was breathing every laboured breath with him. We gently sat on chairs on the other side of the bed. I had met Fiona on a previous admission, she was eager to take Phillip home for end-of-life care and was "holding it all together." She had described some family tensions — she was Phillip's second wife. They met 10 years ago, when his children were in their late teens. It hadn't always been a smooth time and relationships with Phillip's children and their mother had been fraught. His diagnosis had not resolved the tension but sent it underground, making for an atmosphere where everyone was on edge. This made any end-of-life planning difficult. Fiona looked as if she was in constant arousal. She was, as often happens when families are experiencing conflict, working hard to "keep the peace", survive, and "get through it."

Fiona was glad to see us. Phillip acknowledged us as best he could. He opened his eyes and raised his eyebrows. I noticed Fiona squeezed his hand, and he pressed back. This tiny gesture seemed incredibly intimate and bigger under the circumstances of dying in this quiet, grey hospital room.

Fiona addressed Phillip first. She was gently getting his permission to talk to us.

"We've been talking about what Phillip wants", Fiona is calmer now, as if starting this sentence was a first hurdle, and she takes a breath and looks at us.

"Phillip wants to donate his body to science. Can we do that, please?"

Yes, we gently say, and then we begin a conversation.

We know that Phillip will likely die in the next 24 hours.

These tender conversations, as Kathryn Mannix has so finely called them, alongside people who are dying cannot be ambiguous or avoid the reality of their situation.[4] To serve Phillip and Fiona best, we had to lean into the situation and promptly and compassionately support them in articulating their plans.

And so, we ask about the plans they have already made, quickly assessing if the paperwork has been completed, knowing that body donation is impossible without it.

We see the disappointment register on Fiona's face.

There's also something else. Shame? As Fiona asks about the cost of the funeral. I see my colleague gently shift again skilfully asking and providing bite-sized information about options. In this case, they had not considered using his superannuation. I see a growing sense of relief on Fiona's face, and towards the end of our conversation, Phillip signals his approval for the plan, which includes donating his corneas and having a direct cremation, when he looks directly at Fiona and squeezes her hand.

It was probably a 20-minute interaction.

We see that this conversation, while important, has taken precious energy and time and we let them both know we were here the rest of the day and leave.

About 30 minutes later Phillip died.

It was our prior conversations that made the outcomes of this one possible. At its most effective, ACP is a series of conversations, questions, and discussions. The informal discussions in the corridor and the kitchen are as important as ones by the bedside and with the team. In healthcare though, a higher value is placed on exchanges that produce results — like a form being signed or a plan written down. I've come to believe that ACP conversations belong everywhere and can happen at any time. In our community places, in schools, and in our homes. They certainly exist already if we look for them — in death cafes, in books, in plays, in paintings, on the news, and in our local newspapers. And all kinds of micro conversations are happening in families and communities and away from health professionals and institutions. So, how can we get better at paying attention to, leaning into, and supporting the end-of-life conversations that are already happening in our healthcare institutions and communities? How else can we make end-of-life conversations count? Here are my thoughts and learnings:

1. Ask about the strengths and knowledge patients and families bring into our clinics and ward. This means asking "have you been with someone who is dying?" "have you cared for someone dying" and "what experiences are you bringing here?" We know death literacy is related to experience, so explore past experiences and lean into conversations about fears AND strengths.[5]

2. All of us, nursing, allied, and medical, have a part in advance care planning discussions and information sharing. All of us working in healthcare will also benefit from doing our own planning and having the personal experience of asking and talking about your own end-of-life wishes. Then, practice asking your family members too. It can be both a humbling and informative experience, especially when people respond with "you are too young to talk about this."

3. Take time to reflect on your personal experiences of dying and death, caring, and grief. Those beyond your health professional role. Gain insights into your own blind spots and consider professional development, community workshops, and connecting with a clinical supervisor.

4. Advance care planning started as a community movement, became a legal/medical rights issue, and became mainstreamed into healthcare practice. ACDs were initially a "living will", and for some patients, this language may be preferable. If you are interested in learning more about the history of ACP, I've referenced a few articles worth reading.[6–8] Consider informal and social ways of talking about values and care preferences.

5. Take time to explore pain management and symptom management as part of advance care planning conversations. This includes medical and non-medical options, the patient's past experiences with pain symptoms, and what works and what doesn't. Explore with patients both pain and suffering. Explore what it means to you. Read the books written by Palliative Care Specialist Dr Kathryn Mannix.[4,9]

6. An ACP or directive is just the beginning. End-of-life plans can't be executed without friends, family, care providers, volunteers, and neighbours. Be curious, ask gentle questions, and ask about informal support and informal care. Take your time to sit with patients and their families to create a roadmap of the care needed. Who are the people who can help bring this plan to life?

Learning Objectives[1]:

- Advance Care Planning (ACP) can be a series of conversations and micro-interactions. Give space for people to explore their values about dying and their fears about symptoms or care. When we ask people to rate the severity of their symptoms out of 10, also ask about past experiences with pain and suffering. Also, ask about past experiences with caregiving, dying, and death.
- ACP conversations can begin anywhere — funerals, after-death care, equipment needs, questions about spirituality/religion, and past experiences with pain or other people dying/deaths. It doesn't need to be a linear process. So if you use a formal process or a "form", don't make it a "tick a box" exercise".
- Don't underestimate the non-medical aspect of advance care planning. Funeral planning, for example, can be a way to introduce ACP. It also includes social support, music, and food.
- An ACP needs to be shared and communicated with the people who will execute the plan. Ask family members, "Who can support you with your plan?" and then have a conversation about this support and the care networks. Often people haven't considered the next step — taking action.

References

1. Buck K., Detering K.M., Sellars M., Sinclair C., White B., Kelly H., *et al.* (2019). Prevalence of Advance Care Planning Documentation in Australian Health and Residential Aged Care Services, Melbourne.
2. Leonard R., Noonan K., Horsfall D., Kelly M., Rosenberg J.P., Grindrod A., *et al.* (2022). Developing a death literacy index. *Death Stud.* **46**(9): 2110–2122.
3. Noonan K., Read N., Lawson M., and Appleby K. (2021). Advance Care Planning, Funerals and Palliative Care: Developing Death Literacy in older Australians. Concurrent Presentation. Oceanic Palliative Care Conference, 8–10th September 2021.

---

[1] This article has modified identifying information such as names, locations, and specific experiences to safeguard privacy and confidentiality. Although the narratives are inspired by actual events, they should be viewed as fictional accounts created for academic purposes.

4. Mannix K. (2021). *Listen: How to Find the Words for Tender Conversations*. London: William Collins.

5. Noonan K., Horsfall D., Leonard R., and Rosenberg J. (2016). Developing death literacy. *Prog. Palliat. Care* **24**(1): 31–35.

6. Fagerlin A., and Schneider C.E. (2004). Enough: The failure of the living will. *Hastings Cent. Rep.* **34**(2): 30–42. Available from: https://about.jstor.org/terms.

7. Informed Consent and the Dying Patient (1974); **83**(8): 1632–1664. Available from: https://www.jstor.org/stable/795550.

8. Lovell A., and Yates P. (2014). Advance care planning in palliative care: A systematic literature review of the contextual factors influencing its uptake 2008–2012. Palliat. Med. (SAGE Publications Ltd.) **28**: 1026–1035.

9. Mannix K. (2018). *With the End in Mind: Dying, Death and Wisdom in an Age of Denial*. London: William Collins.

Index

Printed in the USA
CPSIA information can be obtained
at www.ICGtesting.com
LVHW020405050524
779260LV00004B/497